Radiology

PreTest®
Self-Assessment
and Review

Radiology

PreTest®
Self-Assessment
and Review

Editor

David M. Hovsepian, M.D.
Senior Fellow
Division of Cardiovascular and Interventional Radiology
Department of Radiology
Thomas Jefferson University Hospital
Philadelphia, Pennsylvania

McGraw-Hill, Inc.
Health Professions Division/PreTest Series

New York   St. Louis   San Francisco   Auckland
Bogotá   Caracas   Lisbon   London   Madrid
Mexico   Milan   Montreal   New Delhi   Paris
San Juan   Singapore   Sydney   Tokyo   Toronto

Radiology: PreTest® Self-Assessment and Review

1 2 3 4 5 6 7 8 9 0   KGPKGP   9 9 8 7 6 5 4 3

ISBN 0-07-052007-0

The editors were Gail Gavert, Susan Finn, and Mary Gibbons Farrell.
The production supervisor was Gyl A. Favours.
This book was set in Times Roman by Compset, Inc.
Arcata Graphics/Kingsport was printer and binder.

Library of Congress Cataloging-in-Publication Data

Radiology : PreTest self-assessment and review / editor,
   David M. Hovsepian.—1st ed.
         p.   cm.
   Includes bibliographical references.
   ISBN 0-07-052007-0
   1. Radiography, Medical—Examinations, questions, etc.
I. Hovsepian, David M.
   [DNLM: 1. Radiology—examination questions.
WN 18 R1299]
RC78.15.R3   1993
616.07′572′076—dc20
DNLM/DLC
for Library of Congress   92-48942
                                                                              CIP

Contents

Contributors

Linda R. Aboody, M.D.
Associate Director of Mammography
Department of Radiology
St. Barnabas Medical Center
Livingston, New Jersey

David P. Friedman, M.D.
Clinical Assistant Professor of Radiology
Division of Neuroradiology
Thomas Jefferson University Hospital
Philadelphia, Pennsylvania

David M. Hovsepian, M.D.
Senior Fellow, Division of Cardiovascular and
  Interventional Radiology
Department of Radiology
Thomas Jefferson University Hospital
Philadelphia, Pennsylvania

Robert M. Jaffe, M.D.
Attending Radiologist
Department of Radiology
Somerset Hospital
Somerville, New Jersey

Lester Kalisher, M.D.
Clinical Director
Department of Radiology
St. Barnabas Medical Center
Livingston, New Jersey
Clinical Professor of Radiology
University of Medicine and Dentistry of New Jersey
Newark, New Jersey

Terry L. Levin, M.D.
Assistant Professor of Radiology
Division of Pediatric Radiology
Albert Einstein College of Medicine
Bronx, New York

Chris Ng, M.D.
Attending Radiologist
Centennial Medical Center
Nashville, Tennessee
Assistant Clinical Professor of Radiology
Vanderbilt University Medical Center
Nashville, Tennessee

Rajesh I. Patel, M.D.
Chief Resident, Department of Radiology
Thomas Jefferson University Hospital
Philadelphia, Pennsylvania

Carrie B. Ruzal-Shapiro, M.D.
Assistant Professor of Radiology
Division of Pediatric Radiology
Columbia-Presbyterian Medical Center
New York, New York

Linda M. Sanders, M.D.
Associate Director of Ultrasound
Department of Radiology
St. Barnabas Medical Center
Livingston, New Jersey

Charles S. White, M.D.
Assistant Professor of Radiology
Division of Thoracic Radiology
University of Maryland Medical System
Baltimore, Maryland

Acknowledgments

This text could not have been completed without many people's help. I am greatly indebted to each of the contributors. I am sure that none of us realized just how much time this would take, and am grateful that each was so dedicated. Gail Gavert and the staff at McGraw-Hill deserve special credit for adding Radiology to the PreTest family (it was their idea in the first place), and they have taken great care to ensure that the book includes enough images of appropriate quality to make this a useful study aid.

I would like to thank Dr. Jeffrey Newhouse and Dr. E. Stephen Amis, Jr., for their help in providing images and reviewing the genitourinary section of the manuscript, as well as for the exceptional training I received from them as a resident at Columbia-Presbyterian Medical Center. I also wish to thank Dr. Newhouse, Dr. John Austin, and Dr. Peter Wright, who first showed me, as a medical student, that radiologists are real doctors and that radiology provides the most fun that one can have in medicine. Thanks, too, to all my colleagues and friends at Columbia who reinforced this conviction time and again.

Thanks to my current teachers and colleagues at Thomas Jefferson University Hospital, especially Dr. Geoffrey Gardiner, Dr. Joseph Bonn, Dr. Marcelle Shapiro, and Dr. Kevin Sullivan, for their instruction, input toward the book, and patience while I burned the candle at both ends during my fellowship in interventional radiology.

Most of all, thanks to my wife, Adrienne, for her love and support.

Introduction

As a resident preparing for the In-Service and American Board of Radiology (ABR) written examinations, I was disappointed when I realized that only a few practice question-and-answer texts were available for this subject. Now that I have taken on the challenge, I have a much clearer understanding of why this is so.

First, the breadth of the material which radiologists must master is daunting; moreover, to give a thorough discourse on a particular topic and yet remain concise and readable requires a great deal of work. Second, and perhaps more importantly, the many authors who contribute to the radiologic literature often have wide ranges of experiences and opinions, making it difficult to provide a single "correct" viewpoint.

In this text, the question formats resemble the Radiology In-Service examination, which is composed of single-answer, multiple-choice, and multiple true-false questions. Although the ABR written board examination includes additional types of questions, they are so varied that it would be inappropriate to try to represent them all in a text of this size.

The purpose of this book is not only to provide a means for self-assessment of strengths and weaknesses but also to convey a high density of information on a given subject. The reader should come away with an understanding of the facts in a given question, as well as additional relevant points of information. The fundamental, practical aspects of each subject are emphasized, and trivia is kept to a minimum. This text should also serve in the future, when the exams are over, as a quick refresher or reference when one's memory needs a little jogging. Medical students and nonradiologist trainees may also benefit from this text, since board-type examinations often include questions about diagnostic tests or images to be analyzed.

The field of radiology is propelled by the fast pace of technologic advances. Some modalities and concepts included within the text are currently considered valid but have not yet withstood the test of time. Notions undoubtedly will change with further experience. Above all, we have strived to make the questions unambiguous and free of controversy.

Since the reader's time is limited, this book has been designed to be used profitably one section at a time. By allowing no more than two-and-a-half minutes to answer each question, you can simulate the time constraints of the actual exams. When you finish answering all the questions in a section, spend as much time as necessary verifying answers and carefully reading the accompanying explanations. If you then feel you need more extensive and definitive discussions, consult the references listed *by section,* in the Bibliography.

The McGraw-Hill/PreTest® staff and I invite your comments and suggestions.

Radiology
PreTest®
Self-Assessment
and Review

Chest Radiology

DIRECTIONS: Each question below contains five suggested responses. Select the **one best** response to each question.

1. The arrow in the lateral chest radiograph in the figure designates which of the following structures?

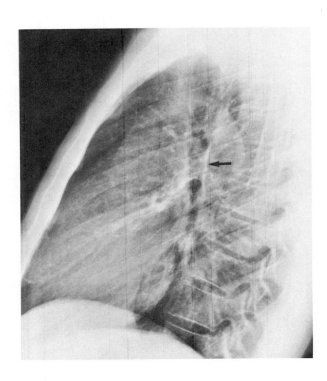

    (A) Posterior wall of the trachea
    (B) Anterior wall of the esophagus
    (C) Posterior wall of the bronchus intermedius
    (D) Posterior wall of the right upper lobe bronchus
    (E) Anterior scapular border

2. A 52-year-old man presented with back pain. A sagittal MR image is shown in the accompanying figure. What is the MOST likely diagnosis?

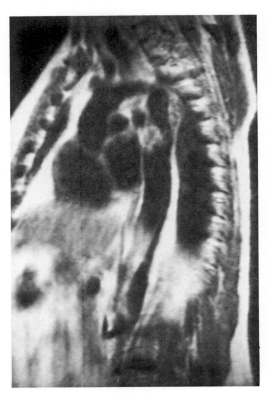

    (A) Aortic dissection
    (B) Adult-type coarctation
    (C) Aortic aneurysm
    (D) Penetrating atherosclerotic aortic ulcer
    (E) Aortic duplication

3. A 29-year-old man with a history of intra-venous drug abuse was admitted to the hospital with shortness of breath and fever. The chest radiograph in the figure was obtained 4 days after admission. What is the MOST likely diagnosis?

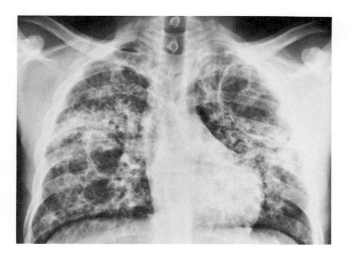

    (A)   Septic emboli
    (B)   Lymphocytic interstitial pneumonitis
    (C)   Lymphoma
    (D)   Kaposi's sarcoma
    (E)   *Pneumocystis carinii* pneumonia

4. Which ONE of the following types of bron-chiectasis is MOST severe?

    (A)   Cystic
    (B)   Varicose
    (C)   Cylindrical
    (D)   Obstructive
    (E)   Irreversible

5. Which ONE of the following is the MOST anterior structure to pass through the dia-phragm?

    (A)   Esophagus
    (B)   Aorta
    (C)   Thoracic duct
    (D)   Vagus nerve
    (E)   Inferior vena cava

6. A 26-year-old man had mild shortness of breath and an abnormal chest radiograph which prompted the accompanying CT scan (see figure). What is the MOST likely diagnosis?

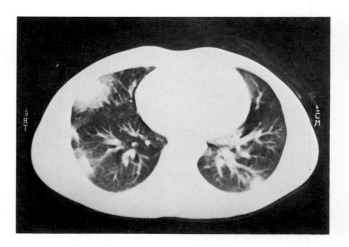

    (A)   Usual interstitial pneumonitis (UIP)
    (B)   Loeffler syndrome
    (C)   Pulmonary infarctions
    (D)   *Hemophilus influenza* pneumonia
    (E)   Sarcoidosis

7. The CT scan of a 25-year-old woman with chest pain is shown in the figure. Which disease is MOST likely?

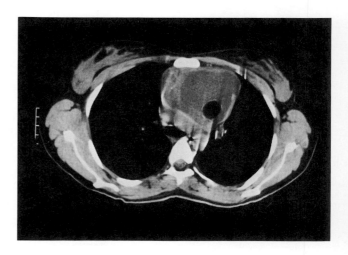

    (A)   Thymic carcinoid
    (B)   Malignant seminoma
    (C)   Nodular sclerosing Hodgkin lymphoma
    (D)   Benign mediastinal teratoma
    (E)   Rebound thymic hyperplasia

8. A 65-year-old woman presented with left chest tightness. Utilizing the chest x-ray shown in the figure, which of the following would you say is the MOST likely diagnosis?

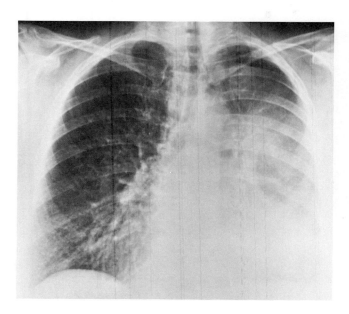

(A) Chylothorax
(B) Bronchogenic carcinoma
(C) Klebsiella pneumonia
(D) Malignant mesothelioma
(E) Fibrosarcoma of the chest wall

9. Which ONE of the following causes of pulmonary arterial hypertension is commonly associated with pulmonary edema?

(A) Thromboembolic disease
(B) Pulmonary venoocclusive disease
(C) Chronic obstructive pulmonary disease
(D) Eisenmenger syndrome
(E) Pulmonary vasculitis

10. Bulky mediastinal adenopathy is MOST characteristic of which ONE of the following subtypes of lung cancer?

(A) Adenocarcinoma
(B) Squamous cell carcinoma
(C) Small-cell carcinoma
(D) Mucoepidermoid carcinoma
(E) Pulmonary blastoma

11. In the CT scan shown in the figure, which structure is marked by the arrow?

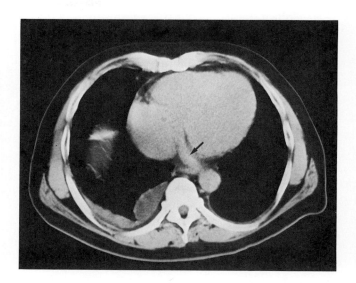

(A) Posterior descending coronary artery
(B) Persistent left superior vena cava
(C) Left inferior pulmonary vein
(D) Coronary sinus
(E) Left superior pulmonary vein

12. A 43-year-old hypertensive man presented with the chest radiograph shown in the figure. What is the MOST likely diagnosis?

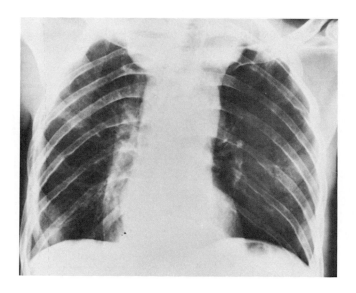

(A) Neurofibromatosis
(B) Thoracic aortic aneurysm
(C) Thymoma
(D) Thyroid goiter
(E) Aortic pseudocoarctation

13. The chest radiograph shown in the figure is that of a 65-year-old man with slowly progressive shortness of breath. Which of the following is the MOST likely diagnosis?

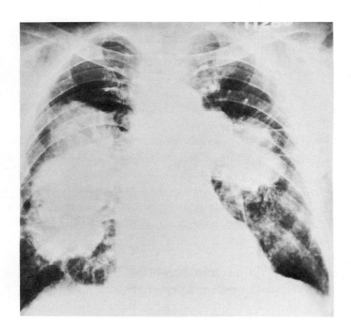

(A) Sarcoidosis
(B) Bilateral bronchogenic carcinoma
(C) Echinococcal disease
(D) Wegener granulomatosis
(E) Progressive massive fibrosis

14. Which ONE of the following lesions is MOST likely to cause hypoglycemia and a pleural-based density?

(A) Lipoma
(B) Peripheral adenocarcinoma of the lung
(C) Metastatic thymoma
(D) Thoracic splenosis
(E) Localized mesothelioma

15. Which of the following structures corresponds to the "aortic nipple" shadow on chest radiographs?

(A) Accessory hemiazygous vein
(B) Hemiazygous vein
(C) Left superior intercostal vein
(D) Left pericardiophrenic vein
(E) Left recurrent laryngeal nerve

16. A 32-year-old man presented with a cough and an abnormal chest radiograph. A high-resolution CT scan is shown in the figure. Which of the following is the MOST likely diagnosis?

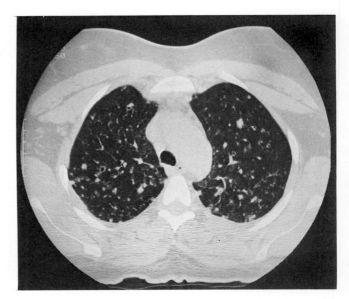

(A) Extrinsic allergic alveolitis
(B) Lymphangitic carcinomatosis
(C) Eosinophilic granuloma
(D) Usual interstitial pneumonitis
(E) Asbestosis

17. Which ONE of the following cases of bronchogenic carcinoma would be considered surgically incurable by the AJCC 1985 TNM classification?

(A) N1 lymph node metastases
(B) Stage IIIA tumor
(C) A tumor whose proximal margin is 3 cm from the carina
(D) Ipsilateral supraclavicular lymph node metastasis
(E) A tumor with invasion of the visceral, but not parietal, pleura

DIRECTIONS: Each group of questions below consists of lettered headings followed by a set of numbered items. For each numbered item select the **one** lettered heading with which it is **most** closely associated. Each lettered heading may be used **once, more than once,** or **not at all.**

Questions 18–21

Match each radiographic description of pulmonary metastatic disease with the primary lesion most likely responsible.

(A) Breast cancer
(B) Seminoma
(C) Cervical cancer
(D) Thyroid cancer
(E) Chondrosarcoma

18. Miliary nodules

19. Cavitary parenchymal masses

20. Calcified pulmonary nodules

21. Endobronchial lesions

Questions 22–25

Match each of the following radiographic descriptions with the infectious agent with which it is most closely associated.

(A) Nocardia
(B) Echinococcus
(C) Klebsiella
(D) Actinomyces
(E) Varicella

22. "Water-lily" sign

23. Small, calcified pulmonary nodules

24. Pulmonary gangrene

25. Pulmonary edema pattern due to alveolar proteinosis

Questions 26–29

Match each of the following radiographic findings with the most closely associated occupational lung disease.

(A) Byssinosis
(B) Coal worker's pneumoconiosis
(C) Asbestos-related lung disease
(D) Silo-filler's disease
(E) Berylliosis

26. Benign pleural effusions

27. Necrobiotic pulmonary nodules

28. Bronchiolitis obliterans

29. Hilar adenopathy

DIRECTIONS: Each group of questions below consists of four lettered headings followed by a set of numbered items. For each numbered item select

A	if the item is associated with	(A) **only**
B	if the item is associated with	(B) **only**
C	if the item is associated with	**both** (A) and (B)
D	if the item is associated with	**neither** (A) nor (B)

Each lettered heading may be used **once, more than once,** or **not at all.**

Questions 30–33

  (A)   Abscess
  (B)   Empyema
  (C)   Both
  (D)   Neither

30.   Round shape

31.   Uniform wall thickness

32.   No displacement of vessels or bronchi

33.   Pneumonia in adjacent lung parenchyma

Questions 34–37

  (A)   Hodgkin lymphoma
  (B)   Non-Hodgkin lymphoma
  (C)   Both
  (D)   Neither

34.   Parenchymal disease without mediastinal adenopathy in untreated patients

35.   Frequent posterior mediastinal adenopathy

36.   Low-density lymphadenopathy

37.   Ill-defined parenchymal nodules

DIRECTIONS: Each question below contains five suggested answers. For **each** of the **five** alternatives listed, you are to respond either YES or NO. In a given item, **all, some,** or **none of the alternatives may be correct.**

38. Which of the following statements are correct concerning thoracic imaging with magnetic resonance (MR) imaging as compared to computed tomography?

    (A) MR is better for detailing parenchymal lung disease
    (B) MR better demonstrates invasion of the subclavian vessels by superior sulcus tumors
    (C) MR provides a significant advantage in demonstrating mediastinal lymphadenopathy in patients with bronchogenic cancer
    (D) MR has better spatial resolution
    (E) MR has better contrast resolution

39. Which of the following statements concerning percutaneous transthoracic needle biopsy (PTNB) is (are) correct?

    (A) The frequency of pneumothorax in fluoroscopically guided procedures is approximately 25%
    (B) Chronic obstructive pulmonary disease is the most important factor contributing to pneumothorax
    (C) PTNB provides an accuracy of approximately 70% for the diagnosis of bronchogenic carcinoma.
    (D) The diagnostic accuracy of PTNB for lymphoma is less than that for bronchogenic carcinoma
    (E) The use of smaller-gauge (19-gauge or higher) needles for PTNB results in a decrease in diagnostic accuracy

40. Which of the following radiographic findings favor(s) elevated hydrostatic pressure as the cause of pulmonary edema over that due to increased capillary permeability?

    (A) Air bronchograms
    (B) Pleural effusions
    (C) Central predominance of the parenchymal opacity
    (D) Blood flow diversion to the upper lung zones
    (E) Simultaneous onset of infiltrates and clinical symptoms

41. Which of the following statements concerning pulmonary sarcoidosis is (are) correct?

    (A) Fiberoptic bronchoscopy is usually not diagnostic in patients with radiographs showing only hilar adenopathy
    (B) Approximately 10% of patients with sarcoidosis have normal chest radiographs
    (C) Posterior mediastinal adenopathy is unusual
    (D) Nodular sarcoidosis frequently cavitates
    (E) Pleural effusions occur in less than 5% of patients

42. TRUE statements regarding the solitary pulmonary nodule include which of the following?

    (A) High kVp technique optimizes visualization of calcification in a nodule
    (B) A lesion which has a doubling time of less than 1 month or greater than 2 years is unlikely to represent bronchogenic carcinoma
    (C) A spiculated border is highly specific for bronchogenic cancer
    (D) The presence of cavitation is of limited value in distinguishing a benign nodule from a malignant one
    (E) Malignant neoplasms, granulomas, and hamartomas account for nearly 95% of solitary pulmonary nodules

43. Which of the following statements regarding pulmonary tuberculosis is (are) correct?

    (A) Primary tuberculosis most often involves the upper lobe
    (B) Reactivation tuberculosis frequently affects the lingula
    (C) Cavitation in reactivation tuberculosis indicates a high probability of active disease
    (D) Tuberculous pleurisy may lead to empyema necessitans
    (E) AIDS patients who acquire tuberculosis rarely have cavitary disease

44. Which of the following statements is (are) TRUE regarding invasive aspergillosis?

    (A) Invasive aspergillus forms mycetomas in preexisting cavities
    (B) The "halo" sign, demonstrated by CT scanning, precedes the appearance of airspace disease
    (C) The presence of precipitating antibodies to aspergillus is necessary for the diagnosis
    (D) Cavitation of pulmonary infiltrates occurs during the recovery phase following neutropenia
    (E) The "gloved finger" shadow is a characteristic plain film finding

45. Which of the following statements regarding bleomycin lung toxicity is (are) true?

    (A) Toxicity is dose-related
    (B) Toxicity is increased with the concomitant use of hyperbaric oxygen therapy
    (C) Diffuse alveolar damage is the most common histologic finding
    (D) The initial radiographic abnormalities predominantly involve the upper lobes
    (E) Pulmonary nodules, which mimic metastatic disease, are uncommon

46. TRUE statements regarding radiation effects on the lung include

    (A) The effect of a given dose of radiation is greater when the dose is given in larger fractions
    (B) Radiation pneumonitis typically develops within 1 month of radiation therapy
    (C) Radiation fibrosis changes continue for up to 18 months after therapy
    (D) Parenchymal opacities in radiation fibrosis are confined to the radiation port
    (E) MR imaging can distinguish radiation pneumonitis from recurrent tumor

47. Which of the following statements regarding bronchial carcinoid is (are) correct?

    (A) It occurs more commonly in females
    (B) There is an increased incidence in cigarette smokers
    (C) Tumor location is more often peripheral
    (D) Atypical carcinoid is associated with a better prognosis than typical carcinoid
    (E) Carcinoid syndrome is present in about 10% of cases

48. Upper lung zone predominance is a feature of which of the following?

    (A) Polymyositis-associated interstitial pneumonitis
    (B) Primary tuberculosis
    (C) Bronchocentric granulomatosis
    (D) Pulmonary fibrosis associated with ankylosing spondylitis
    (E) Bronchial atresia

49. Correct statements concerning Wegener granulomatosis include which of the following?

    (A) It is more common in females
    (B) The upper respiratory tract is more frequently affected at presentation than is the lung
    (C) Nodular masses are the most common form of lung involvement
    (D) The parenchymal disease has a lower lung zone predominance
    (E) Tracheal enlargement is characteristic of airway involvement

50. TRUE statements regarding pneumothorax include

    (A) Primary spontaneous pneumothorax has a strong male predominance
    (B) In asthmatics, pneumothoraces occur more commonly in adults than in children
    (C) Malignant melanoma is the most common metastatic tumor to cause pneumothorax
    (D) Catamenial pneumothorax typically favors the right lung
    (E) Radiographically evident apical bullous disease or fibrosis is present in the majority of patients with Marfan syndrome who develop pneumothoraces

51. Which of the following conditions is (are) associated with tracheal narrowing?

    (A) Mounier-Kuhn syndrome
    (B) Scleroma
    (C) Tracheopathia osteoplastica
    (D) Relapsing polychondritis
    (E) Tuberculosis

52. TRUE statements about rheumatoid lung disease include

    (A) There is a slight female predominance
    (B) Pleural effusion is the most common radiographic manifestation
    (C) Rheumatoid lung nodules have a predilection for the lower lung zones
    (D) Rheumatoid interstitial pulmonary fibrosis is indistinguishable from idiopathic pulmonary fibrosis
    (E) Rheumatoid vasculitis is the primary cause of pulmonary arterial hypertension in most patients with rheumatoid lung disease

53. TRUE statements concerning variant lung anatomy include

    (A) The azygos fissure contains four pleural layers
    (B) The azygos lobe contains branches of the right upper lobe bronchi
    (C) The inferior accessory fissure separates the medial basal segment from the remaining lower lobe segments
    (D) The superior accessory fissure separates the superior segment of the lower lobe from the remaining lower lobe segments
    (E) The left minor fissure is usually located higher than its right lung counterpart

54. TRUE statements regarding traumatic injury to the thorax include

    (A) Fracture of the upper three ribs usually indicates significant intrathoracic injury
    (B) Pneumothorax is the most common radiographic abnormality found in tracheobronchial rupture
    (C) Hematomas typically take from weeks to months to resolve
    (D) Pneumatocele formation implies superinfection of injured lung, usually by *S. aureus*
    (E) The aortic isthmus and aortic root are the two most common sites of aortic transection

55. Which of the following is (are) true regarding thymoma?

    (A) Associations include hypogammaglobulinemia and pure red cell aplasia
    (B) Myasthenia gravis is present in about 35% of patients
    (C) It is uncommon after the age of 40
    (D) Calcification is visible in approximately 10% of tumors imaged by chest x-ray or CT
    (E) CT is able to distinguish benign from malignant thymoma, even in the absence of mediastinal invasion

56. TRUE statements regarding high-resolution computed tomography (HRCT) include:

    (A) The technique requires narrow collimation scans (1- to 2-mm slice thickness)
    (B) A small field-of-view is desirable to maximize spatial resolution
    (C) A low spatial frequency algorithm is the best type for image reconstruction
    (D) Nodules are easier to differentiate from vascular structures by HRCT than conventional CT
    (E) By HRCT, the major fissures typically appear as areas of lucency

57. Which of the following statements regarding lymphangioleiomyomatosis (LAM) is (are) correct?

    (A) It occurs with equal frequency in males and females
    (B) Inheritance is autosomal recessive
    (C) On chest radiographs, decreased lung volumes are characteristic
    (D) High-resolution CT typically demonstrates markedly thickened septal lines
    (E) Chylous pleural effusions are frequently associated

58. Which of the following is (are) characterized by peripheral lung opacities?

    (A) Amiodarone toxicity
    (B) Churg-Strauss syndrome
    (C) Non-Hodgkin lymphoma
    (D) Cardiogenic pulmonary edema
    (E) Bronchioloalveolar carcinoma

59. Correct statements about thoracic amyloidosis include:

    (A) Parenchymal amyloidosis most commonly causes diffuse interstitial thickening
    (B) Calcification occurs in approximately 40% of cases of nodular pulmonary amyloidosis
    (C) Rapid growth is characteristic of amyloidosis-related nodules
    (D) It is a cause of diffuse tracheal narrowing
    (E) Atelectasis is common in the tracheobronchial form of disease

60. Correct statements concerning bronchogenic cysts include which of the following?

    (A) They are lined by squamous epithelium
    (B) Most are incidentally discovered on routine chest radiographs
    (C) They are characteristically well-circumscribed
    (D) An air-fluid level indicates a high likelihood of infection
    (E) By CT, the cyst fluid usually measures water density (0 to 20 Hounsfield units)

Chest Radiology

Answers

1. **The answer is C.** *(Armstrong, pp 27, 37.)*   The structure labeled by the arrow in the lateral radiograph in the figure is the posterior wall of the bronchus intermedius. The bronchus intermedius is the continuation of the right main bronchus after the origin of the right upper lobe bronchus. It courses inferiorly and rightward to terminate at the origin of the right middle lobe bronchus.

   On the lateral chest radiograph, the posterior wall is often visible as a vertical-line shadow which angles somewhat anteriorly. The width of the posterior wall should not exceed 2 to 3 mm. Adjacent lymphadenopathy and parenchymal neoplastic or infectious processes may cause the thickness to increase.

2. **The answer is A.** *(Petasnick, Radiol 180(2): 297–305, 1991.)*   A sagittal view from a magnetic resonance (MR) study of the chest demonstrates a vertically oriented line of increased signal within the flow void of the descending aortic lumen. This represents an intimal flap; a finding diagnostic for aortic dissection. Adult-type coarctation, aortic aneurysm, penetrating atherosclerotic ulcer, and aortic duplication, unless complicated by an aortic dissection, would not result in an intimal flap.

   In patients who are not critically ill, MR imaging provides much useful information without the need for intravenous contrast material. The multiplanar capability of MR allows for assessing long segments of the aorta in the same image as well as detecting extension of the flap into the arch vessels. The advent of cine-MR technology now allows aortic regurgitation to be readily diagnosed.

3. **The answer is E.** *(Goodman, J Thor Imag 6(4): 16–21, 1991.)*   The chest radiograph demonstrates multiple thin-walled cysts superimposed on a background of diffuse parenchymal opacity. In intravenous drug abusers, a group at extremely high risk for AIDS, the most likely cause for these abnormalities is *Pneumocystis carinii* pneumonia with cyst formation. Of the remaining choices, only septic emboli routinely cause cystic lesions, but these usually have thicker walls, are peripherally located, and have surrounding focal opacity. Thin-walled cysts are not characteristic of lymphocytic interstitial pneumonitis, lymphoma, or Kaposi sarcoma.

   Cysts in patients with *Pneumocystis carinii* pneumonia are reported to occur in 10% of patients. Their origin is obscure, but it has been postulated that they represent small pneumatoceles.

4. **The answer is A.** *(Armstrong, pp 821–829.)* Bronchiectasis is characterized by chronic, irreversible dilatation of the bronchi. Bronchiectasis may be obstructive or nonobstructive and is frequently associated with inflammation. Through bronchography, cylindrical, varicose, and cystic varieties have been described, ranging from least to most severe, respectively.

   Cystic bronchiectasis is well-evaluated by CT scanning, which has largely replaced bronchography. CT findings include a "string of beads" appearance, due to contiguous cysts; a continuity of some cysts and the more central airways; and a "signet ring" shape which occurs when there is an accompanying vessel.

5. **The answer is E.** *(Fraser, ed. 3, pp 2921–2923.)* The diaphragm is a musculotendinous structure which consists of sternal, costal, and crural muscular components that insert into a central tendon. Three openings in the diaphragm allow passage of major structures from the thorax to the abdomen. The inferior vena cava passes through the most anterior aperture, at the level of the eighth thoracic vertebra. The esophagus and the vagus nerve traverse the middle opening at the T10 level. The most posterior opening allows passage of the aorta and the thoracic duct at the T12 level.

6. **The answer is C.** *(Armstrong, pp 350–373.)* The transaxial chest CT in the figure demonstrates several peripheral, pleural-based densities which resemble truncated cones, an appearance most characteristic for pulmonary infarctions from embolism. Peripheral opacities may be present in patients with usual interstitial pneumonia, Loeffler syndrome, *Hemophilis influenza* pneumonia, and sarcoidosis, but these usually do not take the form of multiple truncated cones. This patient had protein-C deficiency, a hematologic disorder which predisposes to vascular thrombosis, which sometimes results in pulmonary embolism.

   Chest radiograph findings in patients with pulmonary emboli include regional oligemia, with or without central pulmonary artery enlargement (Westermark's sign), wedge-shaped densities at the pleural margins, bandlike atelectasis, and pleural effusions. These findings are seen to best advantage on contrast-enhanced CT, and occasionally there is direct visualization of thrombus in the central pulmonary arteries, outlined by contrast.

7. **The answer is D.** *(Armstrong, pp 717–720.)* The thoracic CT scan in the figure demonstrates an anterior mediastinal mass which contains a well-defined area of fat density. In a young woman, a benign mediastinal teratoma is the most likely diagnosis. The chest pain in this case was caused by inflammation of pancreatic tissue in the lesion. Thymic carcinoid, nodular sclerosing Hodgkin lymphoma, and rebound thymic hyperplasia do not contain areas of fat density. Malignant seminoma is usually ill-defined.

   Benign teratoma is the term used to denote a tumor which contains more than one embryonic cell layer. The lesion has a slight female predominance and occurs most often in adolescents or young adults. Nearly all are located in the anterior mediastinum and are usually well-defined. Fat density is present in 25 to 50% of lesions and calcification—even teeth—may be identified.

8. **The answer is B.** *(Armstrong, pp 102–106.)* The chest radiograph in the figure shows a hazy opacity in the left chest which spares the left lung apex. There is a loss of visualization of the left heart border, the left hemidiaphragm, and the aortic arch. The mediastinum is slightly shifted to the left suggesting volume loss. This combination of abnormalities is most consistent with left upper lobe atelectasis. Expansion and reorientation of the left lower lobe accounts for the aerated lung in the left apex. In an older patient with left upper lobe atelectasis, central endobronchial lesions such as bronchogenic carcinoma or bronchial carcinoid are the primary considerations.

9. **The answer is B.** *(Armstrong, pp 373–383.)* Pulmonary arterial hypertension is defined as a systolic pulmonary artery pressure of 30 mmHg or higher or as a mean pulmonary artery pressure of greater than 18 mmHg. There are numerous causes of pulmonary arterial hypertension, but only

those which operate at the postcapillary level, such as mitral stenosis, pulmonary vein stenosis, and pulmonary venoocclusive disease, result in pulmonary edema.

The etiology of pulmonary venoocclusive disease is unknown, but a viral cause has been postulated. Pulmonary venous thrombosis and intimal fibrosis leads to capillary hypertension, pulmonary edema, and pulmonary artery hypertension. The left atrium is not enlarged, a finding helpful for differentiating this condition from mitral stenosis.

10. **The answer is C.** *(Armstrong, pp 282–283.)* Bulky mediastinal adenopathy is common in sarcoidosis, lymphoma, granulomatous disease, and intrathoracic or extrathoracic metastatic disease. In patients with lung cancer, massive mediastinal nodal enlargement is characteristic of the small-cell subtype. Often, the primary pulmonary lesion is so small that it is not visible, even by CT. These features are useful in distinguishing small-cell carcinoma from adenocarcinoma and squamous cell carcinoma, which are treated differently.

Mucoepidermoid carcinoma and pulmonary blastoma are rare lung tumors which are not typically associated with bulky mediastinal adenopathy.

11. **The answer is D.** *(Lee, ed. 2, p 388.)* The CT scan of the thorax in the figure shows a tubular structure coursing anteriorly and to the right to enter the right atrium, which is the coronary sinus. The coronary sinus provides the venous drainage for the bulk of the coronary circulation. Enlargement may occur with a variety of congenital cardiac anomalies, especially those associated with a persistent left superior vena cava, which usually empties into the coronary sinus. The vessel is frequently seen on CT scans at the level of the inferior right atrium.

12. **The answer is A.** *(Armstrong, pp 576–579.)* The chest radiograph in the figure demonstrates bilateral superior mediastinal masses, slight generalized widening of the mediastinum, and bilateral rib notching. This constellation of abnormalities is most consistent with neurofibromatosis. Thoracic aortic aneurysm, thymoma, thyroid goiter, and aortic pseudocoarctation may cause a superior mediastinal mass, but would not affect the ribs.

Neurofibromatosis is a systemic autosomal dominant neurocutaneous disorder which affects multiple organs. Central nervous system and skin lesions are particularly common. Systemic hypertension may result from a pheochromocytoma or, as in this case, renal artery stenosis.

In the thorax, patients may present with mediastinal lesions including neurofibromas (as in the case shown), lateral thoracic meningoceles, and pheochromocytomas. Chest wall abnormalities include cutaneous fibromas, thoracic kyphoscoliosis, and rib notching. In the lungs, interstitial fibrosis occurs in 20% of patients.

13. **The answer is E.** *(Armstrong, pp 407–411.)* Although sarcoidosis, bilateral bronchogenic cancer, echinococcal disease, or Wegener granulomatosis could conceivably result in the widespread pulmonary abnormalities in the figure, only progressive massive fibrosis (PMF) characteristically produces large, ill-defined mid-upper-lung-zone masses bilaterally. PMF is most often associated with coal worker's pneumoconiosis and is related to the quantity of dust exposure. PMF usually starts in the lung periphery, slowly enlarges, and migrates centrally. A helpful differential characteristic of PMF is the tendency for the lesion to have a transverse diameter which is much larger than its anteroposterior diameter. Mortality is due to the severe emphysema which usually accompanies the condition.

14. **The answer is E.** *(Armstrong, pp 323–324.)* All the listed choices can produce pleural-based densities, but only localized pleural mesothelioma has a recognized association with hypoglycemia. The term *localized* mesothelioma is preferred to *benign fibrous* mesothelioma, because 10 to 15% of tumors are malignant. Seventy-five percent of lesions arise from the visceral pleura and approximately half are pedunculated. The average age at presentation is 51 years and about half the patients are symptomatic, usually with cough, chest pain, or dyspnea. Symptomatic hypoglycemia occurs in about 40% of patients. Hypertrophic osteoarthropathy is another recognized association.

15. The answer is C.   *(Fraser, ed. 3, pp 218–219.)*   The designation *aortic nipple* refers to a focal convexity which protrudes laterally from the aortic arch on posteroanterior (PA) chest radiographs. It is visible in approximately 5% of technically adequate studies. It is caused by the left superior intercostal vein passing anteriorly across the aortic arch, as it courses to the left brachiocephalic vein. It occasionally serves as a collateral vessel, causing the "aortic nipple" shadow to enlarge, in which case it may be mistaken for a mediastinal mass.

16. The answer is C.   *(Armstrong, pp 573–576.)*   The most likely diagnosis to account for the upper lobe nodules and cysts in the figure is eosinophilic granuloma (EG). EG is part of the spectrum of histocytic diseases. Pulmonary eosinophilic granuloma usually presents in the third or fourth decade, most commonly with cough, dyspnea, and chest pain. Pneumothorax is a rare initial symptom. Chest radiographs characteristically reveal hazy, bilateral reticulonodular infiltrates, which favor the upper lobes. High-resolution computed tomography (HRCT) shows either a combination of multiple small nodules and cysts, or multiple cysts, some of which can be quite large.

By HRCT, extrinsic allergic alveolitis (hypersensitivity pneumonitis) most often causes a "ground-glass" appearance of the interstitium, which does not obscure the vasculature. Lymphangitic carcinomatosis is characterized by septal thickening, often with a beaded appearance. Usual interstitial pneumonia and asbestosis have a basilar predominance, with subpleural cysts often revealed by HRCT.

17. The answer is D.   *(Stitik, pp 619–630.)*   The need for a uniform staging procedure to account for advances in diagnosis and management of bronchogenic carcinoma led to the development of a new TNM staging system by the American Joint Committee on Cancer (AJCC) in 1985.

In the new system, *T* describes the *primary tumor*. Tumors in the T1, T2, and T3 categories are considered resectable. T4 tumors involve vital structures such as the heart, aorta, trachea, and esophagus, and are not amenable to surgical cure. A lesion that extends within 3 cm of the carina or a lesion with invasion limited to the visceral pleura would be classified as a T2 tumor. *N* refers to *lymph node metastasis*. N0 is the absence of nodal involvement. N1 indicates metastasis to the ipsilateral hilum, whereas N2 refers to ipsilateral *mediastinal* nodal involvement. N3 disease means that there is involvement of ipsilateral supraclavicular or scalene nodes, or contralateral nodal disease. Patients with N3 disease are unresectable. *M* designates *metastasis* (M0 = no metastasis, M1 = metastasis). M1 disease indicates unresectability.

Assessment of the TNM status allows staging of bronchogenic carcinoma. Patients with tumor stages 0, I, II, and IIIA are potentially resectable. Those with stage IIIB (T4, any N, M0 *or* any T, N3, M0) or stage IV (any T, any N, M1) disease are usually unresectable.

18–21. The answers are: 18-D, 19-C, 20-E, 21-A.   *(Armstrong, pp 329–335.)*   Pulmonary metastases are more common than primary lung cancer, and most often present nonspecifically as single or multiple parenchymal nodules. Nevertheless, certain patterns allow one to narrow the list of differential possibilities.

A micronodular pattern, similar to miliary tuberculosis, is occasionally encountered. Thyroid cancer is one of the principal sources, and iodine radionuclide scanning often reveals diffuse lung uptake. Other primary cancers associated with this pattern include renal cell carcinoma and melanoma.

Cavitating pulmonary nodules occur in about 5% of patients with metastases. The most common primary lesions are cervical cancer and head and neck tumors. The size of the lesion appears unrelated to its propensity to cavitate.

Calcified metastases are unusual. The most common primary tumors are osteosarcoma and chondrosarcoma. Calcification may also be identified in nonsarcomatous metastases following treatment.

Endobronchial metastases are quite uncommon, with an incidence of 2% in one large autopsy series. The most common primary tumors are breast, kidney, and colon. Presenting clinical symptoms are indistinguishable from those caused by central bronchogenic cancer.

22–25. The answers are: 22-B, 23-E, 24-C, 25-A. *(Armstrong, pp 152–257.)* The chest radiograph is very sensitive for detecting pneumonia, but usually does not allow precise identification of the offending organism. Nevertheless, certain radiographic abnormalities are helpful to narrow the differential diagnostic possibilities.

The "water-lily" or "camelote" sign is pathognomonic of pulmonary echinococcal infection. Most commonly, pulmonary echinococcal disease presents as one or more well-defined, pliant masses which rarely calcify and have a mid- or lower lung zone distribution. The lesion is composed of the endocyst and ectocyst (the parasite) which are surrounded by the pericyst, consisting of compressed lung tissue. If the lesion ruptures but the pericyst remains intact, the crumpled cyst wall may be seen floating in fluid, resulting in the unique radiographic appearance termed the "water-lily" sign.

Multiple small calcified pulmonary nodules are most often associated with prior disseminated histoplasmosis or tuberculosis, but are a well-documented sequela of varicella pneumonia. Over 90% of varicella pneumonia infections occur in adults, particularly in immunocompromised hosts. The radiographic appearance is different from the small patchy consolidations present in most viral pneumonias in that there are often multiple small nodules during the acute infection, which later calcify in a minority of patients.

Pulmonary gangrene results from thrombosis of pulmonary vessels as they course through an area of pneumonia. The most common offending agents are *Klebsiella* sp. and *S. pneumonia*. Radiographically, pulmonary gangrene appears as an area of cavitation containing necrotic lung debris.

Pulmonary nocardiosis is an indolent bacterial infection which often occurs in patients with immunologic deficiencies. The most common radiographic finding in that case is pulmonary consolidation, which is often cavitary. For reasons which are obscure, patients with alveolar proteinosis are prone to superinfection with nocardia. In these patients, the nocardial superinfection is not distinguished from the underlying condition.

26–29. The answers are: 26-C, 27-B, 28-D, 29-E. *(Armstrong, pp 405–440.)* Radiographic imaging plays a major role in determining the presence and severity of occupational lung disease.

In many parts of the country, asbestos exposure is the single largest contributor to occupational lung illness. Malignant pleural effusions may be seen in the most dreaded of asbestos-related complications—malignant mesothelioma and bronchogenic carcinoma. Benign pleural effusions are frequently the earliest manifestations of asbestos exposure. The effusions may be unilateral or bilateral and often recur. They are typically small and asymptomatic. Many patients who have benign pleural effusions later develop diffuse basal pleural thickening.

The combination of rheumatoid arthritis and multiple pulmonary nodules in coal workers is called *Caplan syndrome*. Pathologically, the nodules are similar to the necrobiotic rheumatoid nodules found in the subcutaneous tissues. The nodules are usually bilateral and range from 0.5 to 5 cm in size. They may occur in coal miners who have no evidence of pneumoconiosis.

Silo-filler's disease is caused by nitrogen dioxide fumes emitted from fresh silage. Typically, there is a two-part reaction. The initial phase, which occurs soon after exposure, is characterized by cough and dyspnea, often accompanied by pulmonary edema. After a recovery period of two to three weeks, the symptoms recur and radiographs will often reveal a fine nodular pattern corresponding to the development of bronchiolitis obliterans.

The chronic form of berylliosis has a remarkably similar clinical and radiographic appearance to sarcoidosis. Hilar and mediastinal adenopathy are common, as is a reticulonodular chest x-ray pattern, which can progress to "honeycomb" lung. Berylliosis may involve the skin, liver, and spleen. Unlike sarcoidosis, it spares the skeleton and central nervous system.

30–33. The answers are: 30-A, 31-B, 32-A, 33-C. *(Armstrong, pp 240–248.)* The therapeutically important distinction between lung abscess and empyema is the difference between antibiotics and chest drainage, respectively. Many complex processes are difficult to assess from the chest radiograph, and though CT scanning is often helpful, occasionally the problem eludes even cross-sectional imaging.

The wall of an empyema consists of uniformly thickened visceral and parietal pleura separated by infected pleural fluid. The thickened pleural surfaces may enhance following intravenous contrast administration, giving rise to the "split-pleura" sign. Abscess walls are usually thicker and shaggier than those of empyemas. Abscesses are usually round, whereas empyemas conform to the pleural space and are more often oval.

Empyemas often compress adjacent lung, which may cause distortion or displacement of adjacent parenchymal vessels and bronchi. Abscesses, by contrast, cause tissue destruction. Since there is usually no mass effect, vessels and bronchi in the adjacent normal lung are not displaced.

The presence of adjacent pneumonia is of limited use in differentiating lung abscess from empyema, because it may occur with both conditions. Most empyemas result from seeding of the pleural space by adjacent pneumonia. An abscess is usually the result of cavitation within an area of pneumonia.

34–37. The answers are: 34-B, 35-D, 36-C, 37-C. *(Armstrong, pp 302–315.)* Intrathoracic involvement by lymphoma occurs more commonly with Hodgkin disease than it does with non-Hodgkin lymphoma. Despite many similarities, there are some characteristic differences between the radiographic presentation of the two.

The most important distinction between the two diseases is their mode of spread. Hodgkin disease spreads by extension to contiguous nodal chains, whereas non-Hodgkin lymphoma often skips adjacent nodes. The tendency for contiguity may explain the observation that in untreated patients with Hodgkin disease, parenchymal pulmonary involvement nearly always occurs in the presence of mediastinal lymphadenopathy. Isolated pulmonary involvement is considerably more frequent in patients with non-Hodgkin lymphoma. Patients with Hodgkin lymphoma and treated nodal disease *may* have a recurrence which is confined to the lung.

The most frequently involved nodal groups are in the anterior mediastinum and paratracheal regions. Posterior mediastinal involvement is decidedly uncommon for either type of lymphoma. When present, it suggests the likelihood of retroperitoneal involvement.

CT may demonstrate low-density lymph nodes, which indicates cystic necrosis. Low-density lymphadenopathy may occur in either form of lymphoma and may persist after successful treatment.

Parenchymal involvement in lymphoma has a variable appearance. The patterns are nonspecific, however, and include focal consolidation, ill-defined parenchymal nodules which may cavitate, and widespread reticular-nodular opacities.

38. The answers are: A-N, B-Y, C-N, D-N, E-Y. *(Templeton, Contemp Diag Radiol 14(11): 1–6, 1991.)* Computed tomography (CT) is the primary cross-sectional imaging modality used for evaluating thoracic disease. Magnetic resonance (MR) imaging is frequently employed to provide confirmatory or complementary information. CT remains preeminent because of its superior ability to visualize lung parenchyma and calcifications, and also because of its lower cost and easier accessibility. The spatial resolution of CT is also superior.

MR is advantageous in some situations because it permits imaging through any plane. The sagittal plane optimizes characterization of superior sulcus tumors, detailing invasion of the subclavian vessels and brachial plexus. MR has better contrast resolution, which may be important in areas such as the chest wall, which has poor tissue contrast by CT.

A number of studies have failed to document a significant overall advantage of either CT or MR for the assessment of mediastinal lymphadenopathy in patients with bronchogenic carcinoma.

39. The answers are: A-Y, B-Y, C-N, D-Y, E-N. *(Westcott, pp 593–601.)* Percutaneous transthoracic needle biopsy (PTNB) has proved extremely effective for obtaining diagnostic tissue samples in patients whose lesions are not accessible to fiberoptic bronchoscopy. In masses which ultimately prove to be bronchogenic cancer, PTNB provides a diagnostic accuracy of greater than 90%. Unfortunately, the yield of PTNB in patients with lymphoma or benign lesions is significantly lower.

PTNB can be performed under either fluoroscopic or CT guidance. For large lesions at the periphery, fluoroscopy is preferred because it is faster, simpler, and less expensive. CT is particularly useful for lesions which are centrally located or smaller than 1 cm. The frequency of pneumothorax in fluoroscopically guided procedures is about 25% and is somewhat higher for CT-guided PTNB, probably due to the predominance of deeper lesions. The highest risk for pneumothorax is in patients with chronic obstructive pulmonary disease. Other complications of PTNB include local bleeding, hemoptysis, and air embolism. The smaller-gauge needles (19 gauge or higher) which are used to minimize these complications have not resulted in decreased diagnostic accuracy.

40. The answers are: A-N, B-Y, C-Y, D-Y, E-Y. *(Armstrong, pp 385–397.)* Pulmonary edema is divided into two categories: *hydrostatic,* in which the pulmonary venous pressure is elevated, and that due to increased capillary permeability, as exemplified by *adult respiratory distress syndrome (ARDS).* The radiographic findings do not allow absolute distinction between the two types of pulmonary edema, but certain abnormalities are more characteristic of hydrostatic edema than of increased-capillary-permeability edema.

Patients with hydrostatic edema more often demonstrate a central predominance of the parenchymal opacity, as well as diversion of blood flow to the upper lung zones and pleural effusions. The onset of clinical symptoms typically coincides with the appearance of the radiographic abnormality. Patients with increased-capillary-permeability edema more frequently have air bronchograms, a uniform or peripheral predominance of lung opacity, and a delay between the pulmonary injury and the appearance of parenchymal chest x-ray abnormality. Also, the chest x-ray clears much less rapidly with ARDS than it does with hydrostatic edema, though the patient may be clinically improved.

41. The answers are: A-N, B-Y, C-Y, D-N, E-Y. *(Armstrong, pp 551–573.)* Sarcoidosis is a systemic disorder of unknown etiology characterized by multiorgan involvement by noncaseating granulomas. A pathologic diagnosis may be obtained by fiberoptic bronchoscopy (FOB) in approximately 90% of patients, even when only hilar adenopathy is found on chest x-ray. About 10% of patients with sarcoidosis have normal chest radiographs, but noncaseating granulomas are still discovered by FOB.

Seventy-five percent of patients with sarcoidosis have lymph node enlargement at some time during the course of the disease, most commonly in the form of bilateral and symmetrical hilar and (unilateral or bilateral) paratracheal adenopathy. Posterior mediastinal adenopathy is unusual. Calcification of lymph nodes, which occurs in about 20% of patients, may assume a characteristic eggshell pattern. Parenchymal abnormalities, excluding fibrosis, occur in about one-third of patients and consist of reticulonodular opacities, alveolar consolidation, or large nodular shadows which rarely cavitate. About one-third of patients develop pulmonary fibrosis, which typically has a mid- and upper lung zone predominance. Pleural effusions associated with sarcoidosis are distinctly uncommon, with an incidence of under 2%.

42. **The answers are: A-N, B-Y, C-Y, D-Y, E-Y.** *(Armstrong, pp 118–128.)* According to the definition given by the Fleischner Society, a solitary pulmonary nodule must be the only pulmonary lesion and cannot be larger than 3 cm. The differential diagnosis of the solitary pulmonary nodule is extensive. Malignant neoplasms, granulomas, and hamartomas account for 95% of cases, with the remaining uncommon causes including pulmonary infarction, arteriovenous malformation, "round" pneumonia, and rounded atelectasis.

   Distinguishing benign from malignant lesions is often difficult, but bronchogenic cancer doubling times typically range between one month and two years. The presence of multiple strands extending from the edge of the lesion into the parenchyma, the corona radiata, is a highly specific sign of malignancy. Cavitation occurs in both benign and malignant disease. Cavitary neoplasms tend to have thicker walls, but the overlap with benign lesions is sufficient to preclude this as a differentiating feature. Calcification which is lamelated or has a "popcorn"-like appearance nearly always indicates a benign lesion and is best visualized when low kVp technique (60 to 70 kV) is used.

43. **The answers are: A-N, B-N, C-Y, D-Y, E-Y.** *(Armstrong, pp 174–192.)* The incidence of pulmonary tuberculosis has increased in recent years for two reasons: AIDS and widespread urban decay with inadequate health care.

   The primary infection may be acquired during childhood or as an adult. Radiographically, the most common feature is hilar or mediastinal adenopathy. A focal pneumonitis, which does not have a lobar predilection, may occur and is indistinguishable from typical bacterial pneumonia. Pleural effusions are present in about 25% of cases.

   In an immune-competent host, reactivation tuberculosis results from endogenous disease and commonly involves the posterior portions of the upper lobes and superior segments of the lower lobes. Cavitation occurs frequently and is a strong indicator of active disease.

   Pleural effusion caused by tuberculosis may occur even in the absence of other intrathoracic disease. *Empyema necessitans* is the term given to pleural tuberculosis which extends into the subcutaneous tissues to form an abscess. A therapeutically resistant bronchopulmonary fistula may result.

   AIDS patients who develop pulmonary tuberculosis have radiographic findings similar to primary tuberculosis, probably because of an impaired or absent hypersensitivity reaction, and do not usually develop cavitary disease.

44. **The answers are: A-N, B-N, C-N, D-Y, E-N.** *(Armstrong, pp 210–214, 229–230.)* There are three main clinical forms of aspergillosis. Invasive aspergillosis occurs in immunocompromised patients, particularly those with leukemia or lymphoma. A positive test for precipitation of antibodies to aspergillus is neither sensitive nor specific. Characteristically, the chest radiograph demonstrates one or more ill-defined rounded opacities which cavitate during recovery from neutropenia. The CT "halo" sign is a circular lucency which develops around an area of airspace disease, which is felt to represent a zone of impending cavitation.

   The saprophytic form of aspergillus colonizes preexisting cavities, producing mycetomas.

   Allergic bronchopulmonary aspergillosis occurs in patients with asthma and atopy. Mucoid impaction is common. Radiographically, the affected bronchi appear as branching structures extending from the hilum, which have a "gloved-finger" appearance.

45. **The answers are: A-Y, B-Y, C-Y, D-N, E-Y.** *(Armstrong, p 451.)* Bleomycin is a cytotoxic antibiotic which is used for chemotherapy. It causes lung toxicity in up to 40% of patients, in a dose-related fashion. Concurrent hyperbaric oxygen or radiation therapy, impaired renal function, and advanced patient age are all risk factors for increased toxicity.

Histopathologically, diffuse alveolar damage is the most frequent pattern of disease, although an acute hypersensitivity reaction also occurs. Radiographically, the initial manifestation is that of reticulonodular basilar opacities which progress to massive airspace consolidation. Occasionally, pulmonary nodules form, which simulate metastatic disease.

46. **The answers are: A-Y, B-N, C-Y, D-N, E-N.** *(Armstrong, pp 457–462.)* Radiation effects on the lung are dependent on a number of factors, including the volume of lung irradiated, concomitant therapy, and dose fractionation. In general, for a given total radiation dose, the larger the dose per fraction, the greater the damage to the lung.

The radiographically evident pulmonary effects are divided into radiation pneumonitis, which occurs between 1 and 6 months after treatment, and radiation fibrosis, which follows and may last up to 18 months. In the pneumonitis phase, hazy parenchymal opacities are present, which are nonsegmental and geometric and which are confined to the radiation port. In the ensuing fibrotic phase, the opacities become more linear and may extend outside the radiation port. Volume loss and bronchiectasis may also develop.

MR imaging is potentially useful in differentiating radiation fibrosis (low signal intensity on T2-weighted images) from recurrent tumor (high signal intensity on T2-weighted images). However, radiation *pneumonitis,* which also exhibits high signal intensity on T2-weighted images cannot be reliably distinguished from recurrent tumor.

47. **The answers are: A-Y, B-N, C-N, D-N, E-N.** *(Fraser, ed. 3, pp 1477–1494.)* Bronchial carcinoid is an indolent but malignant neoplasm arising from the Kulchitsky (APUD) cells of the airway epithelium. A slight female predominance has been observed in several studies. Though the etiology of carcinoid tumors is uncertain, there is no established link with cigarette smoking. Eighty percent of bronchial carcinoids are centrally located and frequently cause obstructive atelectasis. The remainder are peripheral and usually present radiographically as solitary parenchymal masses.

"Atypical" carcinoid tumor is a variant of bronchial carcinoid which has increased mitotic activity and nuclear pleomorphism by histologic examination, when compared to typical carcinoid. The lesion is associated with a more aggressive course and a poorer prognosis. Carcinoid syndrome rarely complicates bronchial carcinoid, with an incidence of 0 to 3%. Cushing syndrome, acromegaly, and Zollinger-Ellison syndrome are other associated endocrinopathies.

48. **The answers are: A-N, B-N, C-Y, D-Y, E-Y.** *(Armstrong, pp 518–520, 583–585, 604–605.)* Diseases with an upper lung zone predominance may be diffuse or focal. Well-known conditions which are typically diffuse include sarcoidosis, eosinophilic granuloma, and silicosis. Ankylosing spondylitis is a seronegative spondyloarthropathy which has a strong male predilection and typically leads to spinal and sacroiliac joint fusion. The pulmonary manifestations include apical fibrosis, pleural thickening, and cyst formation. The radiographic findings of primary tuberculosis (TB) include parahilar adenopathy, parenchymal consolidation, and pleural effusion. Unlike reactivation tuberculosis, which favors the upper lung zones (specifically the apical and posterior segments), primary TB has no lobular predilection. The interstitial pneumonitis associated with polymyositis is radiographically indistinguishable from idiopathic pulmonary fibrosis, and has a basilar lung zone predominance.

Bronchial atresia is an example of a focal disease. It typically involves a segmental bronchus and is associated with emphysema and hypoperfusion of the affected lung segment. There is a marked upper lobe predilection, especially on the left.

Bronchocentric granulomatosis is due to fungal infection and affects only that portion of lung which is served by the affected bronchi. Radiographically, it consists of areas of consolidation which are more common in the upper lung zones and tend to be peripheral.

49. The answers are: A-N, B-Y, C-Y, D-N, E-N. *(Armstrong, pp 473–475.)* Wegener granulomatosis is characterized pathologically by the triad of a necrotizing, granulomatous vasculitis of the upper and lower respiratory tracts, a small-vessel vasculitis of both arteries and veins, and focal glomerulonephritis. There is a slight male predominance. At presentation, upper respiratory tract involvement including sinusitis, rhinitis, and otitis is more frequent than lung involvement.

The most common radiographic appearance of parenchymal involvement is that of multiple nodular masses, which cavitate in 40% of cases and have no zonal predilection. Tracheal involvement, usually subglottic stenosis, occurs in up to 15% of patients. Tracheal enlargement does not occur. Pleural effusions and pneumothoraces have occasionally been reported.

50. The answers are: A-Y, B-N, C-N, D-Y, E-Y. *(Armstrong, pp 673–679.)* Spontaneous pneumothorax, that is, occurring without precipitating trauma, may be either primary or secondary. Patients with primary spontaneous pneumothorax probably have had an apical bleb that ruptured, but without any other underlying lung disease. There is a 5:1 male predominance and the peak age is between 20 and 40.

Secondary spontaneous pneumothorax occurs in the setting of preexisting lung disease. For example, airflow obstruction and air trapping caused by chronic obstructive pulmonary disease or asthma may occasionally cause pneumothorax. Asthma is a far less common cause, and the patients are usually in the pediatric age group.

Metastatic lesions have been reported to account for 0.5% of pneumothoraces. Osteogenic sarcoma is the tumor type most frequently responsible. Catamenial pneumothorax is a manifestation of endometriosis in the chest; pneumothoraces usually occur at the time of menses. They may be recurrent and, for unknown reasons, occur almost exclusively on the right.

Patients with Marfan syndrome and other connective tissue disorders are prone to pneumothoraces, which are often bilateral and recurrent. In the majority of affected patients, chest radiographs reveal evidence of apical bullous disease or fibrosis.

51. The answers are: A-N, B-Y, C-Y, D-Y, E-Y. *(Armstrong, pp 815–819.)* Tracheal narrowing is defined by a sagittal or coronal diameter of less than 13 mm in men and 10 mm in women.

Scleroma is a chronic granulomatosis infection caused by *Klebsiella rhinoscleromatis* which affects the sinuses and airways. Tracheal involvement occurs in about 5% of patients and is manifested as nodular or smooth stenoses. Tracheopathia osteoplastica (or tracheobronchopathia osteochondroplastica) is characterized by formation of cartilaginous and bony submucosal nodules in the upper airway. The nodularity may result in airway narrowing and tracheal calcification, which is best detected by CT scanning. Relapsing polychondritis is an inflammatory disease which involves multiple cartilaginous structures, particularly the pinna, nose, and airways. Airway involvement occurs in over 50% of patients and results in narrowing of the larynx, trachea, and/or proximal bronchi. Tuberculosis of the trachea, now rare, causes airway narrowing, usually in association with cavitary lung disease.

Mounier-Kuhn syndrome (or tracheobronchomegaly) is an idiopathic abnormality of the major airways which causes marked enlargement of the trachea and proximal bronchi. There is a strong male predominance, and the clinical history is usually that of chronic cough and recurrent pulmonary infections. Chest radiographs show a dilated trachea, which has a corrugated appearance because of mucosal prolapse through the tracheal rings.

52. The answers are: A-N, B-Y, C-N, D-Y, E-N. *(Armstrong, pp 481–486.)* Rheumatoid arthritis is associated with abnormalities of the lungs and pleura in as many as 50% of patients. Unlike rheumatoid arthritis limited to the joints, which is more common in females, rheumatoid lung disease has a striking male predominance.

The most frequent intrathoracic radiographic abnormality is pleural effusion, which occurs in approximately 3% of patients and characteristically has a low glucose level.

Rheumatoid lung nodules are pathologically identical to the necrobiotic nodules found in the subcutaneous tissues. They are most often located in the mid and upper lung zones and may occasionally cavitate.

Rheumatoid interstitial pulmonary fibrosis occurs in under 2% of patients with rheumatoid disease. Radiographically, it is indistinguishable from idiopathic pulmonary fibrosis and carries a similarly poor prognosis. Pulmonary arterial hypertension is occasionally attributable to rheumatoid vasculitis, but is more often caused by rheumatoid interstitial pulmonary fibrosis.

53. **The answers are: A-Y, B-Y, C-Y, D-Y, E-Y.** *(Fraser, ed. 3, pp 169–174.)*   Accessory pleural fissures are present in up to 50% of lungs examined anatomically. The best known of these is the azygos fissure, which is visible in 0.4% of chest radiographs as a curvilinear arc extending down from the apex of the right lung, and continues medially to the teardrop opacity of the azygos vein. Developmentally, it results from the growth of the lung outward around the azygos vein, creating two apposing layers of parietal and visceral pleura. The resulting fissure is the lateral border of a portion of the right upper lobe which is then called an *azygos lobe*. The azygos lobe contains branches of the apical and posterior right upper lobe segmental bronchi. The four pleural layers of the azygos fissure contrast with the other types of accessory fissures, which have only two pleural layers.

The inferior accessory fissure extends upward from the medial third of the diaphragm and separates the medial basal segment of the lower lobe from the remaining lower lobe segments. It is present on approximately 10% of chest radiographs, more commonly on the right. The superior accessory fissure separates the superior segment of the lower lobe from the rest of the lower lobe segments.

The left minor fissure separates the lingula from the remainder of the left upper lobe. It appears in fewer than 2% of chest radiographs and is located more cephalad than the right minor fissure.

54. **The answers are: A-Y, B-Y, C-Y, D-N, E-Y.** *(Armstrong, pp 857–880.)*   Thoracic trauma may involve the skeleton, airways, lung parenchyma, and/or mediastinum. Fracture of the upper three ribs is often associated with significant trauma to the underlying soft tissues, particularly the aorta and great vessels. Often, there are additional clinical and radiologic clues to vascular injury.

Tracheobronchial rupture results from severe blunt trauma or penetrating injury and has a 30% mortality. The most common radiographic abnormality is pneumothorax, which occurs in 60% of cases. The affected lung may settle inferiorly in the chest cavity, giving rise to the "fallen lung" sign, which is a somewhat more specific, though less common, sign of airway disruption.

Complications of injuries to the lung parenchyma include contusion, hematoma, and pneumatocele. Contusions appear radiographically as ill-defined alveolar opacities which usually clear within 48 hours. By contrast, hematomas are well-circumscribed and may require weeks or months to resolve. Pneumatoceles are thought to result from escape of air into a sheared portion of lung parenchyma and are not typically associated with infection.

Transection of the aorta is among the most lethal of the thoracic injuries. Ninety-five percent occur at the aortic isthmus, where the aorta is tethered by the ligamentum arteriosum. The remainder arise in the aortic root.

55. The answers are: A-Y, B-Y, C-N, D-Y, E-N. *(Armstrong, pp 710–715.)* Thymomas are tumors of the thymic epithelium which contain a variable amount of lymphocytic infiltration. Although some are found incidentally, most patients present with symptoms related to compression of structures in the anterior mediastinum or some form of autoimmune disorder. Of the latter, myasthenia gravis is the most common, occurring in about 35% of patients. Other associations include hypogamma-globulinemia, pure red cell aplasia, and collagen vascular disease.

The most common age at presentation is between 40 and 50 years. In patients under the age of 20, thymoma is rare and is difficult to distinguish from normal thymic tissue, even on cross-sectional imaging. Calcification appears in approximately 10% of thymomas imaged by plain film or conventional tomography, and may be punctuate or curvilinear.

Tumors which extend beyond the thymic capsule are termed *invasive*. Invasive tumors spread to the mediastinum, pericardium, and may occasionally metastasize, especially to the pleural space. Unless there is mediastinal invasion, benign and malignant neoplasms are indistinguishable by CT.

56. The answers are: A-Y, B-Y, C-N, D-N, E-N. *(Mayo, Sem Roentgenol 26(2), pp 104–109, 1991. Webb, Sem Roentgenol 26(2), pp 110–117, 1991.)* High-resolution computed tomography (HRCT) permits a more detailed evaluation of the lung parenchyma than conventional CT because of increased spatial resolution. Proper application of HRCT requires the use of narrow collimation (1- to 2-mm slice thickness), a small field-of-view, and a high-spatial-frequency reconstruction algorithm. Narrow collimation reduces partial volume averaging, and a small field-of-view decreases pixel size; the result is improved spatial resolution. A high-frequency algorithm, such as that used for bone, is chosen because the low-spatial-frequency reconstruction algorithm used for most conventional body CT scans smooths out tissue interfaces, though it does so at the expense of resolution.

On conventional CT scans, the region of the major fissure is usually visualized as a zone of lucency, because the lung is rarified at the periphery and the pleura is too thin to resolve. The superior spatial definition of HRCT usually does resolve the pleural edge. A disadvantage of the thinness of the slices, though, is that vessels (which may be appreciated as linear structures on conventional CT scans) appear as round nodules and may be difficult to follow precisely from slice to slice.

57. The answers are: A-N, B-N, C-N, D-N, E-Y. *(Armstrong, pp 580–583.)* Lymphangioleiomyomatosis (LAM) is a lung disorder characterized by abnormal proliferation of perilymphatic smooth muscle. Some authors consider it a variant of tuberous sclerosis. It occurs almost exclusively in females of child-bearing age. No inheritance pattern has been established.

On chest radiographs, the lung volumes are typically normal or increased, even in advanced stages of the disease. High-resolution CT shows a characteristic pattern of diffuse thin-walled cysts, with sparing of the intervening parenchyma early in the disease. Uni- or bilateral chylous pleural effusions occur in 75% of patients, and pneumothoraces are also common.

58. The answers are: A-Y, B-Y, C-N, D-N, E-N. *(Fraser, ed. 3, pp 1251–1253, 2438–2441.)* Eosinophilic lung disease is the prototype for conditions which predominantly affect the peripheral lung zones. It may be idiopathic (e.g., chronic eosinophilic pneumonia) or may be associated with drugs, parasitic infection, or hypersensitivity. It may also result from a vasculitic condition, such as the Churg-Strauss syndrome (allergic granulomatosis), which consists of the triad of asthma, eosinophilia, and a systemic vasculitis.

Amiodarone, an antiarrhythmic medication with substantial pulmonary toxicity, also causes peripheral lung opacities in the absence of blood or tissue eosinophilia, for reasons which are not understood. By contrast, cardiogenic pulmonary edema is commonly associated with a "batwing," or perihilar predominance of parenchymal opacity and a relative normal periphery.

The pulmonary opacities in patients with non-Hodgkin lymphoma and bronchioloalveolar carcinoma do not have a regional predilection.

59. **The answers are: A-N, B-Y, C-N, D-Y, E-Y.** *(Armstrong, pp 526–532.)* The term *amyloid* is used to describe the deposition of one of a number of different abnormal proteins (usually immunoglobulins) in tissues. Thoracic amyloidosis may be part of a systemic process, or it may be localized to the lung parenchyma or tracheobronchial tree.

Parenchymal amyloidosis most commonly causes single or multiple discrete lung nodules, ranging in size from 5 mm to 5 cm, which occasionally cavitate. Calcification is reported in 30 to 50% of patients with nodular pulmonary amyloidosis. The nodules usually remain stable, but may grow slowly over a period of years.

Tracheobronchial amyloidosis consists of submucosal deposits of amyloid which progress slowly and cause diffuse airway narrowing. Obstructive atelectasis occurs in over 50% of patients.

60. **The answers are: A-N, B-Y, C-Y, D-Y, E-N.** *(Armstrong, pp 601–603.)* Bronchogenic cysts result from branching abnormalities during foregut development, and may occasionally occur in conjunction with spinous malformations. They are lined by pseudostratified columnar (respiratory) epithelium and occur most commonly in the mediastinum and hilar regions. Most bronchogenic cysts are discovered incidentally, though they may sometimes present because of infection, hemorrhage, or airway obstruction. An air-fluid level within the cyst suggests a superimposed infectious process.

On chest radiographs, bronchogenic cysts are typically located in the mediastinum or hila, and are smoothly marginated. CT better defines the relationship of the cyst to adjacent structures. By CT, the cyst fluid is usually denser than water, measuring between 20 and 80 Hounsfield units, which is presumed to result from the presence of proteins in the cyst fluid.

Gastrointestinal Radiology

DIRECTIONS: Each question below contains five suggested responses. Select the **one best** response to each question.

61. Referring to the figure, what would you judge to be the MOST likely diagnosis in a 49-year-old patient with jaundice and abdominal pain?

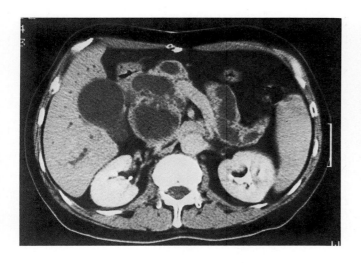

(A) Serous cystadenoma
(B) Acute pancreatitis
(C) Von Hippel-Lindau syndrome
(D) Lymphangioma
(E) Mucinous cystadenoma/carcinoma

62. A 55-year-old man complained of weight loss and epigastric pain. In the study shown in the figure, the MOST likely diagnosis is

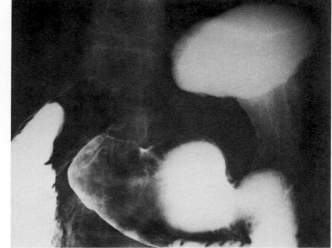

(A) Ménétrier disease
(B) Crohn disease
(C) eosinophilic gastritis
(D) gastric carcinoma
(E) leiomyosarcoma

63. Judging from the figure, what would you say is the MOST likely diagnosis in a 30-year-old patient?

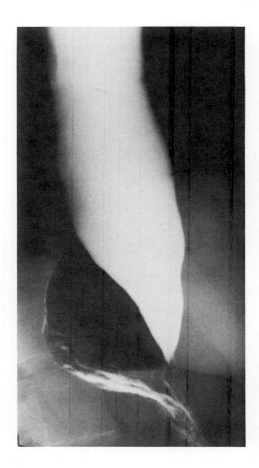

(A) Peptic stricture
(B) Presbyesophagus
(C) Esophageal carcinoma
(D) Achalasia
(E) Corrosive esophagitis

64. All the following may produce "bull's-eye" lesions in the stomach EXCEPT

(A) metastatic melanoma
(B) lymphoma
(C) Crohn disease
(D) ectopic pancreas
(E) Kaposi sarcoma

65. A jaundiced 60-year-old man had the study shown in the figure. The MOST likely diagnosis is

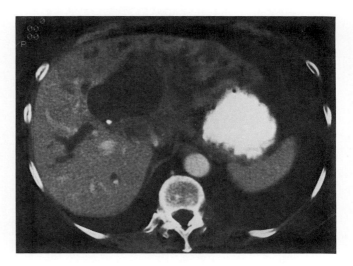

(A) hepatoma
(B) echinococcal cyst
(C) cholangiocarcinoma
(D) lymphoma
(E) polycystic liver disease

66. The risk of malignancy in a colonic polyp which measures 1 cm or less is approximately

(A) 1%
(B) 5%
(C) 10%
(D) 20%
(E) 50%

67. The MOST common cause of colonic obstruction in adults is

(A) diverticulitis
(B) volvulus
(C) primary carcinoma
(D) metastatic disease
(E) hernia

68. On the basis of the figure, the MOST likely diagnosis in an AIDS patient is

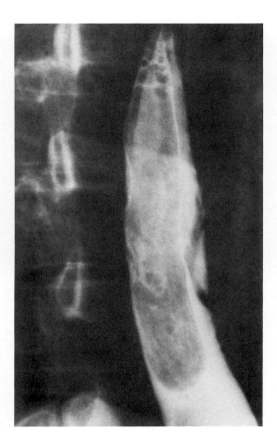

(A) CMV esophagitis
(B) herpes esophagitis
(C) lymphoma
(D) candida esophagitis
(E) Kaposi sarcoma

69. On a nonenhanced CT examination, which of the following organs is the MOST dense?

(A) Pancreas
(B) Kidney
(C) Spleen
(D) Liver
(E) Adrenal gland

70. The most common cause of colovesical fistula is

(A) radiation therapy
(B) diverticulitis
(C) Crohn disease
(D) colonic malignancy
(E) ulcerative colitis

71. A 45-year-old man was discovered to have guaiac-positive stools. Referring to the figure, what would you say is the MOST likely diagnosis?

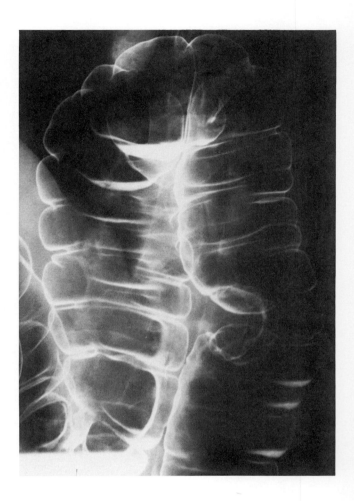

(A) Hyperplastic polyp
(B) Villous adenoma
(C) Lipoma
(D) Endometrioma
(E) Adenocarcinoma

72. All the following neoplasms are associated with Thorotrast exposure EXCEPT

(A) hepatoma
(B) hepatic lymphoma
(C) cholangiocarcinoma
(D) splenic angiosarcoma
(E) hepatic angiosarcoma

73. The 30-year-old man in the figure complained of chronic right lower quadrant pain. The MOST likely diagnosis is

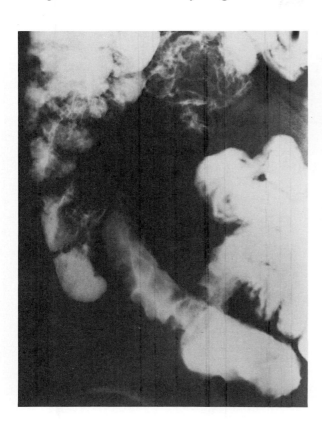

(A) Crohn disease
(B) ulcerative colitis
(C) tuberculosis
(D) amebiasis
(E) lymphoid hyperplasia

74. The MOST common malignant neoplasm in the distal small bowel is

(A) lymphoma
(B) adenocarcinoma
(C) carcinoid
(D) liposarcoma
(E) leiomyosarcoma

75. The figure shows a study of a 65-year-old patient. The MOST likely diagnosis is

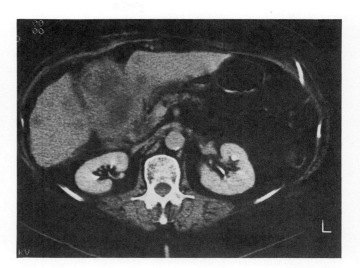

(A) gallbladder carcinoma
(B) emphysematous cholecystitis
(C) lymphoma
(D) adenomyomatosis
(E) metastatic colon carcinoma

76. Referring to the accompanying figure, what would you judge to be the MOST likely diagnosis?

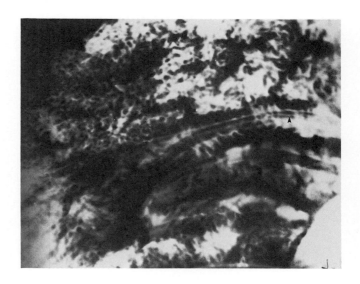

(A) Ascariasis
(B) Blood clot
(C) Bezoar
(D) Inverted Meckel diverticulum
(E) Duplication cyst

77. In the accompanying figure, the MOST
     likely diagnosis in a 40-year-old patient
     with abdominal pain and 20-lb weight loss
     is

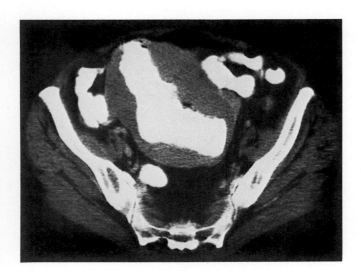

(A) adenocarcinoma
(B) carcinoid
(C) leiomyosarcoma
(D) lymphoma
(E) metastasis

DIRECTIONS: Each group of questions below consists of lettered headings followed by a set of numbered items. For each numbered item select the **one** lettered heading with which it is **most** closely associated. Each lettered heading may be used **once, more than once,** or **not at all.**

Questions 78–80

Match each of the following disease entities with the feature with which most closely related.

  (A)   Rectosigmoid stricture
  (B)   Pseudomembranous colitis
  (C)   Radiographic imitator of ulcerative colitis
  (D)   Thickened and nodular folds in the terminal ileum
  (E)   Primarily involves the duodenum and jejunum

78.   *Yersinia enterocolitica*

79.   Lymphogranuloma venereum

80.   *Salmonella*

Questions 81–83

Match each of the following disease entities with the feature with which it is most closely associated.

  (A)   Alternating constriction and dilatation of the intrahepatic bile ducts
  (B)   Long diffuse tapering of the common bile duct
  (C)   Obstruction at the junction of the right and left hepatic ducts
  (D)   Cystic dilatation of the intrahepatic bile ducts
  (E)   Abrupt obstruction of the distal common bile duct

81.   Caroli disease

82.   Klatskin tumor

83.   Sclerosing cholangitis

Questions 84–86

Match each of the following disease entities with the feature with which it is most closely associated.

  (A)   Normal esophageal motility
  (B)   Patulous gastroesophageal junction
  (C)   Prominent nonpropulsive contractions
  (D)   Prolonged cricopharyngeus muscle contraction
  (E)   Incomplete relaxation of the lower esophageal sphincter

84.   Scleroderma

85.   Achalasia

86.   Diffuse esophageal spasm

Questions 87–89

Match each of the following disease entities with the feature with which it is most closely associated.

  (A)   Regular thickening of small-bowel folds
  (B)   Pseudosacculations
  (C)   Stricture formation
  (D)   Sandlike filling defects in the small bowel
  (E)   Transient intussusception

87.   Adult celiac disease

88.   Henoch-Schönlein purpura

89.   Waldenström macroglobulinemia

Questions 90–92

Match each of the following disease entities with the feature with which it is most closely associated.

(A) Associated with pancreatitis
(B) Increased risk of lymphoma
(C) Massively thickened rugal folds
(D) Multiple gastric ulcers
(E) Linitis plastica

90. Ménétrier disease

91. Zollinger-Ellison syndrome

92. Gastric varices

DIRECTIONS: Each question below contains five suggested answers. For **each** of the **five** alternatives listed, you are to respond either YES or NO. In a given item, **all, some,** or **none of the alternatives may be correct.**

93. Gas in the portal veins

 (A) is a benign condition
 (B) is often seen with primary pneumatosis intestinalis
 (C) often results from biliary surgery
 (D) can occur following barium enema in patients with inflammatory bowel disease
 (E) is usually seen in the central portions of the liver

94. "Downhill" varices develop in cases of

 (A) cirrhosis
 (B) Budd-Chiari syndrome
 (C) fibrosing mediastinitis
 (D) portal vein thrombosis
 (E) congestive heart failure

95. Zenker diverticula

 (A) originate posteriorly in the midline
 (B) contain all layers of the wall of the esophagus
 (C) arise caudal to the cricopharyngeus
 (D) result from a defect in the longitudinal muscle of the esophagus
 (E) are commonly found in children

96. Concerning acute splenic infarcts,

 (A) splenic rupture commonly results
 (B) they appear as high-attenuation lesions by CT
 (C) in patients over age 50, thromboembolism from the heart is the most common cause
 (D) AIDS patients are at increased risk for spontaneous splenic infarcts
 (E) they lack peripheral enhancement on contrast-enhanced CT

97. Regarding acute pancreatitis,

 (A) sonography characteristically shows decreased echogenicity in the pancreas
 (B) CT typically shows focal involvement, rather than diffuse disease
 (C) infiltration of the pararenal spaces can result in the "renal halo" sign
 (D) CT evidence of hemorrhage is a poor prognostic sign
 (E) CT examination of the pancreas nearly always reveals an abnormality

98. Regarding segmental ischemia of the colon,

 (A) gas in the portal venous system is a common plain-film finding
 (B) progression to stricture is frequent
 (C) occlusion of a major mesenteric arterial trunk is the most common cause
 (D) the segment of colon most commonly affected is the cecum
 (E) it may resemble inflammatory bowel disease on barium examination

99. Regarding cavernous hemangioma of the liver,

 (A) it is the most common benign hepatic neoplasm
 (B) it is usually symptomatic
 (C) sonographically it is echogenic relative to normal hepatic parenchyma
 (D) complete opacification on dynamic contrast-enhanced CT distinguishes it from other lesions
 (E) marked hyperintensity on heavily T2-weighted images distinguishes it from metastatic disease

100. Regarding gastric neoplasms,

(A) most gastric polyps are adenomatous
(B) lipomas are the most common benign submucosal tumor of the stomach
(C) non-Hodgkin disease is the most common form of gastric lymphoma
(D) metastatic breast carcinoma typically produces a linitis plastica pattern
(E) gastric stump carcinomas usually appear within 5 years of surgery

101. Regarding spontaneous esophageal tears,

(A) they are usually caused by persistent vomiting
(B) complete rupture usually results in a right pleural effusion
(C) most Mallory-Weiss tears occur at the gastroesophageal junction
(D) the esophagus usually has underlying disease
(E) Boerhaave syndrome is usually self-limiting

102. Regarding sigmoid volvulus,

(A) it occurs in a younger population as compared to cecal volvulus
(B) barium enema is contraindicated
(C) the majority recur
(D) colostomy is the preferred therapeutic procedure
(E) the twisted bowel loop typically projects into the right upper abdomen

103. Regarding Crohn disease of the colon,

(A) aphthous ulceration is specific for this condition
(B) inflammatory polyps and pseudopolyps are similar to those found in ulcerative colitis
(C) toxic megacolon is a frequent complication
(D) mucosal granularity is commonly visible on double-contrast examinations
(E) involvement of the terminal ileum is indistinguishable from "backwash ileitis" of ulcerative colitis

104. Regarding abdominal hernias,

(A) lesser sac hernias are the most common intraabdominal type
(B) right-sided inguinal hernias usually contain small bowel
(C) a spigelian hernia results from a defect along the linea semilunaris
(D) traumatic diaphragmatic hernias occur more commonly on the right side
(E) most congenital diaphragmatic hernias occur through the foramen of Bochdalek

105. Concerning Barrett esophagus,

(A) it is associated with gastroesophageal reflux
(B) it can be diagnosed by technetium pertechnetate scintigraphy
(C) the esophageal ulcerations are typically shallow
(D) there is an increased incidence of squamous cell carcinoma
(E) stricture formation is common

106. Hepatic adenomas

(A) are frequently complicated by hemorrhage
(B) show little change following cessation of oral contraceptives
(C) are typically hypodense on dynamic CT
(D) have specific MRI features
(E) are premalignant

107. Etiologic factors of hepatocellular carcinoma include

(A) aflatoxin
(B) chronic hepatitis B infection
(C) hemochromatosis
(D) fatty infiltration of the liver
(E) Echinococcus granulosus

108. Insulinomas

    (A) are tumors arising from the alpha cells of the pancreatic islets of Langerhans
    (B) are the most common functioning tumor of the pancreas
    (C) are usually larger than 5 cm at presentation
    (D) are typically hypervascular
    (E) are most commonly located in the head of the pancreas

109. Hypervascular hepatic metastases include those from

    (A) pheochromocytoma
    (B) lung carcinoma
    (C) melanoma
    (D) breast carcinoma
    (E) renal cell carcinoma

110. Adenomatous gastric polyps

    (A) are usually multiple
    (B) may become malignant
    (C) are associated with achlorhydria
    (D) occur in patients with familial polyposis
    (E) are a diagnostic feature of Peutz-Jeghers syndrome

111. Gas in the bowel wall (pneumatosis intestinalis) is associated with

    (A) ischemic necrosis
    (B) scleroderma
    (C) chronic obstructive pulmonary disease
    (D) steroid therapy
    (E) inflammatory bowel disease

112. Regarding splenic trauma,

    (A) subcapsular hematomas are typically hypodense on contrast-enhanced CT
    (B) a normal splenic CT excludes clinically significant splenic injury
    (C) fluid in the paracolic gutter may be diagnosed by plain films
    (D) splenectomy is indicated in most cases
    (E) an elongated left hepatic lobe may resemble a subcapsular hematoma on CT

113. Regarding echinococcal (hydatid) disease,

    (A) it is caused by a parasitic tapeworm infestation
    (B) it is the most common cause of hepatic cysts worldwide
    (C) the hepatic cysts rarely calcify
    (D) percutaneous cyst aspiration is contraindicated
    (E) initial presentation may be related to biliary obstruction

114. Regarding pancreatic carcinoma,

    (A) dilatation of both the biliary and pancreatic ducts (the "double duct" sign) is pathognomonic
    (B) there is an increased incidence of carcinoma in patients with chronic pancreatitis
    (C) patients with pseudocysts, arising de novo, should be evaluated for carcinoma
    (D) CT demonstration of soft tissue surrounding the celiac and superior mesenteric vessels is a diagnostic sign
    (E) obliteration of the normal peripancreatic fat is a common CT feature

115. True statements regarding hemochromatosis include which of the following?

    (A) It may be inherited
    (B) Repeated blood transfusions are a frequent cause
    (C) Patients may present with diabetes mellitus
    (D) The CT features are specific
    (E) MRI evaluation of the liver is diagnostic

116. Causes of toxic megacolon include

    (A) Crohn disease
    (B) ischemic colitis
    (C) colitis cystica profunda
    (D) amebic colitis
    (E) cholera

117. A micronodular small-bowel pattern is typical of

   (A) mastocytosis
   (B) histoplasmosis
   (C) neurofibromatosis
   (D) Whipple disease
   (E) lymphoma

118. Malignancy is associated with

   (A) Peutz-Jeghers syndrome
   (B) familial polyposis
   (C) Gardner syndrome
   (D) Cronkhite-Canada syndrome
   (E) Turcot syndrome

119. A Meckel diverticulum

   (A) occurs on the mesenteric side of the small bowel
   (B) is typically located within 15 cm of the ileocecal valve
   (C) may contain enteroliths
   (D) can appear as a filling defect on barium exam
   (E) results from persistence of the omphalomesenteric duct

120. Etiologic factors associated with esophageal carcinoma include

   (A) smoking
   (B) hot tea
   (C) lye ingestion
   (D) untreated achalasia
   (E) Plummer-Vinson syndrome

Gastrointestinal Radiology

Answers

61. **The answer is E.** *(Lee, Sagel & Stanley, pp 560–564.)* The contrast-enhanced CT in the figure demonstrates a multilocular, thick-walled, cystic pancreatic head mass, causing both pancreatic and biliary ductal obstruction. The appearance of the mass is most consistent with a (mucinous) cystadenoma or cystadenocarcinoma. Cystadenomas are subclassified according to cyst size. This particular example is a typical *macro*cystic adenoma. It is multilocular, encapsulated, and has cystic areas larger than 2 cm in size. The walls of these tumors are thick and often nodular. They occur most frequently in the head of the pancreas and produce mucin, which fills the cysts. They do have a malignant potential, though benign and malignant differentiation is often difficult in the absence of metastasis.

In contrast, *micro*cystic (or serous) cystadenomas are rich in glycogen, have no malignant potential, and typically contain numerous tiny cysts. They occur more frequently in the body and tail of the pancreas and often have a central scar which may be calcified. Serous cystadenomas and simple pancreatic cysts are often seen in patients with von Hippel-Lindau syndrome.

Lymphangiomas are rare pancreatic tumors and typically have thin walls. Acute pancreatitis may present with low-density areas, but the peripancreatic fat is usually infiltrated.

62. **The answer is D.** *(Eisenberg, pp 205–218.)* The air-contrast GI study in the figure demonstrates fixed, concentric narrowing and thickening of the rugal folds in the proximal body of the stomach. The nonspecific term for this is *linitis plastica* (*L.*, "leather bottle"). The most common cause of this radiographic appearance is scirrhous carcinoma of the stomach. Tumor invasion stimulates a desmoplastic response which produces thickening and fixation of the gastric wall. Extention of tumor into the mucosa can produce nodular or irregular mucosal folds.

Granulomatous diseases and eosinophilic gastritis can produce a linitis plastica appearance, but typically involve the gastric antrum. Other causes of linitis plastica include lymphoma, metastases, corrosive agents, and gastric freezing. Ménétrier disease causes diffuse nonfixed gastric thickening of the proximal stomach. Leiomyosarcomas appear as intramural masses that frequently ulcerate.

63. The answer is D. *(Eisenberg, pp 17–18.)* The single-contrast esophagogram in the figure demonstrates smooth, conical narrowing in the distal esophagus, which on subsequent radiographs showed intermittent opening, allowing some barium passage into the stomach. This radiographic "beak" appearance is typical of achalasia. However, the pattern is caused by failure of relaxation of the lower esophageal sphincter and is nonspecific. It is also seen in Chagas disease, central and peripheral neuropathy, and malignancy.

The clinical and radiographic features usually help to distinguish between benign and malignant causes of the achalasia pattern. Patients with classic benign achalasia typically are less than 40 years old and have had symptoms for a year or more, while "pseudoachalasia" occurs in patients with carcinoma of the esophagus or gastric cardia who are usually over 60 years of age and have had symptoms for less than 6 months. Radiographically, the distal esophagus in achalasia is pliable; it tapers gradually and has an intact mucosa. In cases of carcinoma, the distal esophagus is rigid; it has a narrow transition zone between normal esophagus and tumor and has areas of mucosal nodularity and destruction. The presence of a mass in the fundus should also suggest carcinoma.

In peptic stricture and corrosive esophagitis, the length of involved esophagus is longer than in achalasia and signs of inflammation are usually present. Patients with presbyesophagus typically demonstrate nonpropulsive tertiary contractions.

64. The answer is C. *(Eisenberg, pp 865–868.)* "Bull's-eye," or target, lesions of the stomach are the result of central ulceration or umbilication in a mass. Multiple bull's-eye lesions may be seen with Kaposi sarcoma, lymphoma, or hematogenous metastases such as metastatic melanoma. As these vascular, or aggressive, tumors outgrow their blood supply, necrosis and central ulceration occur.

The solitary bull's-eye appearance of ectopic pancreatic tissue represents opacification of a rudimentary pancreatic duct rather than central ulceration. Crohn disease in the stomach initially presents as aphthous ulcers or erosions, but each has no associated mass.

65. The answer is C. *(Moss, Gamsu, & Genant, pp 833, 849.)* The contrast-enhanced CT scan in the figure demonstrates a mass in the porta hepatis, which is infiltrating the adjacent liver tissue and obstructing the bile ducts. The choledochal cyst in this case, a dilated intrahepatic bile duct which contains a stone, should suggest the diagnosis of cholangiocarcinoma; since a significant percentage of patients develop biliary tract neoplasms in this setting. Hepatomas and hepatic lymphoma typically appear as solid masses which may resemble cholangiocarcinoma, but are not associated with choledochal cysts.

Other cystic entities which may occur in the porta hepatis, such as hydatid disease and polycystic liver disease, may be occasionally mistaken for choledochal cysts, but the lack of cystic intrahepatic lesions in this case argues against hydatid disease, and renal cysts would be expected to be present in most cases of polycystic liver disease.

Cholangiocarcinoma exists in three distinct forms: as an infiltrative, stricturing process; a bulky exophytic tumor; or a polypoid intraluminal mass. On CT, tumor mass at the level of biliary obstruction is seen in approximately 70% of patients. However, when tumor arises in the portal hepatis and extends into the hepatic parenchyma, distinction between primary cholangiocarcinoma, lymphoma, and metastatic disease may not be possible.

66. The answer is A. *(Margulis & Burhenne, p 1030.)* The single, most important feature in estimating the probability of malignancy in a colonic polyp is its size; the smaller ones are less likely to contain malignancy. Polyps less than 0.5 cm in diameter are rarely malignant, while those less than 1 cm in diameter still have only a 1 to 2% risk of malignancy. Polyps between 1 and 2 cm in diameter have an increased incidence of about 10%, whereas up to 50% of polyps greater than 2 cm in size are malignant.

67. The answer is C. *(Margulis & Burhenne, pp 345–346.)* Approximately 25% of all intestinal obstructions occur in the large bowel. The patients involved are predominantly in the older age groups, and primary carcinoma accounts for approximately 60% of mechanical large-bowel obstructions. Tumors arising in the pelvic viscera may also directly invade or compress the rectum or sigmoid colon and cause obstruction. Serosal implants from gastric or ovarian carcinoma, as well as hematogenous metastases to the colon, occasionally cause obstruction.

68. The answer is A. *(Megibow, Balthazar, & Hulnick, p 31.)* The single-contrast esophagram in the figure demonstrates a deep esophageal ulceration in an otherwise normal mucosa. In an AIDS patient, this finding is most consistent with CMV esophagitis. The deep ulceration is due to ischemic necrosis which results from a virus-induced vasculitis. CMV esophagitis may also present with focal linear ulcerations which have well-defined, edematous borders.

Patients with herpes esophagitis usually have solitary or multiple small ulcerations and an otherwise normal mucosa. *Candida* affects large portions of the esophagus and typically produces shaggy plaques and superficial erosions. Though it may occasionally cause large ulcers, like CMV, a diffusely abnormal mucosa should suggest the proper diagnosis. Patients with esophageal lymphoma or Kaposi sarcoma may develop ulcerations, but these are excavations into tumor masses and are usually distinguishable from the mucosal processes discussed above.

69. The answer is D. *(Moss, Gamsu, & Genant, p 741.)* Liver parenchyma has a higher density than that of the pancreas, spleen, kidney, or adrenal gland. The average liver-spleen difference, though, is only 7 to 8 Hounsfield units. The relative higher density of hepatic parenchyma is felt to result from the high concentration of glycogen in the tissues.

70. The answer is B. *(Eisenberg, pp 925–928.)* Internal fistulae are a frequent complication of diverticulitis, which is responsible for more than 50% of all colovesical fistulae. Recurrent urinary tract infections, pneumaturia, and fecaluria are commonly associated. A radiographic clue to the presence of a colovesical fistula is gas in the lumen of the urinary bladder. The fistulae themselves are often difficult to opacify. Cystography and/or barium enema may outline the connection. Occasionally, it is visualized by excretory urography or contrast-enhanced CT scanning.

Radiation therapy, Crohn disease, and colonic malignancy may result in fistula formation to the bladder. Ulcerative colitis, which is not a transmural process, does not typically create fistulae.

71. The answer is E. *(Eisenberg, pp 668–669.)* The double-contrast barium enema in the figure demonstrates a large, polypoid mass which has a lobular surface. Retraction of the colonic wall, in this case toward a large sessile mass, almost invariably indicates submucosal invasion by malignancy. Benign polyps can also deform the colonic wall, but the indentation that results is from tugging at the base of the stalk by the mass. In further distinction, benign polyps usually have smooth surfaces, while those masses with lobulated surfaces are more likely to be malignant.

Lipomas are typically oval, sharply defined, and radiolucent. They occur frequently at the ileocecal valve. Endometriomas are intramural lesions which predominantly involve the sigmoid colon.

72. The answer is B. *(Levy, pp 997–1004.)* Thorotrast, which was used primarily for cerebral angiography, was discontinued in the 1950s. The average latency from exposure to Thorotrast to the development of cancer is 26 years. Most studies list angiosarcomas as at least 50% of the Thorotrast-associated neoplasms, with cholangiocarcinoma and hepatoma accounting for the remainder. Hepatic venoocclusive disease and peliosis hepatis have also been reported with Thorotrast exposure. Lymphoma is not associated.

73. **The answer is A.** *(Eisenberg, pp 548–549.)* The small-bowel study in the figure demonstrates a nodular terminal ileum with multiple aphthoid ulcerations, diagnostic of Crohn disease. The ileocecal valve and cecum are normal. In the "backwash" ileitis of ulcerative colitis, the ileocecal valve is typically patulous and the mucosal inflammatory changes in the ileum are often only mild. In tuberculosis, involvement of the cecum is more prominent than that of the terminal ileum and results in a typical inverted-cone shape. Amebiasis involves the cecum in 90% of chronic cases, but involvement of the terminal ileum would be unusual. Lymphoid hyperplasia of the terminal ileum typically produces a fine nodular pattern, superimposed on an otherwise normal mucosa, provided there is no additional disease.

74. **The answer is C.** *(Margulis & Burhenne, pp 822–832.)* Common primary malignant tumors of the small bowel include adenocarcinoma, malignant carcinoid, lymphoma, and leiomyosarcoma. Adenocarcinomas occur most commonly in the duodenum and proximal jejunum, with diminishing incidence as the distance increases away from the ligament of Treitz. Most carcinoids occur distally in the small intestine, and they are the most common malignancy of the small bowel and appendix. Lymphomas arise where the lymphoid tissue is most abundant; the distal ileum is the most common location. Sarcomas are evenly distributed throughout the small bowel.

75. **The answer is A.** *(Moss, Gamsu, & Genant, pp 836–840.)* The transaxial CT scan in the figure demonstrates a markedly thickened and irregular gallbladder wall, as well as several low-density areas in the liver. These findings are most consistent with gallbladder carcinoma and hepatic metastasis. The majority of patients with gallbladder carcinoma have cholelithiasis and chronic cholecystitis. An increased risk of carcinoma of the gallbladder in patients with porcelain gallbladder is also well-documented.

    The most common CT finding in gallbladder carcinoma is a mass replacing the gallbladder lumen. Less commonly, it presents as a focal intraluminal mass or eccentric thickening of the gallbladder wall. However, these findings may also occasionally be seen in cases of cholecystitis. Gas in the gallbladder wall or lumen, the distinguishing feature of the emphysematous cholecystitis, is not present in this case. The extreme liver involvement in this case also makes that diagnosis less likely.

    Gallbladder lymphoma has not been reported, but one would expect concomitant portal adenopathy. Adenomyomatosis may present as nonspecific diffuse, segmental, or localized gallbladder thickening. Visualization on CT of the Rokitansky-Aschoff sinuses of adenomyomatosis has been reported only when scans were performed in conjunction with oral cholecystography. Rarely, the gallbladder may be involved by metastatic disease; the most common primary tumor is melanoma.

76. **The answer is A.** *(Eisenberg, pp 500–504.)* The small-bowel study in the figure reveals long, linear filling defects. These are typical of parasitic infestation which, in the U.S., is most commonly due to *Ascaris lumbricoides*. If a worm ingests the barium, its gastrointestinal tract may become visible, appearing as it does in this case *(see arrowhead)* as a thin longitudinal density within the radiolucent worm. In endemic areas, *Strongyloides stercoralis, Ancylostoma duodenale* (hookworm), or *Taenia solium* (tapeworm) have a similar appearance.

77. **The answer is D.** *(Margulis & Burhenne, p 971.)* The contrast-enhanced CT scan in the figure reveals a markedly dilated and thick-walled bowel loop in the pelvis of a young patient with lymphoma. In the endoexophytic form of lymphoma, shown here, the tumor often excavates, creating large areas which can mimic a widened and diseased bowel lumen, an "aneurysmal dilatation." These patients typically have bulky lymphadenopathy, as well, though not in this case.

    Metastatic disease and primary adenocarcinoma can produce focal small-bowel thickening but rarely produces aneurysmal dilatation. Leiomyosarcomas typically arise as focal exophytic masses, with or without central ulcerations. Carcinoids invoke a desmoplastic reaction, producing spiculated soft-tissue masses which cause retraction of adjacent bowel loops.

78–80. The answers are: 78-D, 79-A, 80-C. *(Taveras & Ferrucci, vol 4, chap 33, pp 14–17.)* *Yersinia enterocolitica* is a gram-negative bacillus that causes ileitis and colitis. Patients may present with fever, diarrhea, and bloody stools. Barium examination may show a nodular mucosal pattern in the terminal ileum. Colonic ulcers, resembling those of Crohn colitis, may occur.

Lymphogranuloma venereum (LGV) is caused by a species of the genus *Chlamydia*, and is a venereal disease commonly seen in the tropics. Initially, the radiographic findings are of a nonspecific proctocolitis. Fistulous tracts and perirectal abscesses often occur, and as the disease progresses, strictures may develop in the anorectal area and involve the entire rectum and/or sigmoid colon. Gonococcal proctitis, resulting from anal intercourse, has a similar radiographic appearance.

Salmonellosis typically results from food poisoning. In this type of infection, the organisms produce an endotoxin which irritates the mucosa of the stomach, small bowel, and colon. If a barium examination is performed, the findings are nonspecific but may resemble those of ulcerative colitis. These changes are reversible and recovery is complete.

81–83. The answers are: 81-D, 82-C, 83-A. *(Moss, Gamsu, & Genant, pp 836, 849–857.)* Caroli disease is a congenital abnormality characterized by segmental dilatation of the intrahepatic bile ducts. CT typically shows multiple low-density cystic areas throughout the liver which are contiguous with dilated intrahepatic bile ducts and often contain calculi.

Klatskin tumor refers to a cholangiocarcinoma occurring at the junction of the right and left hepatic ducts. By CT, a mass is commonly visible in the porta hepatis, with abrupt termination of a dilated biliary system. However, hepatoma, metastatic disease, benign stricture, and cholesterol gallstone may produce a similar appearance.

Sclerosing cholangitis can occur either as a primary form (either idiopathic or associated with inflammatory bowel disease or retroperitoneal fibrosis) or may be secondary to cholangitis, surgery, or stone disease. It typically appears on cholangiography as multiple strictures in the intra- and extrahepatic biliary tree with pruning of the normal branching pattern, nodular duct walls, and diverticula. Irregular intrahepatic ductal dilatation results in a beaded appearance on both CT and cholangiography. Cholangiocarcinoma is a well-known complication of primary sclerosing cholangitis (PSC), and may be difficult to differentiate when it arises.

84–86. The answers are: 84-B, 85-E, 86-C. *(Eisenberg, pp 11–20.)* In scleroderma, the smooth muscle in the distal half to two-thirds of the esophagus is replaced by fibrosis, resulting in diminished esophageal motility. Because the lower esophageal sphincter tone is severely decreased, gastroesophageal reflux commonly occurs, often resulting in peptic esophagitis and stricture formation. The appearance of the dilated, atonic esophagus may resemble achalasia if the esophagram is performed with the patient in the recumbent position; however, with the patient upright, barium flows rapidly through the patulous lower esophageal sphincter.

Achalasia, thought to be a disorder of the myenteric (Auerbach) plexus of the distal esophagus, results from a combination of abnormal proximal esophageal motility and incomplete relaxation of the lower esophageal sphincter. Most cases occur between the ages of 20 and 40 years. By esophagram, achalasia presents as a gradual, smooth tapering of the distal esophagus, producing a "rat-tail" or "beak" appearance. Incomplete emptying of the esophagus occurs, even when the patient is upright.

Diffuse esophageal spasm is a controversial entity which typically presents as intermittent chest pain. An esophagram demonstrates diffuse esophageal contractions, and manometry reveals an associated increase in intraluminal pressure with each contraction. The segmental contractions create pseudodiverticula and a corkscrew appearance, often called a "rosary bead" esophagus.

87–89. The answers are: 87-E, 88-A, 89-D.   *(Eisenberg, pp 442–446, 459, 506.)*   Adult celiac disease (nontropical sprue) is the classic malabsorptive disease, which is caused by hypersensitivity to gluten. The small bowel has poor peristalsis and becomes flaccid and dilates, especially proximally. Hypersecretion and mucosal atrophy in the jejunum creates the "moulage" pattern on barium examination. Transient intussusception sometimes occurs, and there is an increased incidence of small-bowel lymphoma.

Henoch-Schönlein syndrome is an acute arteritis characterized by purpura, nephritis, and abdominal and joint pain. It commonly predisposes to diffuse hemorrhage into the small bowel, resulting in a radiographic pattern of regular small-bowel-fold thickening described as "thumbprinting" or "stacked coins," which is usually self-limited.

Primary macroglobulinemia is a plasma cell dyscrasia. In this disease, the small-bowel villi become greatly distended, giving the mucosa a granular, sandlike radiographic pattern. These tiny, nodular lucencies are usually also superimposed on a pattern of diffusely thickened mucosal folds.

90–92. The answers are: 90-C, 91-D, 92-A.   *(Eisenberg, pp 223–234.)*   Ménétrier disease is characterized by massive rugal fold enlargement secondary to hyperplasia and hypertrophy of the gastric mucosa. The resultant hypersecretion produces a protein-losing enteropathy. The disease typically involves the fundus and body of the stomach, although the entire stomach may occasionally be involved. A causal relationship with adenocarcinoma of the stomach has been reported.

Zollinger-Ellison syndrome is a hypersecretory condition caused by the hormonal effects of a gastrin-producing tumor, which is usually a non-beta islet cell tumor in the pancreas. Hypersecretion results in large amounts of retained gastric fluid, despite fasting. Thickened gastric folds result from the high level of acid secretion. Ulcers, single or multiple, may occur anywhere in the upper GI tract and, although more common in the stomach and duodenal bulb, large postbulbous ulcers are virtually diagnostic.

Gastric varices have been found in all parts of the stomach, although the majority are found in the fundus and proximal body. They cause thickened mucosal folds which vary in size and shape. The presence of gastric varices without esophageal varices usually indicates splenic vein occlusion, which is most commonly caused by pancreatitis or pancreatic carcinoma.

93. The answers are: A-N, B-N, C-N, D-Y, E-N.   *(Eisenberg, pp 858–861.)*   The presence of gas in the portal venous system is usually a grave prognostic radiographic finding and a sign of imminent death. It indicates a loss of intestinal mucosal integrity as a result of ischemia secondary to mesenteric artery occlusion or intestinal obstruction. Portal venous gas has been demonstrated in a few patients with ulcerative or Crohn colitis after barium enema, though this complication usually does not cause symptoms in the absence of bowel perforation.

Primary pneumatosis intestinalis is a benign condition characterized histologically by gas-filled cysts in the subserosa or submucosa of the bowel wall. Gas in the portal veins may be distinguished from gas in the biliary system by its distribution in the liver. Portal venous blood flow carries the gas away from the porta hepatis into the periphery of the liver, whereas gas in the biliary tree collects in the larger, more centrally located bile ducts.

94. The answers are: A-N, B-N, C-Y, D-N, E-N.   *(Eisenberg, pp 123–126.)*   "Downhill" esophageal varices develop when the superior vena cava is obstructed below the entrance of the azygous vein. The collateral vessels are most developed in the upper half of the esophagus. Mediastinal tumor or inflammatory disease is usually the cause.

"Uphill" varices, on the other hand, form when there is increased flow through the coronary veins, usually the result of portal hypertension (most commonly due to alcoholic cirrhosis in the U.S.), with blood flow toward the azygous vein. Therefore, they predominate in the lower half of the esophagus.

95. The answers are: A-Y, B-N, C-N, D-N, E-N. *(Margulis & Burhenne, pp 396–397.)* Zenker diverticula originate in the midline of the posterior wall of the hypopharynx (not the esophagus), at an anatomic weak point known as Killian's dehiscence. At this location, immediately above the cricopharyngeus, there is a divergence between the fibers of this muscle and the inferior pharyngeal constrictor. During swallowing, increased intraluminal pressure forces mucosa to herniate through. The etiology of Zenker diverticula is not firmly established, but premature contraction or motor incoordination of the cricopharyngeus muscle is thought to play a major role. Their development presumably takes time, however, as they have not been reported in children.

Lateral pharyngeal diverticula, which also occur at an anatomic weak point, are commonly referred to as pharyngoceles.

96. The answers are: A-N, B-N, C-Y, D-Y, E-N. *(Moss, Gamsu, & Genant, p 1074.)* Acute splenic infarctions are readily detectable by contrast-enhanced CT, but care must be taken not to misinterpret the normal inhomogeneity during the very early phase of dynamic scanning as infarcted tissue. Acute infarction usually produces a wedge-shaped area of decreased attenuation that extends to the splenic capsule. There is no enhancement of the involved area, except for the extreme periphery, which is supplied by capsular vessels. Renal infarcts commonly occur in the same patient, when the cause is cardiac thromboembolism; this is the most common cause of splenic infarcts in patients over 50. AIDS patients are also prone to spontaneous splenic infarction. Acute splenic infarction is usually self-limited, but may result in focal atrophy. Chronic splenic infarction, as seen in homozygous sickle cell disease, frequently produces a small, densely calcified spleen.

97. The answers are: A-Y, B-N, C-Y, D-N, E-N. *(Moss, Gamsu, & Genant, p 877.)* Ultrasound examination of pancreatitis typically demonstrates decreased echogenicity in the involved area, whereas CT scanning usually reveals diffuse pancreatic enlargement, blurring of the pancreatic margins, and thickening of the adjacent renal fascia. However, CT and ultrasound examinations may be normal in one-third or more of patients with acute pancreatitis.

Thickening of the renal fascia is a strong indicator of inflammation and is not seen in normal individuals or in those with pancreatic neoplasms. Involvement of the pararenal spaces, with sparing of the perirenal space, can produce the "renal halo" sign on plain films or CT. Focal thickening of the stomach wall is also evident in the majority of patients.

The diagnosis of hemorrhagic pancreatitis is based on clinical findings, including a falling hematocrit, hypocalcemia, or poor response to medical therapy; there is no correlation between CT evidence of hemorrhage and the clinical diagnosis. The finding is nonspecific and, for example, may be due to hemorrhage into a preexisting pseudocyst.

98. The answers are: A-N, B-N, C-N, D-N, E-Y. *(Eisenberg, pp 596–600.)* Acute intestinal ischemia may result from occlusion of small or medium arteries or may simply be due to poor arterial perfusion (e.g., congestive heart failure). It most commonly occurs in the two "watershed" regions: (1) the splenic flexure (superior and inferior mesenteric artery territories); and (2) the rectosigmoid area (inferior mesenteric and hemorrhoidal artery territories).

As the mucosal layer is most sensitive to an interruption of the blood supply, superficial ulceration may mimic ulcerative colitis at barium enema. With more severe disease, deep penetrating ulcers, pseudopolyps, and "thumbprinting" can be seen. Intramural gas and portal venous gas are infrequent findings and usually are poor prognostic indicators. In the majority of cases, the ischemic episode is self-limited, with radiographic findings resolving within a few weeks after the initial event. Fewer than 10% go on to form strictures.

99. The answers are: A-Y, B-N, C-Y, D-N, E-N. *(Moss, Gamsu, & Genant, pp 764–774.)* Hemangiomas are the most common benign hepatic neoplasm, with an autopsy incidence of approximately 4%. They are usually solitary, but can be multiple. Between 50 and 70% of patients with hemangiomas are asymptomatic. By ultrasound, the lesions are classically echogenic, with acoustic enhancement posteriorly, although the appearance may vary. Diagnostic criteria for CT include low density prior to contrast, intense peripheral enhancement early on, and complete filling-in on delayed images. However, these criteria have been judged by some to be too strict, as only 55% of hemangiomas meet all three. Complete opacification of a lesion on dynamic CT is nonspecific and can be seen in hypervascular metastases, hepatomas, focal nodular hyperplasia, and hepatic adenomas. On MRI, hemangiomas typically demonstrate marked hyperintensity on heavily T2-weighted sequences, although hypervascular tumors and cysts may appear similar.

100. The answers are: A-N, B-N, C-Y, D-Y, E-N. *(Taveras & Ferrucci, vol 4, chap 18.)* Hyperplastic polyps account for 75 to 90% of all gastric polyps. They are not true neoplasms and have no malignant potential. Adenomatous polyps account for most of the remainder and may undergo malignant transformation. The most common benign and malignant submucosal tumors of the stomach are leiomyoma and leiomyosarcoma, respectively. These submucosal tumors may grow intraluminally, intramurally, or exophytically and frequently develop central ulceration. Like intramural tumors, they usually form an obtuse angle with respect to the bowel wall when viewed on edge; in contrast to mucosal tumors, which form an acute angle with the adjacent bowel wall.

Non-Hodgkin lymphoma accounts for the majority of gastric lymphoma and radiographically occurs in four forms: infiltrative, ulcerating, polypoid, and endoexophytic. Hodgkin disease typically produces a desmoplastic reaction, resembling scirrhous carcinoma. Metastatic breast carcinoma also similarly produces a linitis plastica pattern, whereas melanoma metastases commonly appear as "bull's-eye" lesions.

Carcinoma arising in patients following partial gastrectomy usually presents as an irregular mass, which may ulcerate, at the anastomotic margin or in the gastric remnant. Patients usually present in excess of 20 years following surgery, while the majority with benign mucosal ulcerations develop them within the first 2 years.

101. The answers are: A-Y, B-N, C-Y, D-N, E-N. *(Eisenberg, pp 137–140.)* Noniatrogenic tears of the esophagus are usually produced by prolonged vomiting and can either be mucosal (Mallory-Weiss tears) or transmural (Boerhaave syndrome). Mallory-Weiss tears are usually seen in alcoholic men over age 50 who have a history of severe vomiting after excessive alcohol intake, followed by hematemesis. An esophagram may sometimes demonstrate filling of the tear as a thin line in the mucosa, usually at the gastroesophageal junction.

Boerhaave syndrome is similarly caused by severe vomiting, and patients develop immediate and severe epigastric pain. Death often occurs unless the rupture is repaired. The tear almost always occurs along the left posterior esophageal wall near the left diaphragmatic crus, usually resulting in a left hydropneumothorax and pneumomediastinum. Gastrograffin should be used for the esophagram, to minimize the risk of mediastinitis if there is extravasation.

102. The answers are: A-N, B-N, C-Y, D-N, E-Y. *(Eisenberg, p 728.)* Sigmoid volvulus results from a redundant loop of sigmoid colon undergoing a twist on its mesenteric axis, forming a closed-loop obstruction. It occurs in an older population relative to cecal volvulus. The most common presenting symptom is abdominal pain.

On plain radiographs, the distended sigmoid loop typically extends into the right upper abdomen, in contrast to cecal volvulus which usually extends into the left mid- or upper abdomen. The volvulus has a single-layer outer wall and a double-thickness inner wall, which terminate at the root of the twisted mesentery. Barium enema reveals the site of obstruction, which is often likened to a bird's beak.

Fluoroscopic or endoscopic decompression by an endoluminal tube is the preferred form of treatment, if there is no evidence of vascular compromise. As the recurrence rate is high (up to 80%), resection of the redundant sigmoid colon is often necessary.

103. **The answers are: A-N, B-Y, C-N, D-N, E-N.** *(Margulis & Burhenne, pp 982–991.)* Unlike ulcerative colitis, Crohn disease of the colon is a transmural process. Discontinuity and asymmetry of disease are typical for Crohn disease, in contrast to the symmetric, continuous, and diffuse involvement of the colon in ulcerative colitis. Crohn disease most commonly involves the cecum and terminal ileum. The earliest radiographic finding is aphthous ulceration, which is nonspecific and can be seen in several infectious processes. Mucosal granularity and "collar button" submucosal ulcerations are typical of ulcerative colitis and not Crohn disease.

In advanced disease, inflammatory polyps and pseudopolyps are commonly seen in both entities. In approximately 10% of patients with ulcerative colitis, "backwash" ileitis of the terminal ileum produces a patulous ileocecal valve and mucosal granularity of the terminal ileum. In Crohn disease of the terminal ileum, aphthous ulceration, nodularity, spasm, deep ulceration, cobblestoning, and fistula formation are typical. Toxic megacolon, seen in 2 to 3% of cases of ulcerative colitis, occurs less frequently in Crohn disease.

104. **The answers are: A-N, B-Y, C-Y, D-N, E-Y.** *(Eisenberg, pp 166–172, 871–879.)* Herniations of the posterolateral foramen of Bochdalek, which account for most congenital diaphragmatic hernias, occur more commonly on the left, probably due to coverage of the right side by the liver. Herniations through the anteromedial foramen of Morgagni occur more commonly on the right side, probably due to a more extensive pericardial attachment to the diaphragm on the left.

Traumatic diaphragmatic hernias are most commonly caused by direct laceration although they may occur following blunt abdominal trauma, and most are on the left.

The majority of internal hernias are paraduodenal and result from a failure of the mesentery to fuse with the peritoneum at the ligament of Treitz. Bowel herniations through the foramen of Winslow into the lesser sac are less frequent. Right-sided inguinal hernias usually contain small bowel, whereas the sigmoid colon usually prolapses into left-sided hernias. Spigelian hernias occur along the semilunar line, where the fascial layers divide, allowing small bowel, colon, or omentum to prolapse.

105. **The answers are: A-Y, B-Y, C-N, D-N, E-N.** *(Eisenberg, pp 50–55.)* Barrett esophagus is an inflammatory condition in which the pseudostratified squamous epithelium of the esophagus is replaced by columnar (gastric) epithelium. It is thought to result from chronic reflux, which is invariably present, and is usually associated with a sliding hiatal hernia. An esophagram reveals a characteristic, finely reticular mucosal pattern. The ulcerations of Barrett esophagus tend to be deep and penetrating, resembling peptic ulcerations in the stomach. They are usually separated from the hiatal hernia by a variable length of normal-appearing mucosa. Strictures form in a small percentage of patients. Technetium pertechnetate examination usually shows increased activity in the affected segment, as the isotope is actively secreted by the gastric-type mucosa. Approximately 10% of patients with this condition have been reported to develop adenocarcinoma.

106. **The answers are: A-Y, B-N, C-N, D-N, E-N.** *(Moss, Gamsu, & Genant, p 775.)* Hepatic adenomas are benign, well-encapsulated neoplasms composed entirely of hepatocytes. They occur predominantly in women taking oral contraceptives or hormonal supplements, and may regress or completely disappear after discontinuation. Hemorrhage is a frequent complication and may be life-threatening.

Following intravenous contrast, these tumors typically demonstrate significant enhancement during the arterial phase that rapidly diminishes on delayed images. A minority of lesions are hypodense during dynamic contrast-enhanced CT scanning. The MRI features are nonspecific and resemble other benign and malignant lesions. However, evidence of hemorrhage may suggest the diagnosis.

107. The answers are: A-Y, B-Y, C-Y, D-N, E-N. *(Friedman, p 220.)* Eighty percent of hepatocellular carcinomas occur in patients with preexisting chronic liver disease such as cirrhosis, hemochromatosis, or alpha-1-antitrypsin deficiency. It occurs in about 10% of patients with chronic active hepatitis (CAH), which is most commonly due to hepatitis B. Blood chemistry in those patients will reveal a positive HBsAg. A strong association exists between dietary aflatoxin and hepatocellular carcinoma in southeast Asia and Africa, and it is a well-known complication of *Schistosoma japonicum,* which is endemic in the Far East.

108. The answers are: A-N, B-Y, C-N, D-Y, E-N. *(Friedman, pp 865–869.)* Insulinomas are neoplasms arising from the beta cells of the pancreas, and are the most common type of functioning islet cell tumor. They are usually small (70% ≤ 1.5 cm) at presentation, since even very small lesions can produce clinically significant hypoglycemia. Unlike the other islet cell tumors (gastrinoma, glucagonoma, somatostatinoma, VIPoma), insulinomas occur in an even distribution throughout the pancreas. They are hypervascular and demonstrate significant enhancement following intravenous contrast. Arteriography and pancreatic venous sampling are currently the best means of localizing insulinomas, though dynamic CT scanning is still capable of detecting many of these neoplasms.

109. The answers are: A-Y, B-N, C-Y, D-Y, E-Y. *(Moss, Gamsu, & Genant, p 794.)* In tumors with increased vascularity, hepatic metastases may not be visible on contrast-enhanced CT, as they often become isodense with normal liver. A recent study reported that 37% of hepatic metastases, which were visible on noncontrast images, rapidly became isodense on dynamic contrast-enhanced scans. These included renal cell carcinoma, pheochromocytoma, and islet cell tumors. Breast carcinoma, melanoma, carcinoid and some sarcomas have also been reported to have similar CT characteristics.

110. The answers are: A-Y, B-Y, C-Y, D-Y, E-N. *(Eisenberg, pp 240–244.)* Adenomatous polyps of the stomach are true neoplasms and have a definite tendency toward malignant transformation, which increases with the size of the polyp. The majority of these polyps are solitary lesions located in the antrum. Both hyperplastic and adenomatous polyps develop in patients with chronic atrophic gastritis and achlorhydria. Radiographically, adenomatous polyps are large (≥ 2 cm) sessile lesions with irregular surfaces and deep fissures.

Patients with familial polyposis and Cronkhite-Canada syndrome also have an increased incidence of adenomatous polyps. Those with Peutz-Jeghers syndrome predominantly develop gastric hamartomatous polyps which have essentially no malignant potential, although they are reported to have a slight increase in the incidence of adenomatous polyps as well.

111. The answers are: A-Y, B-Y, C-Y, D-Y, E-Y. *(Eisenberg, pp 881–890.)* Pneumatosis intestinalis can either be primary or secondary. In primary pneumatosis, no underlying respiratory or other gastrointestinal abnormality is present. Primary pneumatosis usually occurs in adults, mainly involves the colon, may cause pneumoperitoneum, and usually resolves spontaneously without treatment.

Secondary pneumatosis intestinalis more commonly involves the small bowel and is associated with a number of gastrointestinal diseases, with or without bowel necrosis. These include peptic ulcer disease, inflammatory bowel disease, and connective tissue disorders, such as scleroderma. It also occurs in patients receiving steroids, although sometimes it is difficult to determine if the steroids or underlying disease are responsible. Secondary pneumatosis also occurs in obstructive pulmonary disease and may be found in this setting in conjunction with pneumomediastinum and pneumoperitoneum.

Radiographically, the gas collections in the bowel wall in the primary form are usually cystic, whereas they are more linear in the secondary type.

112. The answers are: A-Y, B-N, C-Y, D-N, E-Y. *(Moss, Gamsu, & Genant, pp 1069–1070.)* Blunt trauma may result in frank splenic laceration or may produce a hematoma which remains confined by the splenic capsule. Indirect plain-film findings include rib fractures, mass or mass effect in the left upper quadrant, and medial displacement of the left colon as fluid fills the paracolic gutter. Most subcapsular hematomas are hypodense on contrast-enhanced CT, unless there is active hemorrhage. However, up to 18% of patients with splenic injury have been reported to have hyperdense hematomas, on noncontrast CT, that became isodense after contrast. Although CT scanning is highly accurate in detecting splenic injury, a normal splenic CT therefore does not exclude the possibility of occult splenic injury, which occasionally results in delayed subscapular hemorrhage. Imitators of splenic trauma at CT include congenital clefts, elongated left hepatic lobes, and delayed, decreased splenic enhancement in hypotensive patients. Management of splenic injuries is based more on clinical criteria than on CT findings. Children are most often treated conservatively, because of the potential for asplenic patients to succumb to infection by encapsulated organisms.

113. **The answers are: A-Y, B-Y, C-N, D-N, E-Y.** *(Friedman, pp 164–170.)* Echinococcal (hydatid) disease is most commonly caused by the larval stage of *Echinococcus granulosus,* which favors the liver. *Echinococcus alveolaris (multilocularis)* is less common, but tends to be more aggressive and often becomes widely disseminated. Hydatid cysts are the most common cause of hepatic cysts worldwide. They may also occur in the brain, lung, kidney, and bone.

    Echinococcus granulosus produces uni- or multilocular cysts, with thin or thick walls as seen by CT or ultrasound. Calcifications may occur peripherally or centrally within the septations. Daughter cysts, which appear as smaller septated cysts near in the periphery of the larger mother cyst, should suggest the diagnosis. Cysts near the porta hepatis may obstruct and cause jaundice or portal hypertension. Percutaneous aspiration of suspected hydatid cysts may potentially cause an anaphylactic reaction should cyst fluid enter the bloodstream, but the danger has been greatly reduced by the use of extremely thin (e.g., 22-gauge) needles.

    Echinococcus alveolaris usually involves the liver as a nonspecific low-density, solid, infiltrating mass which resembles malignancy.

114. **The answers are: A-N, B-Y, C-Y, D-N, E-Y.** *(Moss, Gamsu, & Genant, pp 901–916.)* Pancreatic carcinoma usually produces changes in the size and shape of the pancreas, in addition to abnormal CT density. Obliteration of the peripancreatic fat is one of the most common findings and usually indicates extrapancreatic spread of tumor. Infiltration of the fat around the celiac axis and superior mesenteric vessels, initially thought to be specific for pancreatic carcinoma, has also been reported in pancreatitis, lymphoma, and metastatic disease. Dilatation of the pancreatic and biliary ducts frequently occurs, but is nonspecific and may also be seen in cases of chronic pancreatitis. Cystic masses in the body and tail of the pancreas are occasional presentations of pancreatic carcinoma. Therefore, a pseudocyst which occurs in a patient without a history of predisposing factors for pancreatitis should prompt an investigation for an underlying neoplasm.

115. **The answers are: A-Y, B-Y, C-Y, D-N, E-Y.** *(Moss, Gamsu, & Genant, pp 756–760.)* Hemochromatosis, classified as primary and secondary, is a disorder characterized by excessive iron deposition in many tissues. It most commonly involves the liver, spleen, lymph nodes, pancreas, heart, and endocrine organs.

    Primary or idiopathic hemochromatosis is an inherited condition resulting from a mucosal defect in the small intestine which allows abnormally high iron resorption. These patients usually present with cirrhosis, diabetes mellitus, and hyperpigmentation. Secondary hemochromatosis results from repeated blood transfusions and is seen most commonly in patients with thalassemia or sickle cell anemia, though the introduction of iron chelating agents has reduced the severity of disease in many. By CT, the involved hepatic parenchyma has nonspecific, diffuse, and homogeneous increased attenuation. However, this may also be seen in amiodarone toxicity, the glycogen storage diseases, and Wilson disease (hepatolenticular degeneration). By MRI, T2 shortening due to the excessive hemosiderin deposition causes typically low signal on both T1- and T2-weighted images.

116. The answers are: A-Y, B-Y, C-N, D-Y, E-Y. *(Eisenberg, pp 741–745.)* Toxic megacolon is a severe complication of fulminant ulcerative disease of the colon, which is characterized by marked colonic dilatation and systemic toxicity. Ulcerative colitis accounts for the majority of cases. Less frequently, it occurs in patients with Crohn disease, ischemic colitis, shigellosis (bacillary dysentery), salmonellosis (typhoid fever), and cholera. Interestingly, it rarely occurs with pseudomembranous colitis.

Plain films typically demonstrate marked colonic distention (> 5.5 cm in diameter). The normal haustral pattern is thickened or absent in the affected segments. Dissection of gas into deep ulcers occasionally produces pneumatosis intestinalis. Barium enema is contraindicated, due to the high risk of perforation.

117. The answers are: A-Y, B-Y, C-N, D-Y, E-N. *(Eisenberg, pp 506–512.)* The micronodular small-bowel pattern results from massive enlargement of the intestinal villi, which produces myriad fine, punctate lucencies that appear on a barium enema as grains of sand. This pattern is usually superimposed on a diffusely thickened fold pattern. It is most typically seen in cases of macroglobulinemia, mastocytosis, histoplasmosis, nodular lymphoid hyperplasia, intestinal lymphangiectasia, and Whipple disease. In comparison, the nodules of neurofibromatosis and lymphoma are usually larger and less numerous.

118. The answers are: A-Y, B-Y, C-Y, D-N, E-Y. *(Eisenberg, pp 693–698.)* The intestinal polyposis syndromes are a diverse group of conditions that differ in potential for developing malignancy. Patients with familial polyposis and Gardner syndrome have multiple adenomatous polyps in the colon and rectum. Untreated, there is a 100% risk of developing carcinoma, usually by the third decade. Adenomatous polyps also arise elsewhere in the GI tract, especially the duodenum.

In Peutz-Jeghers syndrome, the polyps are typically hamartomatous and occur predominantly in the small bowel. While these polyps themselves have no malignant potential, patients with Peutz-Jeghers syndrome also have adenomatous polyps which develop adenocarcinomas in 2 to 3%, usually in the stomach, duodenum, or colon; and 5% of women with this condition develop ovarian cysts or tumors.

Patients with Turcot syndrome have an increased incidence of colorectal carcinoma, though most patients die of CNS tumors, usually supratentorial glioblastoma, at a young age. In contrast, patients with Cronkhite-Canada syndrome develop inflammatory polyps in the stomach and colon which have no malignant potential. The most common presenting symptom is diarrhea, usually accompanied by anorexia, vomiting, and severe weight loss. Ectodermal abnormalities are usually present and include alopecia, hyperpigmentation, and nail atrophy. In females, death usually results from inanition and cachexia 6 to 18 months after the onset of diarrhea. In males, there is a tendency for remission.

119. The answers are: A-Y, B-N, C-Y, D-Y, E-Y. *(Eisenberg, pp 536–538.)* A Meckel diverticulum results from a persistent rudimentary omphalomesenteric duct, which is the embryonic communication between the gut and yolk sac. It therefore opens onto the antimesenteric side of the ileum, in contrast to other diverticula and duplications, which occur on the mesenteric side. The diverticulum is located approximately 100 cm from the ileocecal valve.

Though most patients are asymptomatic, the most common presentation in children is related to bleeding from heterotopic gastric mucosa within the diverticulum. In adults, the most common symptoms are due to intestinal obstruction, which may be secondary to invagination and intussusception or volvulus of the diverticulum, or inflammation and adhesions. Stasis within the diverticulum may result in calculi, called enteroliths.

Radiographically, the diverticulum appears as a wide-mouth outpouching of the distal ileum. Occasionally, a diverticulum may invert and appear as an oblong filling defect in the distal small bowel.

120. **The answers are: A-Y, B-Y, C-Y, D-Y, E-Y.** *(Eisenberg, pp 75–76.)* Numerous etiologic factors have been identified in the development of esophageal carcinoma. In the United States, a definite association exists between esophageal carcinoma and excessive alcohol intake and smoking. Carcinoma also occurs with significantly higher incidence in patients with lye strictures. Patients with untreated achalasia have a higher incidence, as well, perhaps from long-term stasis of esophageal contents. Hot tea, the major beverage in China and Russia, has been associated with a high incidence of esophageal carcinoma. The Plummer-Vinson syndrome, which consists of dysphagia, iron deficiency anemia, and mucosal lesions of the mouth, pharynx, and esophagus, has also been linked to esophageal carcinoma.

Genitourinary Radiology

DIRECTIONS: Each question below contains five suggested responses. Select the **one best** response to each question.

121. Judging from the contrast-enhanced CT scan in the figure, which ONE of the following would you say is the MOST likely diagnosis?

(Courtesy of ES Amis, Jr., MD)

(A) Psoas hematoma
(B) Xanthrogranulomatous pyelonephritis
(C) Renal cell carcinoma
(D) Retroperitoneal sarcoma
(E) Renal trauma

122. A 50-year-old man had the CT scan shown in the figure. The MOST likely diagnosis is

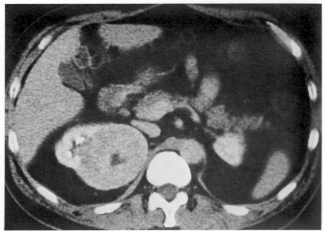

(Courtesy of ES Amis, Jr., MD)

(A) renal cell carcinoma
(B) renal abscess
(C) oncocytoma
(D) complex peripelvic cyst
(E) angiomyolipoma

123. The young trauma victim whose pelvic x-ray is shown in the figure was noted to have several drops of blood in his urethral meatus. In evaluation of the integrity of the urethra, the initial examination should be

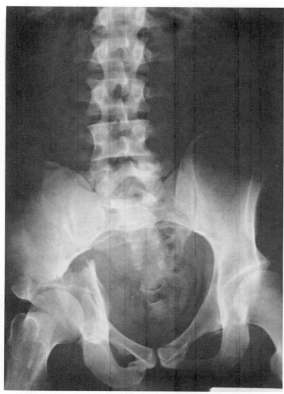

(Courtesy of ES Amis, Jr., MD)

(A) excretory urography
(B) contrast-enhanced CT scan
(C) retrograde examination of the entire urethra
(D) bladder catheterization and voiding cystourethrogram
(E) none of the above

124. Causes of acute cortical necrosis include all the following EXCEPT

(A) abruptio placentae
(B) hemolytic uremic syndrome
(C) burns
(D) phenacitin abuse
(E) snake bite

125. The patient in the figure underwent surgery for bladder cancer. The examination shows a (an)

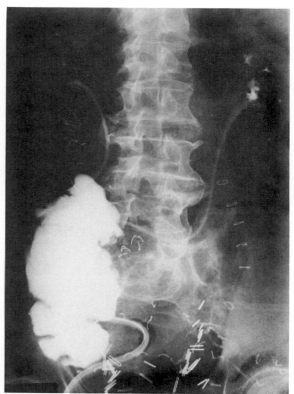

(Courtesy of ES Amis, Jr., MD)

(A) colovesical fistula
(B) ileal conduit
(C) Kock pouch
(D) ureterosigmoidostomy
(E) Indiana pouch

126. Which of the following is the LEAST common cause of medullary nephrocalcinosis?

(A) Type II (proximal) renal tubular acidosis
(B) Oxalosis
(C) Medullary sponge kidney
(D) Hyperparathyroidism
(E) Papillary necrosis

127. The patient in the figure complained of milky-looking urine. The MOST likely diagnosis is

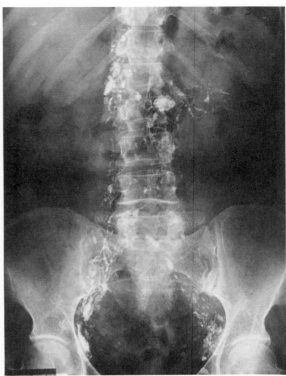

(Courtesy of ES Amis, Jr., MD)

(A) renal vein thrombosis
(B) filariasis
(C) steatorrhea
(D) hypercholesterolemia
(E) none of the above

128. Polycythemia vera or erythrocytosis is associated with ALL the following conditions EXCEPT

(A) renal cell carcinoma
(B) Wilms tumor
(C) polycystic kidney disease
(D) medullary sponge kidney
(E) von Hippel-Lindau disease

129. For the figure shown, the LEAST likely diagnosis is

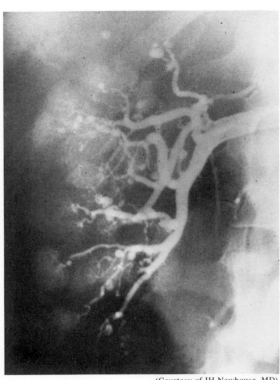

(Courtesy of JH Newhouse, MD)

(A) intravenous drug abuse
(B) polyarteritis nodosa
(C) tuberous sclerosis
(D) scleroderma
(E) Wegener granulomatosis

130. Based on the most likely diagnosis for the patient in question 129, which ONE of the following complications of disease would be LEAST expected?

(A) Hemorrhage
(B) Renal infarction
(C) Hypertension
(D) Renal failure
(E) Neoplasm

131. The patient whose CT scan is shown in the figure MOST likely has

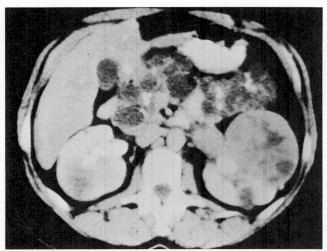

(Courtesy of JH Newhouse, MD)

- (A) tuberous sclerosis
- (B) von Hippel-Lindau disease
- (C) autosomal dominant polycystic kidney disease
- (D) Burkitt lymphoma
- (E) adult Wilms tumor

132. The treatment for the patient in question 131 would primarily include which ONE of the following?

- (A) Radiation therapy
- (B) Chemotherapy
- (C) Hemodialysis
- (D) Surgery
- (E) None required

133. Causes of a striated nephrogram during excretory urography include all the following EXCEPT

- (A) renal vein thrombosis
- (B) acute bacterial nephritis
- (C) Tamm-Horsfall proteinuria
- (D) lymphoma
- (E) medullary sponge kidney

134. The young trauma victim had the CT scan shown in the figure. In the absence of injury to the left kidney or other organs, he might be expected to develop ALL the following EXCEPT

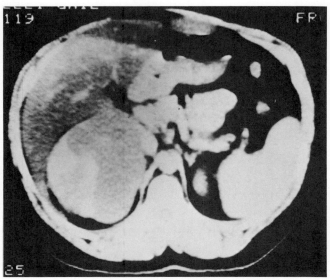

(Courtesy of JH Newhouse, MD)

- (A) urinoma
- (B) hematuria
- (C) electrolyte imbalance
- (D) renal failure
- (E) hypertension

135. Renal masses which may calcify include all the following EXCEPT

- (A) nephrogenic adenoma
- (B) Wilms tumor
- (C) renal cell carcinoma
- (D) tuberculous abscess
- (E) echinococcal cyst

DIRECTIONS: Each group of questions below consists of four lettered headings followed by a set of numbered items. For each numbered item select

A	if the item is associated with	**(A) only**
B	if the item is associated with	**(B) only**
C	if the item is associated with	**both** (A) and (B)
D	if the item is associated with	**neither** (A) nor (B)

Each lettered heading may be used **once, more than once,** or **not at all.**

Questions 136–138

(A)   Autosomal dominant
(B)   Autosomal recessive
(C)   Both
(D)   Neither

136.   Fraley syndrome

137.   Polycystic kidney disease

138.   Ask-Upmark kidney

Questions 139–141

(A)   High resistance to flow in small vessels
(B)   Low resistance to flow in small vessels
(C)   Both
(D)   Neither

139.   Priapism

140.   Hypertension due to Page kidney

141.   Captopril-induced renal failure

Questions 142–144

(A)   Adenocarcinoma of the bladder
(B)   Squamous cell carcinoma of the bladder
(C)   Both
(D)   Neither

142.   Aniline dye exposure

143.   Urachal remnant

144.   Malakoplakia

Questions 145–147

(A)   Wolffian duct
(B)   Müllerian duct
(C)   Both
(D)   Neither

145.   Utricle

146.   Appendix testis

147.   Lower half of vagina

DIRECTIONS: Each group of questions below consists of lettered headings followed by a set of numbered items. For each numbered item select the **one** lettered heading with which it is **most** closely associated. Each lettered heading may be used **once, more than once,** or **not at all.**

Questions 148–150

Match each of the diseases below with the feature with which it is MOST commonly associated.

(A) Uniformly fatal in childhood
(B) Contralateral ureteropelvic junction obstruction
(C) Hepatic fibrosis later in life
(D) Cystic dilatation of distal collecting tubules
(E) Salt-wasting nephropathy

148. Medullary cystic disease

149. Multicystic dysplastic kidney

150. Medullary sponge kidney

Questions 151–153

Which *combination* of the anomalies listed below comprise the following complex endocrine syndromes?

1. Pituitary adenoma   (A) 1,4,5
2. Pheochromocytoma   (B) 1,2,5
3. Medullary carcinoma of thyroid   (C) 2,3,5
4. Pancreatic islet cell tumor   (D) 3,4,6
5. Parathyroid adenoma   (E) 2,3,6
6. Neurofibromata

151. MEN type IIb

152. Sipple syndrome

153. Wermer syndrome

Questions 154–156

Match the appropriate center of activity with the corresponding adrenal hormone.

(A) Zona glomerulosa
(B) Zona fasciculata
(C) Zona reticularis
(D) Adrenal medulla

154. Estrogen

155. Norepinephrine

156. Aldosterone

DIRECTIONS: Each question below contains five suggested answers. For **each** of the **five** alternatives listed, you are to respond either YES or NO. In a given time, **all, some,** or **none of the alternatives may be correct.**

157. Renal vein thrombosis in adults is associated with which of the following?

    (A) Diabetes mellitus
    (B) Glomerulonephritis
    (C) Systemic lupus erythematosus
    (D) Pregnancy
    (E) Dehydration

158. TRUE statements regarding pheochromocytomas include which the following?

    (A) ^{131}I scanning has a sensitivity of 25–30%
    (B) Iodine administered intraarterially may produce profound hypotension in patients with pheochromocytomas
    (C) Approximately 20% arise in the organ of Zückerkandel
    (D) On T2-weighted MR images, the intensity of pheochromocytomas is much greater than liver tissue
    (E) Approximately 10% of cases are familial

159. Retroperitoneal fibrosis may occur secondary to which of the following?

    (A) Ergotamine
    (B) Hyperbaric oxygen
    (C) Aortic aneurysm
    (D) Corticosteroids
    (E) Polyarteritis nodosa

160. Concerning testicular tumors in adult males,

    (A) the most common cell type is seminoma
    (B) embryonal cell tumors frequently produce carcinoembryonic antigen (CEA)
    (C) the 5-year survival for choriocarcinoma is less than 1%
    (D) seminomas are usually hypoechoic at ultrasound examination
    (E) tumor spread is usually to obturator and iliac lymph nodes

161. Concerning infections of the urinary tract,

    (A) emphysematous pyelonephritis is more common in diabetic patients
    (B) an ultrasound examination should be the initial means of evaluation of an infant or child with a urinary tract infection
    (C) stricturing of the infundibula usually precedes papillary necrosis in tuberculous infections
    (D) in patients with schistosomiasis, disappearance of bladder calcification indicates probable adenocarcinoma
    (E) the yellowish patches of malakoplakia are typically umbilicated

162. Which of the following statements regarding contrast-induced nephrotoxicity are TRUE?

    (A) Insulin-dependent diabetes mellitus has been shown to be a risk factor, but only when accompanied by chronic renal failure
    (B) The degree of evaluation of creatinine in chronic renal insufficiency correlates with the resultant severity and duration of contrast-induced renal injury
    (C) It usually produces oliguria
    (D) It is usually transient
    (E) It may occur after cholangiography

163. Concerning hysterosalpingography,

    (A) oil-based contrast (Ethiodol) is associated with fewer complaints of abdominal pain
    (B) the T-shaped uterus is often found in women who were treated with diethylstilbestrol to prevent spontaneous abortion
    (C) salpingitis isthmica nodosa rarely causes infertility
    (D) the diagnosis of Ascherman syndrome includes filling defects which change shape at varying angles
    (E) endometrial hyperplasia may be easily distinguished from leiomyomata

164. Concerning ureteral duplication,

   (A) the Weigert-Meyer rule states that the upper pole moiety in a duplication inserts medially and inferiorly to the lower pole moiety

   (B) most ectopic ureteroceles occur in nonduplicated systems

   (C) the lower pole moiety has a tendency to reflux

   (D) in patients with ectopic ureteral insertion, only females are incontinent of urine

   (E) orthotopic ureteroceles are frequently bilateral

165. Regarding autosomal dominant polycystic kidney disease,

   (A) males are more frequently affected

   (B) there is a higher incidence of upper urinary tract infections

   (C) the cyst walls are commonly calcified

   (D) a density of 60 Hounsfield units in a cyst on a non-contrast CT scan is likely to represent hemorrhage

   (E) the cysts communicate with the collecting system and may opacify during excretory urography

166. True statements concerning xanthogranulomatous pyelonephritis (XGPN) include which of the following?

   (A) It is focal in most adults

   (B) Gram-negative infection is associated in nearly all cases

   (C) Renal calculi are present in approximately three-quarters of cases

   (D) CT scans often reveal gas within the involved areas

   (E) The excretory urogram usually shows preservation of function in the affected kidney

167. Concerning the male urethra,

   (A) approximately 40% of male urethral strictures in the U.S. are due to *N. gonorrhea*

   (B) in patients with chronic indwelling Foley catheters, strictures usually occur near the bladder neck

   (C) most urethral tumors are squamous cell carcinoma and occur in the bulbous urethra

   (D) the glands of Littre arise along the dorsal aspect of the anterior urethra

   (E) in cases of tuberculosis infection, involvement of the urethra may result in scrotal and peroneal fistula formation

168. True statements regarding urinary tract stones include

   (A) CT is useful for distinguishing urate stones from other filling defects

   (B) "mulberry" or "jackstone" bladder calculi are typically composed of calcium oxalate

   (C) urate stones are common in patients who have undergone ileostomy

   (D) the "milk of calcium" found in renal cysts is a calcium carbonate suspension

   (E) cystine stones are completely radiolucent

169. Regarding micturition,

   (A) detrusor external sphincter dyssynergy (DESD) commonly results from spinal cord lesions above the T5 level

   (B) the flaccid type of neurogenic bladder occurs with conus medullaris or sacral spinal cord lesions

   (C) stress incontinence in women most commonly results from loss of external sphincter tone

   (D) uninhibited bladder contractions usually indicate a cerebral etiology

   (E) patients with lower motor neuron lesions usually develop overflow incontinence

170. TRUE statements regarding reninoma include which of the following?

    (A) Peripheral renin levels are usually elevated
    (B) It is more common in women
    (C) Ultrasound typically shows a mass which is hypoechoic
    (D) They are usually 2 to 3 cm in size at the time of diagnosis
    (E) Angiography usually reveals a hypervascular mass

171. Concerning renal cell carcinoma (RCC),

    (A) the papillary cell type is associated with a more indolent tumor
    (B) approximately 50% of tumors have a calcification visible by CT
    (C) growth of tumor into the renal vein, in the absence of distant metastases, signifies Stage IIIA tumor
    (D) most tumors are hypervascular by angiographic examination
    (E) if a CT scan reveals fat in the tumor, the diagnosis of RCC can be safely excluded

172. True statements concerning acute urinary tract obstruction include which of the following?

    (A) The most common place for a stone to impact is at the ureteropelvic junction
    (B) With acute obstruction, an excretory urogram often reveals a dense, delayed nephrogram on the affected side
    (C) Most ruptures occur at the fornices
    (D) An early calyceal rim sign on an excretory urogram is pathognomonic.
    (E) The presence of vicarious excretion indicates chronicity

173. Regarding acute tubular necrosis,

    (A) excretory urography often shows dense, delayed nephrograms
    (B) the kidneys may be normal size or enlarged
    (C) ultrasound examination usually shows an echogenic cortex
    (D) normal perfusion is usually demonstrated by radionuclide scintigraphy
    (E) it may be precipitated by aminoglycosides

174. Calcification of the adrenal gland(s) is commonly associated with which of the following?

    (A) Wolman disease
    (B) Waterhouse-Friderichsen syndrome
    (C) Pheochromocytoma
    (D) Adrenal adenocarcinoma
    (E) Metastatic breast carcinoma

175. True statements concerning leukoplakia include which of the following?

    (A) It is associated with chronic urinary tract infection in most cases
    (B) It is considered to be premalignant
    (C) It arises most often in the elderly
    (D) The bladder is the most common site of involvement
    (E) In the ureter, it cannot be distinguished radiographically from ureteritis cystica

176. Which of the following are calcium-containing urinary crystals?

    (A) Brushite
    (B) Apatite
    (C) Struvite
    (D) Wedellite
    (E) Whewellite

177. Regarding multilocular cystic nephroma (MLCN),

    (A) it occurs most commonly in young girls and elderly males

    (B) the fluid-containing locules usually communicate

    (C) hematuria is a frequent symptom

    (D) the cysts in MLCN frequently enhance with contrast

    (E) the septations occasionally calcify

178. TRUE statements about the zonal anatomy of the prostate gland include which of the following?

    (A) It applies to both MR and ultrasound imaging

    (B) The transition zone is the site of origin of benign prostatic hypertrophy (BPH)

    (C) Carcinomas tend to arise posteriorly in the central zone

    (D) The lobe of Albarrán is situated in the anterior zone

    (E) The peripheral zone is bright on T2-weighted MR images

179. Concerning angiomyolipomas of the kidney,

    (A) most are solitary

    (B) as many as 80% of patients with tuberous sclerosis will have angiomyolipomas

    (C) AV shunting is common

    (D) the larger the tumor, the greater the likelihood of hemorrhage

    (E) for brightly echogenic lesions less than 1 cm in size which are found on USG, confirmatory CT scanning is not recommended

180. Regarding MRI of the adrenal glands,

    (A) pheochromocytomas are similar in intensity to water on T2-weighted images

    (B) adrenal adenomas typically acquire an intensity greater than that of liver on T2-weighted images

    (C) all adrenal masses have similar intensities on T1-weighted images

    (D) adrenal adenomas and carcinomas are rarely distinguishable

    (E) MRI is helpful for differentiating Wilms tumor from neuroblastoma

Genitourinary Radiology

Answers

121. The answer is B. *(Amis & Newhouse, pp 145–152.)* The figure reveals a soft-tissue density in the left retroperitoneum which is infiltrating the psoas muscle and which displaces the left kidney anteriorly. Additionally, there is a calcification in the renal pelvis and there are fluid-containing structures in the kidney. This is a case of xanthogranulomatous pyelonephritis, which is a form of chronic infection that occurs in the setting of long-standing obstruction, usually by a stone. The renal parenchyma is replaced by low-density material (foamy, lipid-laden macrophages that give the cut surface a yellow color), and the inflammatory process extends here, as it frequently does, outside the kidney to involve adjacent tissues.

It is the presence of the calculus that makes trauma, psoas abscess, renal cell carcinoma, and sarcoma less likely.

122. The answer is A. *(Amis & Newhouse, pp 123–127, 129–135.)* The CT scan in the figure reveals a rounded soft-tissue mass in the upper pole of the right kidney which has a central, stellate scar that is typical of an oncocytoma. In this case, a characteristic tumor "pseudocapsule" is created by the adjacent compressed renal tissue. The major differential diagnosis is renal cell carcinoma (RCC) and, in fact, the correct answer to the question *is* RCC, because it is a far more common tumor and most tumors that have the features seen here are actually RCCs.

Both oncocytoma and RCC are more common in men, by a factor of nearly 2 to 1, and both occur more commonly in the older age groups. Pain and hematuria may occur with either tumor, and radiographic features, such as the "spoke-wheel" arteriographic pattern typical of oncocytoma, have significant overlap. Most oncocytomas, however, tend to be homogeneous and have a central stellate scar by CT examination or ultrasound, which enables one to suggest the proper diagnosis. The central scar has the density of fibrous tissue, and should not be mistaken for fat in an angiomyolipoma.

The appearance of this mass would be atypical for an abscess, which is usually a shaggy, thick-walled lesion that may have a debris-filled center. Similarly, the possibility that this is a complex cyst would also be less likely, since there is no component which is clearly cystic.

123. The answer is C. *(Amis & Newhouse, pp 360–365.)* The plain radiograph in the figure shows a typical Malgaigne fracture, in which the pelvic ring is fractured anteriorly across the pubi rami and posteriorly at the sacroiliac joint. This creates a shearing stress on the pelvic contents which most often causes injury to the bladder base or posterior urethra. Although only 10% of patients will have a ruptured bladder, over 80% of patients with extraperitoneal bladder rupture will have associated pelvic fracture(s). In blunt injury to the pelvis, the incidences of intra- and extraperitoneal bladder rupture are roughly equal.

The presence of blood at the urethral meatus is a strong indicator of urethral injury. In such instance, a retrograde urethrogram should be performed. After evaluation, the catheter may then be advanced under fluoroscopic guidance into the bladder for cystography. Contrast-enhanced CT scanning and excretory urography do not sufficiently distend the bladder to rule out even a large tear.

During cystography, in order to rule out bladder rupture, the bladder should be filled with at least 400 cc or 50 cc more than the volume at which patient discomfort becomes moderate. It is then allowed to drain completely, so that a small posterior rupture is not missed. Cystography of extraperitoneal bladder rupture typically reveals a "sunburst" pattern of contrast dispersal around the bladder, whereas the contrast extravasation in an intraperitoneal rupture outlines the viscera and bowel.

124. The answer is D. *(Amis & Newhouse, pp 215–216. Davidson, p 238.)* Acute cortical nephrocalcinosis results when severe renal injury causes dystrophic calcification to form. It occurs most commonly in the setting of profound hypotension, and is seen most often in obstetric patients as a result of placental abruption and/or sepsis. In children, common causes include sepsis, shock, and dehydration, as well as hemolytic uremic syndrome and transfusion reaction.

In adults, sepsis, dehydration, cardiac failure, and burns may all adversely affect renal blood flow. The ingestion of toxins (ethylene glycol) and snake bites may similarly cause shock and resultant multiorgan damage.

Phenacetin abuse is not associated with cortical nephrocalcinosis, but is a common cause of papillary necrosis in some areas of the world.

125. The answer is E. *(Amis & Newhouse, pp 374–379.)* The patient in the figure has undergone a type of continent urinary diversion known as an Indiana pouch (developed at the University of Indiana). With such reservoirs, the patient need only intermittently catheterize the pouch to drain it, eliminating the need for external appliances.

The Indiana pouch is constructed by isolating the cecum and terminal ileum for use as the reservoir and surface conduit, respectively. The bowel is "detubularized" by folding over the open end, so that organized contractions can no longer occur. The ileocecal valve makes the pouch continent, and the ureters are tunneled into the teniae of the colon to prevent reflux.

The Kock pouch utilizes 40 cm of ileum which are fileted open and then resewn together to form a pouch, with both ends intussuscepted into it to provide antireflux valves for the inflow channel and conduit to the surface. The surgery is considerably more complex than the Indiana or similar cecal pouches (Penn, King, etc.). Any foreign body, such as a staple or suture, that protrudes into the pouch lumen may act as a nidus for stone formation.

The ureterosigmoidostomy procedure has been abandoned due to the complication of adenocarcinoma, which develops 15 to 20 years after diversion, typically at the ureteral anastomoses.

This patient does not have an ileal (Bricker) conduit, as the haustral markings of the colon are readily apparent. The position of the colonic loop and lack of bladder opacification exclude a colovesical fistula.

126. The answer is A. *(Amis & Newhouse, pp 213–218.)* Medullary nephrocalcinosis results from deposition of calcium salts in the distal collecting tubules near the papillae. Although renal tubular acidosis (RTA) is responsible for 20% of cases of medullary nephrocalcinosis, it is the distal type (type I) rather than proximal type (type II) which is responsible. Though occasionally familial, it is usually a sporadic disease in which there is an inability to eliminate hydrogen ions (a function of the distal tubules only), causing calcium to precipitate in the less acid urine.

Hyperparathyroidism is the most common cause of hypercalcemia and is responsible for up to 40% of cases of medullary nephrocalcinosis. Other causes of hypercalcemia and stone formation include increased intestinal absorption of calcium (e.g., hypervitaminosis D), paraneoplastic syndromes, and skeletal demineralization.

Medullary sponge kidney (MSK) causes nephrocalcinosis by producing stasis of urine in anatomically dilated distal collecting tubules. Interestingly, in contrast to the other causes of nephrocalcinosis, the involvement in MSK is often patchy and asymmetrical.

Oxalosis, in distinction to the other causes of nephrocalcinosis, more frequently results in cortical nephrocalcinosis. However, it may be so severe as to affect both cortex and medulla. It occurs as a primary disorder in patients with an inherited overproduction of oxalate or secondary to increased absorption secondary to bowel resection or inflammatory bowel disease, because of an insufficient amount of bile salts needed to bind the oxalate for elimination.

Papillary necrosis, as with other forms of tissue necrosis in the body, results in dystrophic calcification. Sometimes the rim of a "ghost" papilla may be visible, though often the necrotic papilla is sloughed and eliminated.

127. The answer is B. (*Amis & Newhouse, pp 82–83.*) The lymphangiogram in the figure shows tortuous and dilated retroperitoneal lymphatic vessels and retrograde filling of lymphatics in the left renal hilum, indicating obstruction. The milky urine is due to chyluria. Worldwide, the most common cause of this is filariasis ("tropical" chyluria). The retroperitoneal lymph nodes are infiltrated by nematode microfilaria (e.g., *Wuchereria bancrofti, Loa loa,* or *Dracunculus medinensis*) and become obstructed.

In the U.S., it is usually due to "nontropical" causes, which include malignancy, surgery, trauma, infection (particularly tuberculosis) and, rarely, lymphangioleiomyomatosis (LAM). The mechanism is the same for each: lymphatic infiltration and obstruction, either by tumor, granulomata, or fibrous or muscle tissue. Lymphangiography typically reveals obstructed lymphatics, lack of nodal opacification, retrograde renal flow, and perhaps eventual contrast accumulation in the collecting system.

Renal vein thrombosis, steatorrhea, and hypercholesterolemia do not explain either the patient's symptom of chyluria or the abnormal lymphangiogram.

128. The answer is D. (*Wilson, ed. 12, pp 226, 1563–1565.*) Polycythemia vera is a disorder of abnormally high myeloid cell production, but splenomegaly and an increased red cell mass dominate the clinical picture. In its primary form, there is no elevation of erythropoietin level, in contrast to the secondary form (e.g., due to chronic hypoxemia) in which erythropoietin production is stimulated.

Certain tumors or conditions may elaborate erythropoietin or a similar substance. These arise predominantly in the posterior cranial fossa (hemangioblastoma is the most common cell type), as well as in the kidney. Of the latter, renal cell carcinoma (RCC) is the most common, but Wilms tumor, oncocytoma, and some sarcomas may also cause erythrocytosis or frank polycythemia. Patients with von Hippel-Lindau disease (possibly related to the increased incidence of RCC), polycystic kidneys, renal artery stenosis, or hydronephrosis may also develop severe erythrocytosis, though not necessarily progress to polycythemia.

Medullary sponge kidney is not associated with erythrocytosis or polycythemia.

129. The answer is C. (*Amis & Newhouse, pp 178–179.*) The renal angiogram in the figure reveals numerous saccular aneurysms arising from the medium- and small-size arteries and occlusions of many small vessels. This is a case of polyarteritis nodosa, but the angiographic pattern of vasculitis is often nonspecific. Though scleroderma often produces myriad tiny aneurysms, it may assume the appearance of the arteritis in this case. Wegener granulomatosis, systemic lupus erythematosus, and intravenous drug use may also develop a similar vasculitis.

Only tuberous sclerosis does not fit the pattern. Though the angiomyolipomas may have aneurysms, they arise from neovessels in masses, and neither are present in this case.

130. **The answer is E.** *(Amis & Newhouse, pp 178–179.)* Any of the collagen-vascular disorders in question 129 may result in aneurysm formation or vasculitic stenosis or occlusion from vasculitis. The aneurysms are prone to rupture and may produce renal or perirenal hemorrhage.

If the subcapsular hematoma is large enough, the kidney may be compressed and become ischemic, which in turn activates the renin-angiotensin system to raise the blood pressure. Similarly, ischemia due to the impairment of blood flow from the vasculitis may lead to hypertension. If severe enough, it can cause renal infarction. The progression of disease may ultimately cause renal failure. There is no associated risk of benign or malignant neoplasia.

131. **The answer is B.** *(Amis & Newhouse, pp 142–143.)* The CT scan in the figure reveals multiple cysts in both kidneys and the pancreas. The diagnosis is von Hippel-Lindau disease (VHL), an autosomal dominant syndrome which usually arises in the second or third decade. It is characterized by frequent occurrence of retinal angiomas, cerebellar hemangioblastomas, pheochromocytomas, cysts in multiple organs (especially the kidneys, pancreas, liver, spleen, and epididymis), and a high incidence of renal cell carcinoma (RCC). In fact, in addition to the renal cysts, there are several solid masses in the left kidney which, indeed, are carcinomas. These tumors tend to occur at an earlier age in patients with VHL than in those with RCC, and although they may be more indolent, they are nonetheless malignant.

The presence of the pancreatic cysts helps to exclude the diagnoses of tuberous sclerosis, autosomal dominant polycystic kidney disease (which *can* have cysts in the liver), Burkitt lymphoma, and Wilms tumor. Although considered strictly a pediatric tumor, Wilms tumor has been reported to occur in young adults.

132. **The answer is D.** *(Amis & Newhouse, pp 142–143.)* The renal cell carcinomas (RCCs) in the left kidney of the patient in question 131 require surgical excision. Since these patients continue to form RCCs throughout their lives, partial nephrectomy or local tumor resection is desirable to preserve as much kidney as possible. Such "bench" surgery, wherein the kidney is removed and later replaced following excision of the tumor, is painstaking. Radiation and chemotherapy are not helpful. Since renal function is preserved, despite severe involvement, hemodialysis is not usually required, although bilateral nephrectomies may ultimately be necessary in cases of tumor. Most patients, unfortunately, usually succumb to other aspects of the disease.

133. **The answer is D.** *(Amis & Newhouse, pp 233–238. Davidson, pp 261, 269, 282.)* The finding of a striated nephrogram on an excretory urogram is nonspecific and usually follows obstruction and dilatation of the collecting tubules, which have a parallel and radial orientation. Although stone disease is the most common cause, Tamm-Horsfall proteinuria and other causes of tubular blockage may also produce a striated nephrogram. Additionally, nonobstructive dilatation of the tubules, as is seen in medullary sponge kidney (MSK), occasionally results in striations.

Renal vein thrombosis causes edema which enlarges and distorts the intrarenal collecting system. It rarely has been reported to cause a striated nephrogram. Striations may also appear in a wedge-shaped distribution in areas affected by acute focal bacterial nephritis (AFBN). Lymphoma, however, has not been associated with a striated nephrogram.

134. The answer is D. *(Amis & Newhouse, p 173.)* The CT scan in the figure reveals a large subcapsular collection in the right kidney. Most likely this represents a hematoma, although occasionally a urinoma may develop in this location. (A urinoma might be expected to be less dense, but immediately following trauma it might also contain blood.) When large (>500 ml), a subcapsular or perirenal collection compresses the kidney to such a degree that it becomes ischemic. Hypertension may develop, a phenomenon known as the Page kidney, which often resolves spontaneously as the collection organizes and is resorbed. Though hypertension may appear in a matter of days, it is often more insidious in onset. Drainage is occasionally necessary. The activation of the renin-angiotensin system, which is responsible for causing hypertension, may also lead to hypernatremia and hypokalemia by elevated aldosterone levels. Renal failure does not occur if the contralateral kidney is functioning properly. There is often microscopic or gross hematuria following blunt trauma.

135. The answer is A. *(Amis & Newhouse, pp 129–138, 164–168, 296–297.)* Of the choices given, not only do nephrogenic adenomas not calcify, but also, contrary to what their name would imply, they are neither adenomas nor of nephric origin. They are proliferative endothelial masses which develop in response to chronic infection, and though they can occur anywhere in the urinary tract, they are most common in the bladder. They have no malignant potential and have gotten their name from their histologic similarity to proximal renal tubular tissue.

Wilms tumor, or nephroblastoma, is the most common abdominal malignancy in children. It is also one of the most treatable; the 5-year survival with chemotherapy and radiation therapy now reaches 85–90%. About 9% of tumors calcify; the pattern is one of dense clumps or arcs, in distinction to the stippled calcification of neuroblastoma and transitional cell carcinoma (TCC).

Renal cell carcinomas, overall the most common primary renal malignancy, calcify in only 10–20% of patients, but since calcification in a renal mass has a 75% chance of malignancy, it warrants investigation. The pattern of calcification varies widely, from central and punctate to curvilinear and peripheral.

Tuberculous abscesses commonly calcify in a variety of ways; the most characteristic pattern is that of calcified caseous material (coalescent granulomata) that creates the "putty kidney" appearance. The shrunken kidney is replaced by an amorphous ground-glass substance and is often referred to as having undergone "autonephrectomy."

Ecchinococcal cysts affect the kidney in only 25% of cases. As elsewhere in the body, the cyst walls calcify with age. The arcuate configuration may become amorphous, should the cysts collapse. Rarely, they communicate with the collecting system and opacify on excretory urography.

136–138. The answers are: 136-D, 137-C, 138-D. *(Amis & Newhouse, pp 58–59, 108–114, 179. Davidson, pp 128–129, 167.)* Of the three disorders listed (Fraley syndrome, polycystic kidney disease, and Ask–Upmark kidney), the only heritable one is polycystic kidney disease. Often classified into "infantile" and "adult" types, it is more correctly viewed in terms of inheritance pattern.

Autosomal recessive polycystic kidney disease (ARPKD) produces innumerable small cysts which arise from the collecting tubules. Though subclassified into four subtypes, the more simplified "infantile" and "juvenile" categories help one to remember that hepatic fibrosis takes time to develop. In children with ARPKD, the younger the disease becomes manifest, the more the renal disease dominates, and the patient usually doesn't live long enough for the liver disease to become severe. Conversely, if the patient presents in his or her teens, it is more likely that the renal disease is milder and the sequela of hepatic involvement have brought them to medical attention.

Autosomal dominant polycystic kidney disease (ADPKD) affects males and females equally. The cysts are usually more numerous than the simple cysts which normally arise with age (50% of people over the age of 50 have one or more cysts). If the cysts become large or numerous enough, they may cause renal failure by compression of the normal intervening parenchyma. Liver cysts are present in over half the patients, but these rarely if ever compromise liver function. Berry aneurysms arise around the circle of Willis in 10% of patients.

Crossing vessels may obstruct an upper pole infundibulum, which may be exacerbated by diuretic substances (e.g., beer, coffee, etc.). When it is painful, it is known as Fraley syndrome.

The Ask-Upmark kidney is characterized by small size and a typical deep groove crossing the lateral surface near the upper pole. It is still debated whether it is a form of true hypoplasia or the result of focal reflux nephropathy, with or without infection. The histologic data supports both theories, but clinical and radiographic evidence points to the latter cause as most likely.

139–141. The answers are: 139-C, 140-A, 141-B. *(Amis & Newhouse, pp 172–175.)* Priapism, a condition in which penile erection persists uncontrolled, may occur in two ways. Most commonly, it occurs in patients with sickle cell disease who develop occlusion of the small venous outflow channels, which results in a painful, engorged penis. Treatment may require (surgical) intracavernosal shunt. Another form is called "high flow" priapism. It occurs because the arterial inflow has been abnormally increased, often due to trauma or stimulation by cocaine use. Treatment in this case may involve embolization of the cavernosal arteries with a nonpermanent agent, such as autologous clot.

Page kidney is a type of renovascular hypertension that occurs as a result of a subscapsular or perirenal space-occupying lesion causing compression and ischemia of the kidney. It most commonly follows blunt abdominal trauma, with the development of a subscapular hematoma; though the time course of the hypertension may vary from immediate to a slow onset over many months. It results from activation of the renin-angiotensin system, and in the case of traumatic hematoma, often resolves spontaneously as the hematoma organizes and is resorbed.

Captopril, an angiotensin-converting enzyme inhibitor, directly reduces efferent anteriolar vasomotor tone in the glomeruli. In individuals with normal glomerular filtration, no change in GFR occurs following captopril administration. However, those who rely on efferent arteriolar vasoconstriction to maintain GFR, such as those with renal artery stenosis, will suffer a precipitous drop in filtration pressure when on captopril. A rise in serum creatinine is an indirect screen for renal artery stenosis which is bilateral.

142–144. The answers are: 142-D, 143-A, 144-D. *(Amis & Newhouse, pp 136–138, 274–275, 298–300.)* Approximately 95% of bladder cancers are transitional cell carcinoma (TCC). They occur most commonly above the age of 60 and are 3 to 4 times more common in males. Risk factors include exposure to aniline dye (and various other petroleum compounds), smoking, phenacetin abuse, and cyclophosphamide used chronically for cancer treatment.

The next most common type is squamous cell carcinoma. It occurs more commonly in the setting of chronic inflammation, including chronic urinary tract infection (UTI) from stone disease, infected diverticula, or simply recurrent UTIs. In endemic areas, schistosomiasis is a well-known cause; the chronic inflammation that results causes squamous metaplasia of the urothelium (leukoplakia), which is premalignant.

Malakoplakia, on the other hand, although due to chronic infection (usually *E. coli*), is not premalignant. The yellowish plaques which appear on the bladder surface are comprised of large histiocytes which contain partially digested bacteria and calcospherules called Michaelis-Gutmann bodies. They look similar to cystitis cystica radiographically, though the latter tends to have rounder lesions and does not cause ureteral dilatation, which occurs with malakoplakia even in the absence of obstruction.

Adenocarcinomas account for only 1% of bladder malignancies. They occur most often near the dome and are associated with urachal remnants or bladder exstrophy. While most patients present with hematuria, 10% of adenocarcinomas produce mucus, which may be visible in the urine.

145–147. The answers are: 145-B, 146-B, 147-D. *(Amis & Newhouse, pp 3–4.)* The development of the urinary tract and sex organs is a complex process. The Müllerian and Wolffian ducts are embryonic structures which undergo a different series of transformations for each sex.

In the male, Müllerian inhibitory factor (MIF) is produced, which suppresses the development of the two Müllerian ducts into the female reproductive organs; only the vestigial appendix testis and utricle remain. Each Wolffian (or mesonephric) duct continues to develop, giving rise not only to the ureteral bud, which eventually forms the ureter and the renal collecting system, but also the ejaculatory duct, vas deferens, and epididymis.

In the female, the only Wolffian duct structures which develop are those which form the urinary tract structures. The Müllerian ducts form the fallopian tubes and fuse caudally to form the uterus, cervix, and upper third of the vagina. The lower part of the vagina is formed by the urogenital sinus.

The testes and ovaries arise from the urogenital ridge and, by differential growth, "migrate" caudally to their final location.

148–150. The answers are: 148-E, 149-B, 150-D. *(Amis & Newhouse, pp 116–120. Davidson, pp 210–213. Pollack, pp 1151–1166.)* Medullary cystic disease, multicystic displastic kidney, and medullary sponge kidney are three very different disorders, with distinct manifestations and associations.

Medullary cystic disease may exist as an autosomal recessive disease, which is referred to as juvenile nephronophthisis. Presenting symptoms include azotemia, polysypsis, polyuria, and salt wasting. The disease often progresses to anemia, hypertension, uremia, and death by age 30, though some have lived into adulthood. The adult-onset form, which is autosomal dominant, is more rapidly progressive, though edema and hypertension are typically absent. Death usually occurs within a few years of onset. Azotemia is again a feature, and the nephrogram reveals a typically "streaky" pattern of persistent striations in the renal medulla. Cysts, when present, are usually only 1 to 2 cm in diameter and therefore difficult to spot by excretory urography.

Multicystic dysplastic kidney is a congenital lesion without any inheritance pattern. It is felt to arise from failure of the ureteral bud to properly connect with the metanephric blastema. It is associated with abnormality of the contralateral kidney in approximately 30% of cases, most commonly ureteropelvic junction obstruction, but anomalies of rotation and horseshoe kidney also occur more frequently. The disease may be bilateral, which is fatal within a few days of life. When unilateral, it is a common cause of an abdominal mass in the newborn, though it is often discovered only as an incidental finding (calcific nubbin on an abdominal x-ray) in the adult.

Patients with medullary sponge kidney (MSK), which is often referred to as *benign tubular ectasia* when no calcification is present, is most often asymptomatic. When stones form because of urinary stasis in the dilated collecting ducts, they may pass and produce typical renal colic and hematuria. The nephrogram reveals "paintbrushed," streaky papillae. MSK is considered by some authors to be part of a spectrum or overlapping disorders that include hepatic cysts and Caroli disease, and has also been linked to hemihypertrophy and hyperparathyroidism.

151–153. The answers are: 151-E, 152-C, 153-A. *(Wilson, ed. 12, pp 1811–1812.)* Wermer syndrome, also referred to as multiple endocrine neoplasia type I (MEN I), is typified by tumors of the pituitary, parathyroid, and pancreas. The lesions in the first two are usually benign adenomas, whereas the islet cell tumors that arise in the pancreas are often malignant. Patients may develop pituitary dysfunction or hyperparathyroidism (eventually most become hyperparathyroid) and often present with symptoms due to hormone production by the islet cell tumor, specifically peptic ulcer, Zollinger-Ellison syndrome, or diarrhea (gastrin) or hypoglycemia (insulin). Other tumors include Schwannomas, multiple lipomas, carcinoids, and thymomas. Symptoms usually arise after childhood, but before the age of 60. The disorder is heritable and all first-degree relatives should be screened. The defective gene which causes MEN I, possibly a form of neurocristopathy, is reported to be localized to chromosome 11.

Multiple endocrine neoplasia type IIa (MEN IIa), or Sipple syndrome, is a disorder of the cells of the adrenal medulla and parafollicular (C) cells which are known to be derived from the neural crest. Consequently, patients develop pheochromocytomas and medullary carcinoma of the thyroid (MTC); half of those afflicted also develop parathyroid hyperplasia. The gene has been mapped to chromosome 10, and the disorder is inherited as autosomal dominant. While the parathyroid disease is often clinically silent, the other features of the syndrome bring the patient to attention. Of patients presenting with pheochromocytomas, which are frequently multiple and bilateral in MEN IIa & IIb, 5% of them will also have MTC. In patients who present with MTC, 10% will have MEN IIa or IIb. Associated tumors include gliomas, glioblastomas, and meningiomas.

MEN IIb, which is sometimes referred to as *mucosal neuroma syndrome,* or MEN III, also features pheochromocytomas and MTC, but has associated neuromas of multiple organs and, in some ways, resembles neurofibromatosis. However, additional features (Marfanoid body habitus, hypotonia, etc.) distinguish this entity. The gene locus has not been identified. The clinical course is worse than with the other disorders, with a mean survival of about 30 years.

154–156. The answers are: 154-C, 155-D, 156-A. *(Wilson, ed. 12, pp 1713–1718.)* The adrenal glands are Y-shaped and are composed of three concentric cortical layers and a medulla. The latter is responsible for the production of epinephrine and norepinephrine.

The three cortical layers are, from outside to inside: the zona glomerulosa, which produces the mineralocorticoids, principally aldosterone; the zona fasiculata, which makes cortisol; and the zona reticularis, which produces the androgens, primarily dehydroepiandrosterone (DHEA), which is a precursor of testosterone. Urinary 17-ketosteroids are used as a means of gauging androgen production.

157. The answers are: A-Y, B-Y, C-Y, D-Y, E-N. *(Amis & Newhouse, pp 185–187.)* Renal vein thrombosis (RVT) in the adult usually occurs in conjunction with underlying renal disease, most commonly due to diabetes mellitus, glomerulonephritis, or papillary necrosis.

Less common associations include pregnancy, burns, trauma, and surgery. Direct compression of the renal vein may cause subsequent thrombosis; bland or tumor thrombus may extend from the inferior vena cava into the renal vein.

Although dehydration is commonly associated with RVT in infants less than 2 weeks old, as is maternal diabetes mellitus, it is not a frequent association in adults. In children, rehydration and/or correction of the underlying metabolic problem is usually sufficient to restore normal renal function. In adults, anticoagulation is necessary, as there is a 50% risk of propagation of clot and pulmonary embolism.

158. The answers are: A-N, B-N, D-N, D-Y, E-Y. *(Amis & Newhouse, pp 85–88.)* Pheochromocytomas, or paraganglioneuromas, arise from the chromaffin cells of sympathetic ganglia or, most commonly, the adrenal medulla (99%). The most common extraadrenal site is the organ of Zückerkandel, which is a ganglion located just below the origin of the inferior mesenteric artery. Rare cases have been reported near the dome of the bladder; these patients developed symptoms during voiding.

Most patients are in the fourth or fifth decade and most present with hypertension, headache, flushing, palpitations, or apprehension. Pheochromocytomas are responsible for 0.5 to 1% of all cases of hypertension. They usually arise de novo, though in some patients they are associated with the multiple endocrine neoplasia syndromes. The *rule of tens,* as it is referred to, gives the following rough approximations:

10% are malignant
10% are familial
10% are extraadrenal
10% are multiple
10% of adrenal pheochromocytomas are bilateral

Intravenous contrast may precipitate a *hyper*tensive crisis in sensitive individuals. In patients with suspected pheochromocytoma, prophylactic alpha blockade has been recommended before contrast examination. Regitine (5 mg IV) may be given in acute cases. ^{131}I-MIBG scanning is very sensitive (80–90%) and is highly specific. On T1-weighted MR scans, pheochromocytomas are slightly less intense than liver, but similar to kidney and spleen. On T2-weighted images, however, they exhibit the brightest signal of any adrenal mass.

159. **The answers are: A-Y, B-N, C-Y, D-N, E-Y.** *(Amis & Newhouse, pp 76–78.)* Idiopathic retroperitoneal fibrosis (RPF), or Ormond disease, accounts for 68% of cases of RPF. The remainder are acquired in both benign and malignant conditions.

When idiopathic, it is most common in middle-aged men. It occurs most commonly in the abdomen, around the abdominal aorta, causing medial deviation of the midureters and ultimately ureteral obstruction. The fibrotic process may extend the entire length of the spine. The disease may be asymmetrical and involve one side more severely than the other. The aorta may be surrounded by fibrosis, but is not usually displaced, in contrast to retroperitoneal lymphadenopathy, in which CT commonly shows the aorta elevated off the spine by an enveloping mass.

RPF may occur secondary to medication, most notably the ergot derivatives. Corticosteroids, rather than cause RPF, have often been employed with some success for treatment of cases which fail to recede after discontinuing the causative drug. Treatment may require surgical dissection and transplantation of the ureters from the retroperitoneum into the peritoneal cavity.

Collagen vascular diseases, including polyarteritis nodosa, have been associated with RPF, as well as aortic aneurysm (with or without leakage). Hyperbaric oxygen is associated with retrolental fibroplasia in neonates, and not with RPF.

160. **The answers are: A-Y, B-N, C-Y, D-Y, E-N.** *(Amis & Newhouse, pp 347–351.)* Germ cell tumors of the testis are the most common malignant solid tumors in young men. About 10% arise in cases of cryptorchidism. Roughly two-thirds of germ cell tumors are purely one cell type; the remainder are mixed. Seminoma is the most common cell type (45%), followed by mixed embryonal carcinoma and teratoma (teratocarcinoma) (25–30%), embryonal carcinoma (20–25%), teratoma (5–10%), and choriocarcinoma (<1%).

By ultrasound, most testicular tumors are hypoechoic. Though usually nonspecific, some cell types have additional features. Embryonal carcinoma and teratoma tend to be inhomogeneous and have cystic areas and highly echogenic foci within them. Sometimes, the bright foci alone are found, without associated tumor. These are felt to possibly represent "burned out" tumors which outstripped their blood supply and infarcted.

Testicular tumors, including the non-germ-cell Leydig and Sertoli cell tumors, spread locally to the epididymis and spermatic cord, and distally by hematogenous spread (usually to the lungs) or more commonly via the retroperitoneal lymphatic channels to the renal hila, bypassing the obturator and iliac nodal chains.

Choriocarcinoma has the worst prognosis, with a 5-year survival of less than 1%. Seminoma, on the other hand, has a high cure rate. The tumor is highly radiosensitive and even large nodal metastases are treatable.

The nonseminomatous tumors, especially embryonal cell carcinoma, often have an elevated alpha fetoprotein (αFP) level, and a number of them will also have elevated HGC levels. Carcinoembryonic antigen (CEA) is not elaborated by testicular tumors, but rather is a marker for metastatic disease to the liver, especially from colon carcinoma.

161. **The answers are: A-Y, B-N, C-N, D-N, E-Y.** *(Amis & Newhouse, pp 153–170, 274–275, 294–295.)* Emphysematous pyelonephritis most commonly occurs in patients with severe diabetes mellitus. Gas may form in and around the kidney as well as in the collecting system, which is produced by the infecting bacteria, typically *E. coli*. Patients are usually extremely ill, with nausea, vomiting, abdominal pain, and fever, and the mortality rate is nearly 50%.

The evaluation of urinary tract infections (UTI) is dependent on the age and sex of the patient. In neonates and young children, although ultrasound is useful in evaluating the upper tracts, the high incidence of vesicoureteral reflux and posterior urethral valves in boys warrants voiding cystourethrography (VCUG). There is some controversy as to whether young girls should be evaluated at the first occurrence of UTI or whether the lower frequency of anomalies should preclude evaluation until the second or third infection. As the age of the patient increases, the workup is tailored to the increased incidence of stone disease, prostatism, or other conditions which predispose to infection.

In cases of tuberculosis, the natural history of renal involvement is for affected papillae to slough, releasing bacilli into the urine. These invade the urothelium and produce inflammation and granuloma formation, leading to ulceration and eventual development of fibrosis and strictures. The kidney becomes partially or completely obstructed, and the closed infection ultimately leads to total destruction (autonephrectomy), producing the so-called putty, or mortar, kidney, as the result is a solid agglomeration of caseous material.

The calcification which develops in the bladder wall in patients with *Schistosoma hematobium* infection most frequently assumes a linear configuration. Although these patients are at risk for bladder cancer, and the disappearance of bladder calcification is a clue to such possible neoplastic change, it is squamous cell cancer, not *adeno*carcinoma.

Malakoplakia, which most commonly affects the bladder, is due to chronic inflammation. When it affects the ureter, it is usually a long segment of the more distal portion. Plaques are formed by aggregates of histiocytes which contain partially digested bacteria (usually *E. coli*) and are typically umbilicated and surrounded by hyperemia.

162. **The answers are: A-Y, B-Y, C-N, D-Y, E-Y.** *(Amis & Newhouse, pp 43–55.)* Many risk factors have been cited which predispose to nephrotoxicity, including acute or chronic renal failure, multiple myeloma, older age, proteinuria, and diabetes. The only ones, however, which are supported by the combined literature are (1) chronic renal failure (CRF), in which the creatinine level is indeed directly related to the likelihood, severity, and duration of contrast-induced nephrotoxicity, and (2) diabetes mellitus with glomerulopathy. The latter group may be a subset of the patients with CRF, as diabetes alone appears not to put patients at higher risk. Contrast-induced nephrotoxicity may follow intraarterial or intravenous injection, as well as nonvascular studies such as cholangiography. Additionally, the incidence of contrast-induced nephrotoxicity does not appear to be dose-related, nor does the use of low-osmolality agents prevent its occurrence.

The course of nephrotoxicity usually follows a pattern of rapidly rising creatinine, which usually peaks at about 3 days, with a return to baseline in a week or so. Urine output, surprisingly, does not usually decrease during this time, which implies that many cases of mild contrast-induced ATN may go unnoticed.

Prophylactic use of lasix and mannitol directly following contrast injection increases excretion of the agent and may avoid nephrotoxicity. Careful replacement of fluid losses should be instituted during the 24-hour period following diuretic administration.

163. **The answers are: A-Y, B-N, C-N, D-Y, E-N.** *(Hunt & Siegler, pp 20–22, 59–94, 128–138.)* Oil-based (Ethiodol) and water-soluble (Sinografin) contrast agents are currently used for hysterosalpingography (HSG). The water-soluble media are rapidly absorbed and excreted by the kidneys. They have the theoretical advantage of decreased pulmonary complications should the agent intravasate, but Ethiodol pulmonary embolism has not been associated with significant morbidity or mortality. The oil-soluble agents reportedly cause less discomfort, but are not readily resorbed, so that material which spills into the peritoneum persists and may invoke granuloma formation.

Hysterosalpingography is commonly performed to evaluate the cause of infertility. Salpingitis isthmica nodosa (SIN) is associated with infertility in about half of cases, and there is an increased incidence of tubal pregnancy. It is a disease which is characterized by nodular thickening of the tubes which may create diverticula.

Diethylstilbestrol (DES) is a synthetic estrogen which was used in the fifties and sixties to treat threatened abortion. The T-shaped uterus results from exposure to DES *in utero* and acquires its distorted shape because of disorganized myometrial hypertrophy. This also affects the cornua, creating circumferential bands, which appear as stenoses when compared to the bulbous cornua beyond. They are not obstructive, however. Whether the uterus appears abnormal by HSG or not, those who were exposed to DES *in utero* have a higher incidence of infertility and complicated pregnancy.

Ascherman syndrome involves a subset of patients with intrauterine adhesions and synechiae, and most commonly develops after uterine curettage. In these patients, the cervical canal is stenotic and abdominal pain occurs in conjunction with menses. The irregular filling defects seen by HSG are characteristic, though overfilling of the uterus may obscure them. Treatment includes curettage and placement of an IUD (or repeated instrumentation at 1 month) and hormone therapy.

Endometrial hyperplasia often appears as nodular thickening of the uterine lining or polypoid protrusions into the lumen. HSG cannot reliably distinguish between conditions which may appear similar, including endometrial polyps, multiple small submucous leiomyomata, and occasionally infiltrating carcinoma.

164.   The answers are: A-Y, B-N, C-Y, D-Y, E-Y.   *(Amis & Newhouse, pp 64, 257–267.)*   Ureteral duplication is a common congenital anomaly, occurring in about 1–2% of the population. Embryologically, it occurs when the ureteral bud divides before it contacts the metanephric blastema. Partial duplication is 4 times as common as complete duplication, because complete duplication requires that two individual ureteral buds arise separately from the mesonephric duct. Duplications are bilateral in up to 20% of cases.

In complete duplication, the ureters insert into the bladder in separate but predictable locations. The ureter from the upper pole moiety enters anteriorly, medially, and inferiorly to the lower pole ureter. This is the Weigert-Meyer rule. The lateral position of the lower pole ureter insertion into the trigone of the bladder compromises the valve mechanism, leading to a tendency to reflux. The upper pole ureter, on the other hand, which inserts ectopically, is prone to ureterocele formation and obstruction. Urographically, when the upper pole moiety fails to opacify, there are clues to the presence of duplication. These include mass effect of the nonvisualized upper pole which alters the renal axis; fewer-than-normal number of visible calyces in the kidney, which often resemble a "drooping lily"; and deviation of the lower pole moiety ureter by the tortuous and dilated upper pole ureter, with which it is intertwined.

Two-thirds of cases of ectopic ureteral insertion are associated with complete duplication of the ipsilateral side. In males, the most common site of insertion is the prostatic urethra. In all cases, the insertion is into structures above the external sphincter and therefore males are always continent of urine. In females, two-thirds of ectopic ureteral insertions are outside the urinary tract (uterus, vagina, and vestibule) and these patients are continuously wet. Both males and females may present with urinary tract infection, as ectopic ureteral insertion outside the urinary tract is often obstructive.

Most ectopic ureteroceles occur in cases of duplication, again arising from the functioning tissue left in the upper pole. Orthotopic ureteroceles, in contrast, occur most commonly in nonduplicated systems, and they may be congenital or acquired ("pseudoureterocele"). The latter is produced when a lesion in the bladder (especially TCC) causes obstruction at the ureterovesical junction and a ballooning out of ureteral mucosa into the bladder lumen.

The contrast-filled ureterocele, outlined by radiolucent mucosa, has a characteristic "cobra head" urographic appearance. Orthotopic ureteroceles are frequently bilateral.

165.   The answers are: A-N, B-Y, C-N, D-Y, E-N.   *(Amis & Newhouse, pp 108–112. Davidson, pp 299–305.)*   Autosomal dominant polycystic kidney disease, which is often called adult-type polycystic kidney disease, affects males and females with equal frequency. Though as many as half the patients with the disease will live into old age without signs or symptoms, a frequent history is the development of hypertension or renal insufficiency in the fourth or fifth decade. Those who present earlier usually have more rapidly progressive disease and ultimately go on to renal failure and require dialysis.

Though the cysts arise from the tubular epithelium, they do not communicate with the collecting system. Therefore, they do not opacify with excretory urography or with retrograde ureteropyelography. Early on, the renal parenchyma functions normally. When the cysts become large enough, they compress the tissues and renal failure develops. The cysts predispose to infection, which occurs more commonly in female patients, and *E. coli* is the most common cause.

The cyst walls sometimes calcify and hemorrhage into the cysts is not uncommon. The CT values in hemorrhagic cysts may reach as high as 100 Hounsfield units. The kidneys enlarge with progression of the disease, and the collecting system may become severely distorted, mimicking diffuse metastatic disease, especially lymphoma.

166. **The answers are: A-N, B-Y, C-Y, D-N, E-N.** *(Amis & Newhouse, pp 163–164.)* Xanthogranulomatous pyelonephritis is a condition in which a chronically obstructed and infected kidney is gradually replaced by yellow *(xantho-)* noncaseating granulomatous material. The histology shows foamy, lipid-laden macrophages in abundance. Since there is destruction of tissue, the affected portion usually has no function. The disease is commonly focal in children, but usually involves the whole kidney in adults.

Most cases are associated with gram-negative infection and an obstructing calculus, typically a staghorn. Though the process is a form of abscess or pyonephrosis, gas in the tissues is not a feature. And although the substance which replaces the kidney has a high lipid content, the CT density is greater than fat. The MR characteristically shows a low-intensity lesion on T1-weighted images, with high signal on T2-weighted images. The inflammatory process may extend outside the kidney to involve adjacent tissues, often the psoas muscle. Treatment usually requires surgical resection.

167. **The answers are: A-Y, B-N, C-Y, D-Y, E-Y.** *(Amis & Newhouse, pp 335–339.)* The male urethra is divided into four parts. The anterior half is comprised of the penile (distal) and bulbous (proximal) segments, which are delimited by the angle which forms at the penoscrotal junction. The glands of Littre typically line the dorsal (upper) aspect of the anterior urethra. They may act as traps for infection, which is why scarring and stricture formation so commonly occur in this portion of the urethra. They do not usually fill during retrograde urethrography until inflammatory dilatation occurs. When opacified, the dilated glands appear as small diverticula. The posterior urethra, which lies between the external sphincter and bladder base, is made up of the membranous (GU diaphragm) and prostatic segments.

Gonococcal urethritis is the cause of approximately 40% of male urethral strictures in the U.S. Chlamydia and mycoplasma are also frequent causes of urethritis, though stricturing is less common. Tuberculosis and schistosomiasis both may cause urethritis and stricturing, as well as fistula formation. The fistulae produced by tuberculosis, in a fashion similar to scrofula in the neck, may be so numerous as to produce the "watering can" perineum.

Urethral injuries commonly result from instrumentation. Though the lumen may be perforated anywhere along the course of the urethra, force is frequently used to pass through the external sphincter, and injuries are common in that location. However, in patients with long-term indwelling catheters, erosion and stricture formation is most common at the penoscrotal junction, where sharp angulation occurs, especially if the penis has been secured in a downward orientation.

Tumors of the urethra are rare. Malignancy is sometimes accompanied by hematuria, which clears during voiding. Most tumors are squamous cell carcinoma, and arise in the bulbous urethra. There is usually a history of chronic urethritis and strictures. Tumor spread is usually via lymphatics to the iliac and obturator lymph nodes, unlike testicular tumors which bypass local chains and track directly to the paraaortic lymph nodes.

168. The answers are: A-Y, B-Y, C-Y, D-Y, E-N. *(Amis & Newhouse, pp 219–226.)* About 90% of urinary tract calculi are visible on x-ray, in contrast to biliary tract stones, which are radioopaque in only 10–15% of cases. By ultrasound and CT, however, nearly all renal calculi are detectable. Most urinary calculi, with the exception of matrix stones which are composed of glycoprotein, have CT attenuation values of 300 Hounsfield units or more. Those which contain calcium may be many times greater.

Most urinary calculi are composed of calcium oxalate or calcium phosphate (apatite), or both. These are the most dense, and stones as small as 2 mm may be visible on x-ray. Struvite (magnesium ammonium phosphate) stones are the next dense, followed by cystine. Cystine stones are not very radiopaque, but once they reach 3 to 4 mm they are almost always visible on x-ray.

Stones which form in the bladder are also usually calcium oxalate. They frequently assume a lobular, spherical shape which is likened to a mulberry. Not infrequently, they grow into a more spiculated configuration which resemble jacks (the children's game), and are therefore called *jack-stones*. Often, a retained foreign body, such as a hair or suture from prior intervention, acts as a nidus for bladder-stone formation.

The "milk of calcium" in renal cysts or calyceal diverticula is composed of calcium carbonate. Decubitus radiographs may help distinguish this type of cyst, as the suspension should layer on an upright film, with a sharply defined upper edge. In calyceal diverticula, small stones are far more common than milk of calcium.

Uric acid stones occur commonly in patients who have undergone ileostomy or in those who are losing bicarbonate for some other reason. The urine becomes intensely acidic and the urate cannot remain in solution. Alkalinization of the urine is a method of treating these stones.

169. The answers are: A-Y, B-Y, C-N, D-Y, E-Y. *(Amis & Newhouse, pp 307–316.)* The subject of the neurogenic bladder is quite complex. It may be broken down into a more simple scheme based on the anatomic site of the lesion, which allows one to understand the mechanisms that produce the wide variety of clinical and uroradiological findings.

Two centers control micturition. The first is in the pons, and the second is located in the sacrum. The pontine center is under the control of the cerebral cortex. Cerebrovascular accidents or other central nervous system (CNS) disease, such as normal pressure hydrocephalus (NPH) or parkinsonism, may release control and result in uninhibited bladder contractions. Because the voiding process occurs as a normal sequence of reflexes, however, the urinary tract is often normal radiographically.

Should a lesion occur below the pons, but above the sacral muturition center (especially above T5), the result is discoordination between the voluntary control of the external sphincter by the CNS and the voiding reflex. This is known as bladder–external sphincter dyssynergia (DESD). The external sphincter obstructs normal emptying, and the bladder becomes thickened and trabeculated ("Xmas tree" bladder). The upper tracts suffer from high pressure or reflux. Common etiologies include multiple sclerosis, spinal cord tumors, and trauma.

The flaccid or hyporeflexive bladder occurs when the lesion involves the conus medullaris or sacral micturition center. Common causes include disk disease, diabetic neuropathy, pelvic trauma, and surgery. The bladder distends imperceptibly until intravesicle pressure builds up enough to cause overflow incontinence. Again, the upper tracts may suffer, too.

Stress incontinence has been postulated to occur because of an improper vesicourethral angle, which produces an incompetent sphincter. More recently, it has been shown that it is not the change in the angle, which typically results from sagging of the pelvic floor, as much as it is the differential pressure between the bladder the urethra, which now lies outside the confines of the pelvis. This type of stress incontinence is far more common than incontinence due to loss of sphincter tone.

170. The answers are: A-Y, B-Y, C-N, D-Y, E-N. *(Amis & Newhouse, pp 127–128.)* Reninomas, or juxtaglomerular tumors, occur most frequently in women, with a mean age of about 30. The tumors may be very small, yet hormonally active. They typically arise near the poles of the kidney in a subcapsular location. At discovery, most are 2 to 3 cm in size. There is usually an elevated plasma renin level and evidence of activation of the renin-angiotensin system; hyperaldosteronism and hypertension frequently bring the patient to attention. Surgery is curative and often provides nearly immediate relief of hypertension.

Ultrasound typically shows the mass to be echogenic, though not of the same intensity as that seen with fat or angiomyolipomas. This is felt to be due to the myriad tissue interfaces that this vascular tumor presents to the ultrasound beam. This vascularity is microscopic, however, and the tumors do not enhance particularly strongly nor does angiography show more than an occasional small feeding vessel.

171. The answers are: A-Y, B-N, C-Y, D-Y, E-Y. *(Amis & Newhouse, pp 129–135.)* Renal cell carcinoma (RCC) accounts for 85% of primary renal malignancies. Histologically, most are of the clear-cell type (80–95%). These are typically hypervascular (65–75%) and are associated with a more aggressive disease; they have a higher stage at presentation and a worse prognosis. The remainder (5–15%) are of the papillary cell type. These tend to be more indolent tumors which are hypo- or avascular by angiography and metastasize infrequently and later in the course of disease.

Only 10–20% of RCCs calcify, and the pattern is nonspecific. It may be amorphous, stippled, or curvilinear. However, 75% of calcified masses turn out to be RCC, and so calcification means malignancy until proved otherwise. RCCs also vary widely in size at the time of diagnosis. Fat detectable within the lesion by CT is felt to safely exclude the diagnosis of RCC.

CT scanning, which is always done pre- and post-contrast, is very useful for staging. Stage I (confinement within renal capsule) and Stage II (confinement within Gerota's fascia) lesions are treated by radical nephrectomy and have a combined 5-year survival of 71%. Stage III (A = spread to renal vein and IVC; B = spread to hilar nodes; C = both) and Stage IV (A = local spread, B = distant metastases) have a combined 5-year survival of 12%, and no effective treatment beyond surgery exists.

172. The answers are: A-N, B-Y, C-Y, D-N, E-N. *(Amis & Newhouse, pp 235–244. Davidson, pp 267–281.)* The causes of acute urinary tract obstruction are varied. The most common of these—blood clot and stone—usually impact at the uretero*vesicle* junction and obstruct. If the obstruction is significant, then the back pressure will be transmitted to the ureter, tubules, and ultimately the glomeruli. The result is a poorly functioning kidney with decreased concentrating ability as shown by excretory urography and CT. The nephrogram may be faint, but usually in cases of incomplete obstruction, transit is slowed so that contrast continues to accumulate, which produces a dense, delayed nephrogram that often persists for many hours.

The caliceal pressure may be so high as to cause rupture of the collecting system, which occurs most frequently at the fornices. However, for the number of cases of obstruction, this is a relatively rare event.

The calyceal rim, or crescent, sign refers to the appearance of thin slivers of contrast that appear in cases of *chronic* urinary tract obstruction. These slivers arise between the unopacified, distended calices and renal parenchyma.

"Vicarious excretion," the appearance of contrast in the gallbladder, is simply an alternate means of elimination of contrast. Although it may occur more rapidly in cases of urinary tract obstruction, it is a nonspecific finding. In fact, it is often found incidentally in patients who undergo CT scanning a day or two after excretory urography.

173. The answers are: A-N, B-Y, C-N, D-Y, E-Y. *(Davidson, pp 233–237.)* Acute tubular necrosis results from a toxic or ischemic injury to the kidney. Patients usually become oliguric a day or so later and the serum creatinine begins to rise, often reaching 5 to 10 mg/dl before the recovery phase begins a week or so later. Full resolution usually follows within 1 to 2 weeks.

Numerous nephrotoxic agents are recognized. These include radiographic contrast (especially if the patient is dehydrated), aminoglycosides (e.g., gentamicin), arsenicals, bismuth, ethylene glycol, carbon tetrachloride, bichloride of mercury, and uranium. Acute tubular necrosis (ATN) commonly occurs in hypotensive patients, following renal transplantation (more common with cadaveric as opposed to living-related donor transplants), and in cases of crush injuries, burns, severe dehydration, and transfusion reactions.

Excretory urography reveals swollen kidneys. The nephrogram phase occurs *rapidly* (as compared to obstruction) and then becomes quite dense. It also persists because contrast has leaked into the interstitium from the injured tubules. Because of poor function and obstruction of tubules by debris, the collecting system opacifies little, if at all.

The interstitial edema makes the kidney appear hypoechoic by ultrasound. Radionuclide scanning also confirms normal perfusion but diminished function.

174. The answers are: A-Y, B-Y, C-N, D-Y, E-N. *(Amis & Newhouse, pp 94–99.)* Although metastatic disease to the adrenal glands is quite common, occurring in roughly one-fourth of patients who die of their malignancy, calcification is rare. Pheochromocytomas occurring in the adrenal gland also calcify infrequently. Adrenal carcinomas, on the other hand, are often large, necrotic, and hemorrhagic; and as a result frequently develop dystrophic calcification. Adrenal adenomas, because they are more often small (and usually nonfunctioning) rarely calcify.

In neonates with meningococcemia, bilateral adrenal hemorrhage and adrenal insufficiency is known as the Waterhouse-Friderichsen syndrome. The hemorrhagic glands frequently develop a rim of calcification in sometimes as little as 2 weeks. The calcification usually persists after the hematoma has resolved. Wolman disease is a rare, fatal disorder of metabolism. There is a virtually pathognomonic pattern of stippled calcification which conforms to the triangular shape of the enlarged gland.

175. The answers are: A-Y, B-Y, C-N, D-Y, E-N. *(Amis & Newhouse, 1991, pp 273–276. Davidson, pp 483–484.)* Leukoplakia is a rare condition in which chronic infection or inflammation transforms the normal uroepithelium into keratinized squamous epithelium, which creates focal or generalized plaques that may desquamate. It is most common in the bladder, but may occur anywhere along the urinary tract. It is most common in the third to fifth decades and has no gender predilection. It is associated with stone disease in half of cases. It is felt to be linked to epidermoid carcinoma, which is present in 20% of patients at the time of diagnosis.

Radiographically, the lesions appear as plaques, or thickening, which may become confluent over large areas. Desquamated keratin may produce lacy filling defects. It does not resemble ureteritis or pyelitis cystica, which typically produces numerous small, rounded filling defects, which are sharply defined, most commonly in the proximal ureter and renal pelvis. If shed into the distal ureter, this material may obstruct and produce a pattern of renal colic, with hematuria and renal impairment mimicking stone disease.

176. The answers are: A-Y, B-Y, C-N, D-Y, E-Y. *(Amis & Newhouse, 1991, pp 213–215.)* Most urinary tract stones contain calcium, and most are also idiopathic. The remainder occur in the setting of hypercalcemia, renal tubular disorders, errors of metabolism, and a variety of other causes. Interestingly, a large percentage of patients with idiopathic stones have hypercalciuria without hypercalcemia.

A third of urinary calculi contain calcium oxalate in either monohydrate (whewellite) or dihydrate (weddellite) form. Another third contain a mixture of calcium oxalate and calcium phosphate (apatite). Brushite is calcium hydrogen phosphate and frequently is mixed with apatite. Brushite and apatite together account for 6% of urinary tract stones. Struvite, or magnesium ammonium phosphate, almost always forms in the setting of infected urine and is the only one of the choices which does not contain calcium. However, the majority of struvite-containing stones also contain apatite and are therefore *calcium* magnesium ammonium phosphate or "triple" phosphate stones.

177. **The answers are: A-N, B-N, C-N, D-N, E-Y.** *(Amis & Newhouse, pp 127–128. Davidson, pp 383–386.)* Multilocular cystic nephroma (MLCN) is a benign neoplasm which has a trimoidal age and gender distribution. It is most common in males under the age of 4 and in females between the ages of 4 and 20 and 40 to 50. It is said to occur more commonly in the lower pole of the kidney and, though usually indolent, can occasionally grow rapidly. It may rarely herniate into the renal pelvis, producing hematuria or obstruction.

Excretory urography may show enhancement of the thick septa separating the cysts, but the cysts themselves do not enhance. Occasionally, the septa may calcify. Angiographically, these tumors are generally hypo- or avascular, though the septa may contain small neovessels. The septa often appear as brightly echogenic bands on ultrasound.

There are no radiographic criteria to distinguish MLCN from a cystic renal cell carcinoma or Wilms tumor.

178. **The answers are: A-Y, B-Y, C-N, D-N, E-Y.** *(Amis & Newhouse, pp 13–14, 317–330.)* Although the prostate is described as having five anatomic lobes (an anterior, posterior, median, and two lateral lobes), MR imaging and transrectal ultrasound have revealed a zonal, rather than lobar, architecture.

The gland is roughly arranged in concentric layers of tissue which envelop the prostatic urethra. The innermost is the transitional zone, which is the smallest and the only one which completely wraps around the urethra. It is this tissue which hypertrophies in benign prostatic hypertrophy (BPH). The next layer is the central zone which, like the outermost peripheral zone, is deficient anteriorly, where the tissue is primarily fibrous. The peripheral zone is the site of origin of prostatic carcinoma and prostatitis. On T2-weighted MR images, it is distinguishable from the intermediate signal transitional and central zones because of its high signal. The peripheral zone is echogenic on ultrasound examination, and is used as the reference tissue; the transitional and central zones are therefore considered *hypo*echoic. Carcinomas are hypoechoic in 60% of cases and isoechoic (hence indistinguishable from the surrounding tissue) in the remaining cases.

Vestigial lobes of prostatic tissue may occur in nearby locations. When the tissue posterior to the bladder neck and trigone hypertrophies, it is referred to as the lobe of Albarrán. It characteristically creates a central, posterior filling defect on the bladder on a urogram. The lobe of Home is a similar rest of prostatic tissue.

179. **The answers are: A-Y, B-Y, C-N, D-Y, E-N.** *(Amis & Newhouse, pp 124–125, 141–142.)* Angiomyolipomas (AMLs) are hamartomas of the kidney and are quite common, being found in 11% of autopsies. They contain abnormal blood vessels *(angio-)*, smooth muscle cells *(myo-)* and fat *(lipo-)* in varying proportions; though all three elements are usually present. Because of the propensity of the vessels to hemorrhage, CT scanning sometimes fails to show the fat because it is volume-averaged in with blood, and the density readings are misleading. Tumors greater than 4 cm in diameter have a greater risk of bleeding, and surgical removal is considered prudent. Despite the increased vascularity, these tumors do not demonstrate AV shunting angiographically. Myriad vessels are the cause of their high echogenicity, rather than their fat content. When a solitary echogenic focus is found incidentally during an ultrasound of the kidney, confirmatory CT scanning is usually recommended when the lesion is larger than 1 cm.

AMLs occur most frequently (75%) as solitary lesions, four times more commonly in middle-aged women, and not in association with tuberous sclerosis (TS). About 5% will be multiple or bilateral, again without any link to TS. Only 20% of patients with AMLs will have TS. Conversely, though, up to 80% of patients with TS will have AMLs, which are usually numerous and bilateral. These also usually appear at a younger age and may grow.

180. The answers are: A-Y, B-N, C-N, D-N, E-Y.   *(Amis & Newhouse, pp 85–102.)*   MR imaging is very helpful in the differentiation of masses in the adrenal gland. While overlap between the lesions exists, as a general rule metastases are slightly less intense than adrenal adenomas on T1-weighted images. On T2-weighted images, however, they become much brighter. Adenomas generally have the same intensity as liver on T1- and T2-weighted images. The difficulty in differentiating between adenomas and metastases arises in cases where adenomas hemorrhage or undergo necrosis or where metastases are unusually well-differentiated and appear homogeneous. Adrenal carcinomas are typically large and unresectable at the time of diagnosis. When small, they may appear similar to adenomas and metastases.

Pheochromocytomas typically have a signal on T1-weighted images which is slightly less than liver, but they become even brighter (same intensity as water) than metastases on T2-weighted images.

Although the tissue characteristics of neuroblastoma and Wilms tumor are similar on T1- and T2-weighted images, the multiplanar capability of MRI often affords distinction between renal and adrenal processes, which is often difficult by axial imaging alone.

Musculoskeletal Radiology

DIRECTIONS: Each question below contains five suggested responses. Select the **one best** response to each question.

181. Based on the figure, which is the MOST likely diagnosis?

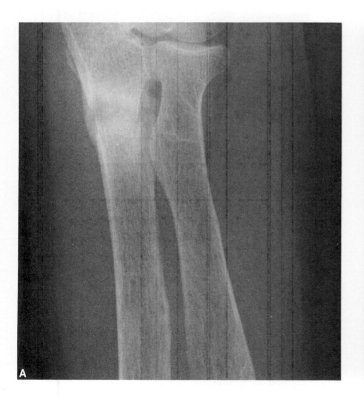 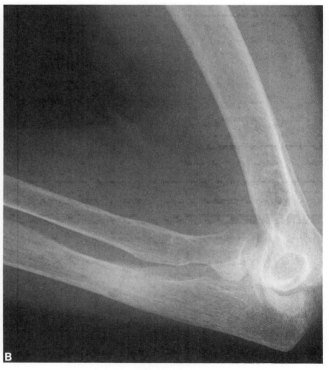

(A) Looser zone
(B) Healing Galeazzi fracture
(C) Nonunion of fracture in patient with neurofibromatosis
(D) Metastatic prostate carcinoma
(E) None of the above

182. Judging from the figure, which of the following would you say is the MOST likely diagnosis?

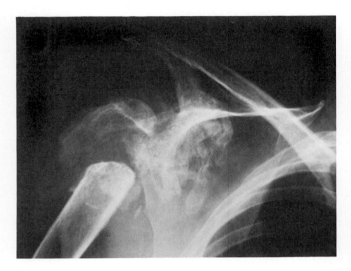

(A)   Giant cell tumor
(B)   Psoriatic arthritis
(C)   Myositis ossificans
(D)   Rheumatoid arthritis
(E)   Neuropathic arthropathy

183. ALL the following are complications of Paget disease of bone EXCEPT

(A)   neurologic impairment
(B)   "banana" fracture
(C)   malignant transformation
(D)   degenerative joint disease
(E)   vertebra plana

184. Involvement of the first carpometacarpal joint is common in ALL the following arthropathies EXCEPT

(A)   osteoarthritis
(B)   gout
(C)   scleroderma
(D)   erosive osteoarthritis
(E)   Reiter syndrome

185. A 9-year-old girl had the MR study of the knees shown in the figure. The differential diagnosis includes ALL the following EXCEPT

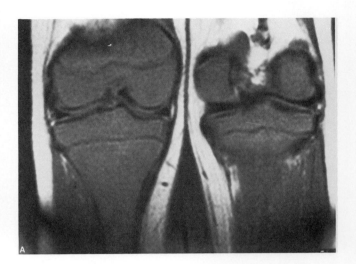

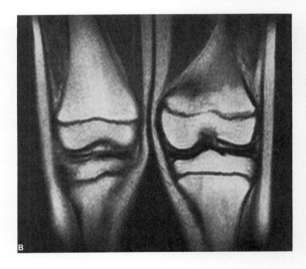

(A)   sickle cell disease
(B)   leukemia
(C)   metastatic neuroblastoma
(D)   normal variation of marrow composition
(E)   Gaucher disease

186. Based on the figure, which of the following is the MOST likely diagnosis?

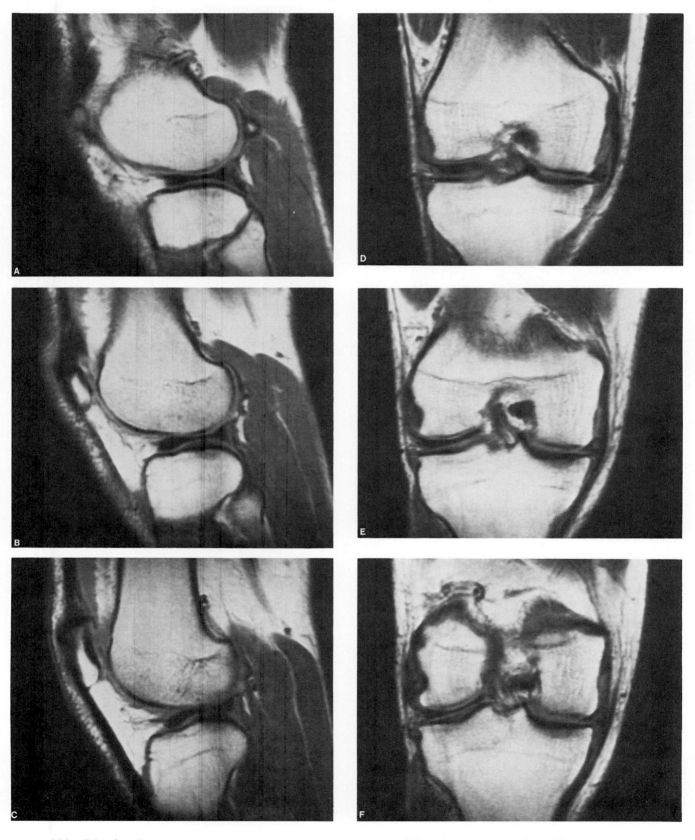

(A)   Meniscal cyst
(B)   Discoid meniscus
(C)   Meniscal tear

(D)   Anterior cruciate ligament tear
(E)   None of the above

187. In the figure ALL the following are fractured EXCEPT

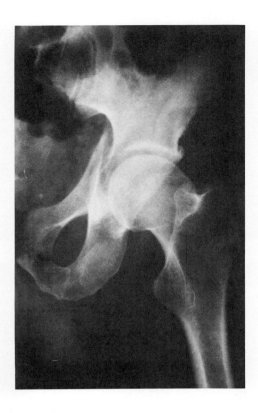

(A) acetabular roof
(B) anterior column
(C) posterior column
(D) femoral neck
(E) symphysis pubis

188. All the following are radiographic manifestations of systemic lupus erythematosus EXCEPT

(A) polyarthritis
(B) soft-tissue calcification
(C) osteonecrosis
(D) "seagull wing" erosions
(E) spontaneous tendon rupture

189. Which of the following is MOST likely to cause the wrist disease shown in the figure?

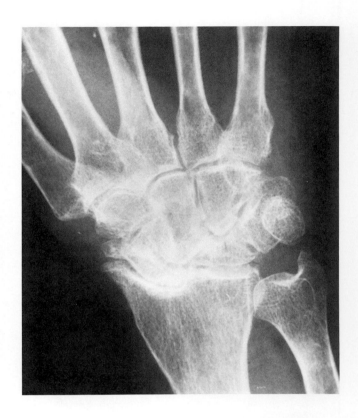

(A) Rheumatoid arthritis
(B) Gout
(C) Psoriasis
(D) Pyrophosphate arthropathy
(E) None of the above

190. All the following are examples of enthesopathies EXCEPT

(A) anklyosing spondylitis
(B) psoriasis
(C) Reiter syndrome
(D) diffuse idiopathic skeletal hyperostosis (DISH)
(E) lipoid dermatoarthritis (multicentric reticulohistiocytosis)

191. The woman in the figure complained of pain at the symphysis pubis. T1- and T2-weighted MR images were obtained (see middle and bottom figures). Which of the following is the MOST likely diagnosis?

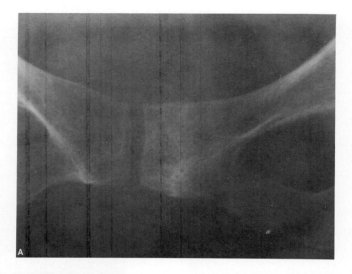

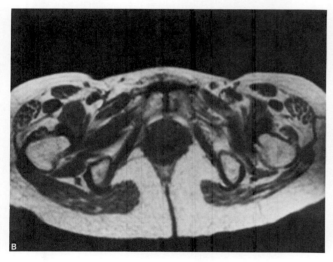

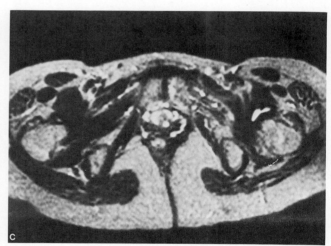

(A)   Insufficiency fracture
(B)   Osteitis condensans pubis
(C)   Fatigue fracture
(D)   Osteomyelitis
(E)   Metastatic breast carcinoma

192. A 19-year-old had the radiograph of the left hip shown in the figure. Which of the following is the MOST likely diagnosis?

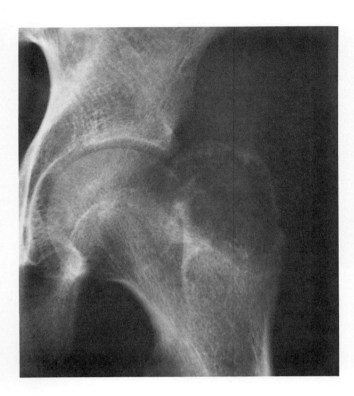

(A) Giant cell tumor
(B) Paget disease of bone
(C) Clear cell chondrosarcoma
(D) Chondroblastoma
(E) Osteoid osteoma

193. The bare area of an articulation is

(A) the intrascapular portion of a bone which articulates with an adjacent bone
(B) a cartilage-covered surface that has been denuded
(C) the site of "marginal" erosion
(D) a region of cartilage fibrillation
(E) the portion of a synovial joint which does not contact a meniscus

194. A patient with a bipolar hip prosthesis had the radiograph shown in the figure. The features are consistent with any of the following EXCEPT

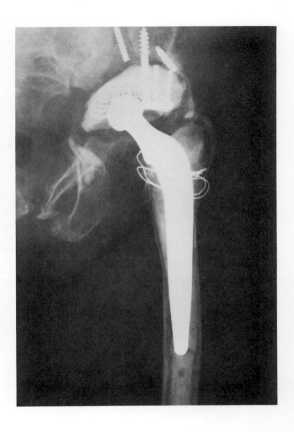

(A) loosening of the prosthesis
(B) infection
(C) osteolysis
(D) myositis ossificans
(E) stress shielding

195. A radiograph of the shoulder of a 50-year-old patient who had no history of trauma reveals joint space narrowing, subchondral sclerosis, subchondral cysts, and spurs. The MOST likely diagnosis is

(A) osteoarthritis
(B) a crystal deposition disease
(C) amyloidosis
(D) multiple myeloma
(E) multicentric reticulohistiocytosis

196. In a child, ALL the following may account for the process shown in the figure EXCEPT

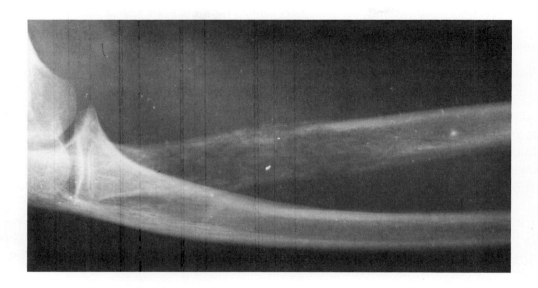

(A) Langerhans cell histiocytosis (histiocytosis X)
(B) osteomyelitis
(C) primary lymphoma of bone
(D) metastatic medulloblastoma
(E) Ewing tumor

---

197. The findings of exophthalmos, clubbing, soft-tissue swelling of the fingers and toes, and periostitis limited to the diaphysis of the tubular bones of the hands and feet BEST suits which diagnosis?

(A) Fluorosis
(B) Pachydermoperiostosis
(C) Hypertrophic osteoarthropathy
(D) Thyroid acropachy
(E) Hypervitaminosis A

198. Which ONE of the following statements regarding neoplasm-associated osteomalacia is TRUE?

(A) There is no direct relationship to the neoplasm
(B) It is related to the treatment of the lesion, and not the tumor itself
(C) There is often an underlying endocrine disorder such as one of the multiple endocrine neoplasia syndromes
(D) It occurs with either primary bone or soft-tissue tumors
(E) It is only seen in tumors of infancy and childhood

DIRECTIONS: Each group of questions below consists of lettered headings followed by a set of numbered items. For each numbered item select the **one** lettered heading with which it is **most** closely associated. Each lettered heading may be used **once, more than once,** or **not at all.**

Questions 199–201

Match the following clinical findings with the disease with which they are most closely associated.

  (A)   plasma cell myeloma
  (B)   osteoporosis circumscripta
  (C)   solitary plasmacytoma
  (D)   brown tumor
  (E)   POEMS syndrome

199. Diffuse skeletal osteopenia and Bence-Jones proteinuria

200. Sclerotic spine lesion and diabetes mellitus

201. Solitary lytic lesion and survival for 12 years without evidence of disease spread

Questions 202–204

Match the following lesions with the most likely tumor type.

  (A)   Classical osteosarcoma
  (B)   Periosteal osteosarcoma
  (C)   Parosteal osteosarcoma
  (D)   Telangiectatic osteosarcoma
  (E)   Paget sarcoma

202. A 40-year-old with a slow-growing, dense mass in the posterior distal femur

203. A 30-year-old with an aggressive lesion in the distal femur anteriorly, which has a spiculated periosteal reaction and no marrow involvement

204. A 12-year-old with a lytic, permeative pattern involving the distal femoral metaphysis. A biopsy was initially interpreted as aneurysmal bone cyst.

Questions 205–207

Match the following lesions with the MOST likely tumor type.

  (A)   Secondary chondrosarcoma (low-grade)
  (B)   Paget sarcoma
  (C)   Dedifferentiated chondrosarcoma
  (D)   Clear cell chondrosarcoma
  (E)   Soft-tissue chondrosarcoma

205. A 40-year-old is found to have a lytic, slow-growing lesion with a wide zone of transition at the proximal end of the humerus

206. A 40-year-old with a 10-cm enchondroma which has increased in size over the past year and now contains heavy "popcorn" calcifications

207. A bone lesion under treatment becomes purely lytic and grows rapidly

Questions 208–210

Match the following clinical features with the MOST likely cause.

  (A)   Gout
  (B)   Pyogenic infection
  (C)   Hemophilia
  (D)   Tuberculosis
  (E)   Rheumatoid arthritis

208. Juxtaarticular osteoporosis, relative joint space preservation, and marginal erosions

209. Subperiosteal abscess and reactive periostitis

210. Osteoporosis, dense effusion, and joint destruction

Questions 211–213

Match the following descriptions with the entity with which each is MOST commonly associated.

(A) Stress riser fracture
(B) Bennett fracture
(C) Hill-Sachs deformity
(D) Stress shielding
(E) Barton fracture

211. Anterior shoulder dislocation

212. Common, often unavoidable, complication of an internal or external fixation device

213. Occurs at the ends of an intramedullary rod or side plate

Questions 214–216

Match the following lesions with the condition with which each is MOST likely associated.

(A) Fibrous dysplasia
(B) Osteofibrous dysplasia
(C) Chondromyxoid fibroma
(D) Adamantinoma
(E) Primary lymphoma of bone

214. A 7-year-old with a well-demarcated lytic and blastic lesion in the proximal tibial cortex and an anterior bowing deformity

215. A 35-year-old with a well-demarcated lytic and blastic lesion involving the anterior one-third of the distal tibial diaphysis

216. A 25-year-old with a central lytic lesion in the midtibia

Questions 217–219

For each of the following pathologic entities, select the descriptive sign which is most closely associated.

(A) Shiny corner
(B) Bone within bone
(C) Dripping wax
(D) Blade of grass
(E) Hair on end

217. Melorrheostosis

218. Osteopetrosis

219. Ankylosing spondylitis

DIRECTIONS: Each group of questions below consists of four lettered headings followed by a set of numbered items. For each numbered item select

A	if the item is associated with	(A) **only**
B	if the item is associated with	(B) **only**
C	if the item is associated with	**both** (A) and (B)
D	if the item is associated with	**neither** (A) nor (B)

Each lettered heading may be used **once, more than once,** or **not at all.**

Questions 220–222

(A) Juvenile chronic arthritis
(B) Adult-onset rheumatoid arthritis
(C) Both
(D) Neither

220. Overtubulation of the long bones

221. Generalized osteopenia

222. Periostitis

Questions 223–225

(A) Osteoid osteoma
(B) Osteoblastoma
(C) Both
(D) Neither

223. A 22-year-old with a 3-cm lytic lesion in the proximal femoral diaphysis

224. A 22-year-old with a 1-cm lytic lesion centered in the medullary cavity of the femoral neck

225. Pain at night, relieved by aspirin

Questions 226–228

(A) Rheumatoid arthritis
(B) Osteomyelitis
(C) Both
(D) Neither

226. Sinus tracts

227. Baker cysts

228. Juxtaarticular osteopenia

DIRECTIONS: Each question below contains five suggested answers. For **each** of the **five** alternatives listed, you are to respond either YES or NO. In a given item, **all, some,** or **none of the alternatives may be correct.**

229. Regarding giant cell tumor of bone,

(A) there is generally a sclerotic rim
(B) the lesion typically involves the end of a bone
(C) it is an indolent lesion that rarely spreads locally or distantly
(D) histologically, it is sometimes indistinguishable from the brown tumor of hyperparathyroidism
(E) resection is always curative

230. Which of the following statements regarding rheumatoid arthritis (RA) are true?

(A) the boutonniere deformity is characterized by flexion of the proximal interphalangeal (PIP) joint and hyperextension of the distal interphalangeal (DIP) joint
(B) the swan neck deformity involves hyperextension of the PIP joint and flexion of the DIP joint
(C) ulnar deviation is pathognomonic for RA
(D) soft-tissue swelling often occurs over the ulnar styloid in the early stages of disease
(E) erosions of the ulnar styloid and distal ulna result from synovial hypertrophy

231. Which of the following is/are true concerning Langerhans cell histiocytosis (eosinophilic granuloma)?

(A) Focal lesions in the flat bones typically have a "beveled-edge" appearance
(B) Some cases cannot be differentiated radiographically from malignancy
(C) In the spine, the vertebral bodies are involved more frequently than the posterior elements
(D) Steroid injection into a lesion may be curative
(E) The flat bones are the most common site of involvement

232. Which of the following is/are radiographic manifestations of hyperparathyroidism?

(A) Articular erosions
(B) Subchondral erosions of the vertebral endplates
(C) Generalized osteopenia
(D) Chondrocalcinosis
(E) Subperiosteal resorption involving the medial proximal tibial metaphysis

233. Which of the following has/have been implicated as etiologic factors in the development of osteoporosis?

(A) Alcoholism
(B) Hyperthyroidism
(C) Pregnancy
(D) Intravenous heparin therapy
(E) Postmenopausal state

234. Which of the following is/are true statements concerning an aneurysmal bone cyst?

(A) It is a form of neoplasm
(B) In the long bones, the metaphysis is the most common site of origin
(C) It originates in a vertebral body more often than in the posterior vertebral arch
(D) It typically involves the long bones in an eccentric fashion
(E) Approximately 50% occur over the age of 50

235. Which of the following disorders may cause the H-shaped vertebra (of Reynold) sign?

(A) Neiman-Pick disease
(B) Gaucher disease
(C) Fibrous dysplasia
(D) Sickle cell anemia
(E) Osteopetrosis

236. Which of the following are characteristic of reflex sympathetic dystrophy syndrome?

(A) Soft-tissue swelling
(B) Marked joint space narrowing
(C) Regional osteoporosis
(D) Large intraarticular erosions
(E) Bilateral distribution

237. Which of the following is/are risk factors for the occurrence of slipped capital femoral epiphysis?

(A) Obesity
(B) Female sex
(C) Sedentary lifestyle
(D) Adolescence
(E) Postmenopausal state

238. Concerning osteonecrosis,

(A) the dead bone is structurally weaker than normal bone
(B) hyperemia is a factor in cases of collapse of the femoral head
(C) it commonly occurs idiopathically in the medial femoral condyle
(D) the "crescent" sign on an x-ray of the femoral head is an indicator of fracture
(E) increased density in an infarcted zone results from accelerated osteoblastic activity

239. The radiographic features of acromegaly include which of the following?

(A) Widened joint spaces
(B) Absence of degenerative joint disease
(C) Bone formation at tendinous and ligamentous insertions
(D) Neuropathic changes
(E) Thickened heel pad

240. Regarding ossification of the posterior longitudinal ligament,

(A) approximately 20% of cases are also found to have diffuse idiopathic skeletal hyperostosis
(B) the most commonly affected site is the cervical spine
(C) the visible thickness of the ossified ligament on plain radiographs correlates well with the severity of spinal cord symptoms
(D) the most common age at presentation is the sixth or seventh decade
(E) it is commonly associated with ankylosing spondylitis

Musculoskeletal Radiology

Answers

181. The answer is A. *(Resnick, ed. 2, pp 2096–2099.)* The figure reveals a transverse lucent line in the left proximal ulna, surrounded by sclerosis. Overall, the bones are osteopenic. This is a patient with osteomalacia and a Looser zone in the ulna. Its characteristic appearance makes the other choices (healing Galeazzi fracture, neurofibromatosis, and metastasis) unlikely.

Looser zones, also called *pseudofractures,* are lucencies that occur in osteomalacia and may, in fact, be its earliest radiographic manifestation. These lucent bands are oriented perpendicular to the bone and extend to involve a cortical surface, though they frequently do not traverse the entire width of the bone.

Looser zones are frequently bilateral and are often surrounded by sclerosis and callus formation. The weight-bearing bones, interestingly, are not commonly involved. Typical sites include the lateral edge of the scapula, ribs, proximal ulna, pubic rami, and proximal femur. Osteomalacia may be difficult to diagnose radiographically, as it may appear indistinguishable from the osteopenia of osteoporosis. Bone biopsy may ultimately be necessary.

182. The answer is E. *(Resnick, ed. 2, pp 3154–3183)* The anteroposterior radiograph of the right shoulder in the figure reveals fragmentation of the humeral head, glenoid deformity, and a sawed-off appearance of the humeral shaft. These features are typical of a neuropathic, or Charcot, joint. In this case, the patient had syringomyelia. Diabetes mellitus, leprosy, and neurosyphilis are other causes of a neuropathic joint, as are myelomeningocele, spinal cord injury, and congenital insensitivity to pain.

Loss of sensation and repetitive abnormal stresses lead to progressive destruction in a neuropathic joint. Bone and cartilage debris litter the synovium. The fragments are nourished by the synovial fluid and can grow. As they irritate the synovium, an effusion is produced, yielding a distended joint cluttered with bone debris, called *detritic synovitis.* Bone sclerosis, callus formation, and frank disorganization of the distended joint commonly result. Superimposed infection may be difficult to rule out in cases in which the bones appear unsharp.

183. The answer is E. *(Resnick, ed. 2, pp 2146–2162, 2433.)* Overgrowth of bone in patients with Paget disease may encroach upon the neural foramina and result in peripheral and cranial nerve symptoms. The middle ear structures and spinal canal may also be involved. Both stress fractures and complete fractures occur in the pagetoid bone, where bone formation is often disorganized and not modeled along lines of stress. The fractures are often transverse and called "banana" fractures. Bowing of the bones of the lower extremity and cortical stress fractures occur frequently. As the bones in Paget disease are affected diffusely, enlargement of the end of a bone may narrow the joint space and distort the articular surfaces. Degenerative joint disease, especially in the weight-bearing bones of the lower extremity, may be severe. Sarcomatous degeneration is rare. It has been estimated to occur in 1 to 5% of patients with Paget disease, though some authors feel that it occurs even less frequently.

The vertebra plana is a sign associated with histiocytosis X. Spinal involvement by Paget disease characteristically produces the densely white "ivory" vertebra, as well as the bone-within-bone appearance called the "picture frame" vertebra.

184. The answer is E. *(Resnick, ed. 2, pp 1206, 1304, 1402–1403, 1465–1466.)*   Osteoarthritis (OA) frequently involves the base of the first metacarpal bone (at the trapeziometacarpal articulation). It is probably caused by capsular and ligamentous laxity, and often occurs in the absence of a specific traumatic history. Both OA and erosive osteoarthritis have the same distribution of affected joints, which, in the hand, are the distal interphalangeal and metacarpophalangeal joints, especially at the base of the first metacarpal bone and the trapezioscaphoid articulation. Erosive osteoarthritis is distinguished from noninflammatory osteoarthritis by the presence of clinical joint inflammation, erosions, and ankylosis. In the early stages of erosive osteoarthritis, however, a radiograph cannot differentiate between the two.

The base of the first metacarpal bone at the trapeziometacarpal articulation is also a preferred site of involvement by scleroderma and gout. Extensive upper extremity involvement with Reiter arthritis is unusual, but when it occurs, the proximal interphalangeal joints are most frequently affected.

185. The answer is D. *(Moore, Radiology 175;219–233, 1990.)*   The coronal T1- and T2-weighted MR scans of the knees reveal a uniform loss of the normal fatty (bright) marrow signal on the T1-weighted images, which is more heterogeneous on the T2-weighted images. This patient had sickle cell disease, and the marrow signal reflects the conversion to red marrow, in response to the anemia.

Marrow MR signal intensity may be discordant with the microscopic evaluation. Tissues that have the MR signal of yellow (fatty) marrow may contain only 10% fat histologically. Within several months of the formation of secondary ossification centers, the MR appearance on T1-weighted images is that of fatty marrow. Homogeneously low or intermediate signal within the epiphyseal ossification centers on T1-weighted spin-echo sequences is always abnormal, but is nonspecific. Neoplasms such as leukemia, neuroblastoma, and rhabdomyosarcoma, as well as metabolic disorders, such as Gaucher disease, sickle cell anemia, polycythemia, and myelofibrosis, may all produce such an alteration.

186. The answer is B. *(Resnick, ed. 2, pp 381–393.)*   The figures aligned vertically on the left are sagittal T1-weighted images of the left knee; those on the right are coronal T1-weighted images. This patient has a discoid meniscus.

The meniscus is a fibrocartilagenous structure that is C-shaped. When cut perpendicularly, the normal meniscus has a triangular shape. A discoid meniscus contains material that partially or completely fills in the central portion of the C (see middle left and right figures). It more commonly involves the lateral meniscus. These patients are at increased risk for meniscal tears, and a discoid meniscus should be considered in all children who present with symptoms of a meniscal tear.

The function of the meniscus is to distribute the forces on the knee evenly. The rounded femoral condyle articulates with a relatively flat tibial plateau. Without a meniscus to make up the gap and provide a broad articular contact surface, the risk of osteoarthritis increases greatly.

Meniscal cysts are intrameniscal mucinous collections that mostly are located peripherally and are associated with meniscal tears. Like the discoid meniscus, they more commonly involve the lateral meniscus.

187. **The answer is D.** *(Resnick, ed. 2, pp 700–713.)* The figure reveals a complex fracture. The left acetabular roof, left anterior and posterior columns, and symphysis pubis are clearly fractured. The accompanying plain film and CT scans below are numbered to reveal the normal landmarks and the true extent of injury, respectively.

The iliopectineal line (1) marks the anterior column, and the ileoischial line (2) marks the posterior column. The roof (3) and anterior (4) and posterior (5) lips of the acetabulum are also clearly visible. The "teardrop" (6) is a guide only to the location of the quadrilateral surface (7), and is not an indicator of its integrity.

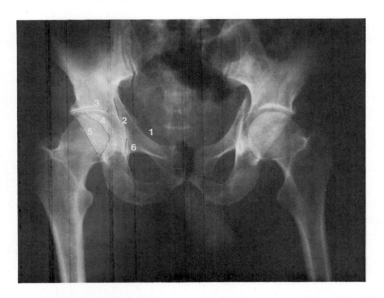

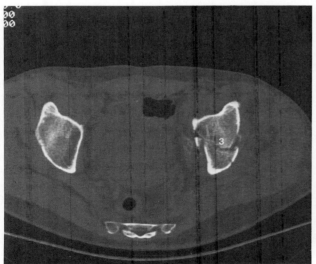
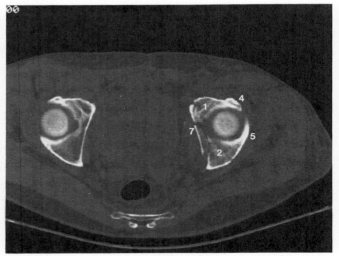

188. **The answer is D.** *(Resnick, ed. 2, pp 1268–1279.)* The arthritis in patients with systemic lupus erythematosus (SLE) is nonerosive. It is most often polyarticular, and patients may also have a polyserositis. Soft-tissue calcifications do occur in patients with SLE. Their morphology is variable, and they may appear similar to those seen in polymyositis, dermatomyositis, and scleroderma.

Osteonecrosis occurs frequently in patients with SLE. Common locations include the hip, knee, shoulder, and metacarpal heads. Confusing the issue, though, is the fact that most patients with SLE who develop osteonecrosis have been on high-dose steroids. However, osteonecrosis has also been reported in a very small number of SLE patients who have not received steroids. Spontaneous tendon rupture may also occur.

189. The answer is A. *(Chen, Radiology 177:459–461, 1990.)* The figure reveals marked narrowing and sclerosis involving the radiocarpal and captiolunate articulations. There is scapholunate dissociation, erosion of the distal radius by the scaphoid, and the capitate has collapsed onto the lunate. The proximal and distal carpal rows overlap. This is a case of scapholunate advanced collapse (SLAC). This appearance, also called the *stepladder configuration,* is typical of calcium pyrophosphate arthropathy (CPPD).

CPPD commonly affects the radiocarpal joint. Helpful plain-film findings that suggest pyrophosphate arthropathy include chondrocalcinosis of the triangular fibrocartilage complex and/or calcification of the scapholunate ligament. The knee is also commonly involved and, typically, the patellofemoral compartment is preferentially affected. The clinical presentation may mimic gout, and has been referred to as *pseudogout.* Interestingly, it, too, responds to colchicine treatment.

190. The answer is E. *(Resnick, ed. 2, pp 1111–1112, 1500–1503, 1165, 2419–2428.)* An enthesis is a tendon-to-bone or a ligament-to-bone junction. Conditions that are commonly associated with osseous proliferation at the entheses are the seronegative spondyloarthropathies, which include ankylosing spondylitis, psoriasis, Reiter syndrome, and inflammatory bowel arthropathy.

Other conditions that are also associated with proliferative changes at entheses include diffuse idiopathic skeletal hyperostosis (DISH), and fluorosis. They cause changes that may be seen throughout the skeletal system, providing a radiologic clue to the category of disease, since the seronegative spondyloarthropathies tend to have preferred sites of involvement.

Lipoid dermatoarthritis, or multicentric reticulohistiocytosis, is characterized by bilateral and symmetrical involvement, with a predilection for the interphalangeal joints of the hands and feet. There is nodular accumulation of histiocytes in the skin and viscera. The erosive changes may radiographically mimic rheumatoid arthritis (RA), but this entity has a propensity for the distal interphalangeal joints, unlike RA, and also lacks the juxtaarticular osteopenia which is characteristic of RA.

191. The answer is A. *(Resnick, ed. 2, pp 2304–2306, 2773–2785.)* The radiograph in the figure at top reveals a vertical line of sclerosis in the left half of the pubic symphysis. The MR scans more clearly show the linear nature of the defect. The area has dark signal on the T1-weighted sequence (see middle figure), which becomes high signal on the T2-weighted image (see figure at bottom). This represents a fracture. The linear nature of the lesion makes osteomyelitis and metastasis unlikely. The appearance of osteitis condensans pubis, which is a condition that affects mostly women who have borne children, is usually sclerosis involving both sides of the symphysis pubis.

In this case, the bones are diffusely osteopenic. The patient, therefore, has suffered an *insufficiency*-type fracture, wherein normal loading has exceeded the strength of inherently weak bone. Other predisposing factors to the development of insufficiency fractures include osteomalacia, Paget disease, and metastatic disease.

Fractures may also occur as the result of excessive loading of an otherwise normal bone. These are termed *fatigue* fractures. They often occur in persons undergoing vigorous exercise, such as the fractures of the second metatarsal bone ("march" fractures) that occur in new recruits during basic training.

Stress fractures, if biopsied, may be difficult to distinguish from neoplasm.

192. The answer is D. *(Resnick, ed. 2, pp 3622, 3688–3697, 3730, 3760.)* The figure demonstrates a lytic, expansile lesion in the greater trochanter of the left hip. Since the trochanter is an apophysis, this is an end-of-bone lesion. It is faintly sclerotic at the periphery, and although it is subtle, the matrix is not purely lytic but contains vague densities. This patient has a chondroblastoma.

Chondroblastoma affects mostly adolescents. Approximately 75% occur between 10 and 20 years of age, with an average age of 19. They are overwhelmingly epiphyseal and commonly originate in the proximal humerus, knee, proximal femur, hindfoot, and acetabulum.

A sclerotic rim is a common feature, as is a predominant lytic matrix. Punctate calcifications within the matrix may be present, but often cannot be seen except by CT. Aneurysmal bone cysts may arise in association, complicating the radiographic and pathologic evaluation of chondroblastoma.

Regarding the other choices, giant cell tumor may look quite similar, although the rim of sclerosis and the dense areas in the matrix make it unlikely. Osteoid osteoma favors the femoral neck when it occurs in the proximal femur. Clear cell chondrosarcoma typically affects older patients, around 40 years of age, and Paget disease is also a disease of adults.

193. **The answer is C.** *(Resnick, ed. 2, pp 638, 964.)* The bare area of an articulation is the intracapsular portion of a bone in a synovial joint where there is normally no cartilage coating the bone. In the bare area, the cortex is directly exposed to synovial fluid and to the synovium. Therefore, it is a region particularly vulnerable to the erosive changes of rheumatoid arthritis (RA) which result from synovial hypertrophy. These "marginal" erosions of RA occur predominantly at the metacarpophalangeal and proximal interphalangeal joints.

194. **The answer is D.** *(Scott, AJR 144:977–982, 1985.)* The figure reveals a bipolar left hip prosthesis. Two screws have sheared off from the acetabular component. There is a crack in the methylmethacrylate cement near the distal tip of the femoral implant, suggesting a loose femoral component. The bones are generally osteopenic, and the pubic bones are disorganized. The proximal femur, especially the calcar, has undergone significant osteolysis. This patient has suffered many of the potential complications that can occur following hip replacement; he also had a staphylococcal infection.

Normally, there may be a 2-mm (or less) band of lucency surrounding a prosthesis, which may represent a fibrous tissue layer or may be due to a Mach effect. A thickness of greater than 2 mm indicates loosening of the prosthesis, which may occur with or without infection being present.

Osteolysis may occur and cause further loosening. It often starts focally, causing endosteal resorption, but may enlarge to such a degree as to become radiographically indistinguishable from infection or neoplasm. The causes of osteolysis are uncertain and may vary, because of the various compositions and means of placement and anchoring that are in use. It may be due, in part, to stress shielding. Foreign body reaction, reactive histiocytosis to methylmethacrylate cement, and the use of prostaglandin E_2 have also been postulated as causes.

195. **The answer is B.** *(Resnick, ed. 2, pp 1408–1409.)* The findings of joint space narrowing, subchondral sclerosis, subchondral cystic changes, and spurring are radiographic manifestations of a degenerative arthritis. To deduce which type of underlying arthropathy is most likely present, one must take into acount the distribution of joints involved, the age and sex of the patient, and any relevant history.

In the absence of trauma, the shoulder joint is infrequently affected by osteoarthritis. It is often said that when osteoarthritic changes are found in the shoulder joint and there is no history of trauma, a search must be made for another cause of the arthropathy. Crystal deposition diseases, including hydroxyapatite deposition disease (HADD) and calcium pyrophosphate arthropathy (CPPD), should be primary considerations.

196. **The answer is C.** *(Resnick, ed. 2, pp 2429–2439, 3604, 3980.)* The figure shows a permeative area of destruction in the proximal radius which has a discontinuous cloak of periosteal reaction. The zone of transition is wide. This patient has Langerhans cell histiocytosis (histiocytosis X).

The lytic, permeative pattern suggests a class of lesions known as *round-cell* lesions. The differential diagnosis for a patient of this age includes Langerhans cell histiocytosis, Ewing tumor, osteomyelitis, and neuroblastoma metastasis. Myeloma is a round-cell tumor that occurs in adults. Primary lymphoma of the bone can occur at any age, but tends to be more common during the third to fifth decades.

All these tumors may behave aggressively. In fact, Langerhans cell histiocytosis and osteomyelitis may sometimes be indistinguishable radiographically from a malignancy, such as a Ewing tumor. Medulloblastoma frequently produces blastic metastases.

197. The answer is D. *(Resnick, ed. 2, pp 2205–2209.)* Thyroid acropachy is a rare disorder which occurs in patients who have been treated for thyrotoxicosis. Most cases arise several years following the onset of hyperthyroidism. The periosteal reaction involves the diaphysis of the metacarpals, metatarsals, and proximal and middle phalanges of the hands and feet. The osseous manifestations of thyroid acropachy are generally not progressive, but they do not remit with treatment. Another clinical feature is pretibial myxedema.

The other conditions listed (fluorosis, pachydermoperiostosis, hypertrophic osteoarthropathy, and hypervitaminosis A) all have a propensity for involving the long, tubular bones with periosteal reaction. Fluorosis also routinely affects the axial skeleton.

198. The answer is D. *(Resnick, ed. 2, p 1995, 2210–2111.)* Oncogenic osteomalacia is a type of osteomalacia which is thought to be caused by the humoral influence of a tumor. Possible mechanisms include inhibition of renal tubular phosphate resorption and/or interference with the hydroxylation of vitamin D at the 1-position. Low serum levels of phosphate and/or 1,25 $(OH)_2$ vitamin D (active vitamin D) have been found in some patients. Oncogenic osteomalacia has been described with many primary bone and soft-tissue tumors, including adenocarcinoma of the prostate.

199–201. The answers are: 199-A, 200-E, 201-C. *(Resnick, ed. 2, pp 2362, 2374, 2381.)* Diffuse skeletal osteopenia that is radiographically indistinguishable from osteoporosis is a recognized manifestation of multiple myeloma. Typically, though, it appears as single or multiple slow-growing lytic lesions. Some cases of untreated myeloma present with sclerotic lesions, which occur most often in patients with lambda-chain disease. Sclerosis of a lesion may also follow a fracture in the underlying area or treatment with radiation or chemotherapy. The prognosis for sclerotic myeloma is the same as that for the lytic form.

POEMS syndrome is a syndrome with chronic progressive polyneuropathy (P), organomegaly (O), endocrinopathies such as diabetes mellitus (E), M-spike proteins (M), and skin thickening and pigmentation (S). *Sclerotic* plasmacytomas, particularly involving the pelvis and spine, are the type more often associated with the POEMS syndrome. In these cases, the bone marrow usually demonstrates no plasma cell infiltration. Proliferation of bone at entheses, especially the posterior elements of the spine, sacroiliac joints, and costovertebral joints, often develops.

Most lesions that are referred to as solitary plasmacytoma are actually just the first visible focus of multiple myeloma. If followed for a sufficient period, usually within 5 years, the myeloma becomes widespread.

202–204. The answers are: 202-C, 203-B, 204-D. *(Resnick, ed. 2, pp 3648–3659, 3661–3663, 3669–3677.)* Parosteal osteosarcoma occurs between the ages of 20 and 50, with a peak incidence at age 30. Most commonly found around the knee, especially in the posterior distal femur, it is a low-grade malignancy that arises from the periosteum and has a very dense center. The tumor is usually confined to one side of the bone, but occasionally wraps around it. Imaging studies, especially MR, may be of value in differentiating parosteal and periosteal osteosarcoma, which both characteristically spare the marrow, from classical osteosarcoma which is extending out through the cortex.

Periosteal osteosarcoma has a wide range of incidence, occurring from ages 9 to 70, with a mean of 22 years. Approximately 85% of periosteal osteosarcomas arise in the femur or the tibia, and they are usually diaphyseal. The lesions are characterized by a lack of marrow involvement, a perpendicular spiculated new bone that occurs in 50% of lesions, and a lenticular, or saucer, shape. A Codman triangle of aggressive periosteal reaction may be seen with periosteal osteosarcoma, unlike parosteal osteosarcoma. Both periosteal osteosarcoma and parosteal osteosarcoma have a better prognosis than the intramedullary forms of osteosarcoma.

Telangiectatic osteosarcoma is a highly lethal form of osteosarcoma. The radiographic presentation is usually that of a lytic lesion, which may be expansile or multilocular but there may be a purely permeative pattern. Matrix mineralization is uncommon. Sites of involvement include the femur, tibia, and humerus, which are also the sites most commonly affected by conventional osteosarcoma. Diagnosis of the telangiectatic type of osteosarcoma is often difficult radiographically, due to its variable appearance. Histologically, the lesion may be confused with benign entities such as aneurysmal bone cyst, simple bone cyst with hemorrhage, or a blood clot.

Classical osteosarcoma is the most common form of osteosarcoma. About 75% occur between the ages of 15 and 25. The lesions are most often metaphyseal and have a mixed sclerotic and lytic matrix. However, a purely sclerosing form or, rarely, even a purely lytic form may be seen; in the latter case the telangiectatic form of osteosarcoma is a diagnostic consideration. "Skip" metastases can occur with osteogenic sarcoma, wherein foci arise elsewhere in the same bone or in an adjoining bone. Marrow involvement of the primary lesion differentiates this lesion from the surface, or juxtacortical, forms of osteogenic sarcoma, namely, periosteal and parosteal osteosarcoma.

205–207. The answers are: 205-D, 206-A, 207-C.   *(Resnick, ed. 2, 2148–2154, 3720–3735, 3737–3739.)*
Clear cell chondrosarcoma most commonly affects either the proximal femur or humerus and the average age is 39. It has an affinity for the end of the bone, as does giant cell tumor, chondroblastoma, and intraosseous ganglion. Most lesions are predominantly or completely lytic and periosteal reaction is uncommon. The clinical course is similar to that of a low-grade malignancy; it will recur if it is not completely removed.

Secondary (central) chondrosarcoma has features that resemble both a benign enchondroma as well as a chondrosarcoma. The secondary chondrosarcoma arises in a preexisting enchondroma and is usually not seen prior to age 20. Primary (central) chondrosarcoma has a mean age of presentation of 50, and indeed these two entities may be the same lesion, with primary (central) chondrosarcoma arising in a solitary, but undetected, enchondroma that has been completely replaced by malignant tissue.

In patients with Ollier disease (nonhereditary multiple enchondromatosis), chondrosarcoma presents at an average age of 30 to 40. The increased risk of malignancy in patients with Ollier disease can be directly attributed to the volume of dysplastic and atypical cartilage present. At sites where the volume of cartilage is small, such as a solitary enchondroma in a digit, the risk of malignant change is far less than 1%. In a large volume condition such as Ollier disease, the risk may be as high as 25%. Usually, the more differentiated the calcifications it contains (popcorn, rings, and broken rings), the lower the histologic grading of the lesion.

A dedifferentiated chondrosarcoma has the worst histologic grade and prognosis. The average age of development of this complication is 60 years, and the diagnosis should be questioned below the age of 30 if not occurring in a patient with multiple enchondromatosis. The radiographic appearance is that of a lytic, aggressive growth within or at the margin of the preexisting lesion. Histologically, it assumes some of the features of other high-grade malignancies, such as fibrosarcoma, malignant fibrous histiocyoma, and high-grade osteosarcoma.

Sarcomatous degeneration of Paget disease of bone is the most-feared complication of the disease. Regardless of the histologic type of malignancy, the prognosis is poor, with the patient's demise occurring 6 to 9 months following diagnosis. The most common form is typical osteogenic sarcoma, and the most common sites of involvement are the femur, pelvis, humerus, and tibia. Notable exceptions to the poor prognosis of Paget-associated neoplasms are the lesions that resemble giant cell tumors that occur in the facial bones and skull. Occasionally, these lesions may be multiple. Although some have likened the histology to giant cell reparative granuloma, aggressive behavior, more typical of giant cell *tumor* of bone, has been reported.

208–210. The answers are: 208-D, 209-B, 210-C.   *(Resnick, ed. 2, pp 2497–2517, 2525–2546, 2674–2685.)*
The classic radiographic appearance of tuberculous arthritis is Phemister's triad, which consists of juxtaarticular osteoporosis, gradual joint space narrowing, and peripheral erosions. In early cases, the nonspecific findings of bone demineralization and soft-tissue swelling may be all that is detectable. Tuberculous dactylitis rarely occurs beyond the age of 10. Cystic tuberculosis, also more common in children, usually involves the appendicular skeleton, and when it occurs in a digit, it causes the bone to balloon out, which is termed *spina ventosa* (*L.,* "wind-blown bone"). Single-bone involvement is most common and arises from hematogenous dissemination of the organisms. Most cases of articular tuberculosis, however, are due to spread from an adjacent osteomyelitis. This is a particularly frequent scenario at the knee.

In hematogenous osteomyelitis, elevation of the periosteum by subperiosteal abscess and the formation of an envelope of new bone is called an *involucrum*. Undermining of cortical bone by pyogenic organisms and separation of a fragment (sequestrum) is called *cortical sequestration*. These cortical sequestra may be extruded out of the bone (and the body) through sinus tracts. In infants and children, prominent involucrum and cortical sequestrum formation are common features, whereas sinus tract formation occurs most often in adult chronic osteomyelitis. Brodie abscesses occur most often in children with subacute pyogenic osteomyelitis. They are radiographically well-defined lucencies in the metaphysis that rarely involve the epiphysis.

In patients with hemophilia, soft-tissue swelling may be the only radiographic finding. The bones then become osteoporotic, and hyperemia causes overgrowth of the epiphyses by accelerated maturation, in a fashion similar to that seen in patients with juvenile chronic arthritis (formerly called JRA). Radiodense effusions and articular and subarticular erosions are followed by joint space narrowing due to cartilage degradation. Joint destruction, reminiscent of neuropathic disease, indicates advanced stage. Although, this sequence is not always followed, the radiographic signs usually underestimate the degree of joint destruction. Hemorrhage beneath the periosteum or within a bone can result in a bizarre radiographic appearance known as *hemophiliac pseudotumor.*

211–213. The answers are: 211-C, 212-D, 213-A.   *(Resnick, ed. 2, p 783–784, 2824, 2832, 2862–2864, 2876.)*   The Bennett fracture typically results from forced abduction of the thumb. The base of the first metacarpal bone is fractured, and the fracture line extends to involve the articular surface.

Mechanical stress is essential for maintaining bone mineralization and strength. When an internal fixation device is placed, the entire bone, or a portion of it, may become shielded from the mechanical stresses normally placed upon it. This results in demineralization and loss of the intrinsic mechanical strength of the bone. This concept is termed *stress shielding.*

Compared to orthopedic hardware, bone has some flexibility. When an orthopedic fixation device is placed, either in the medullary cavity (intramedullary rod) or attached to the external surface on the bone (plate), that portion becomes stiffened. On either side of the hardware, the bone maintains its normal flexibility. The result is an abrupt transition zone that is a common site of fracture, which is called a *stress riser.*

The Hill-Sachs deformity is a posterolateral defect in the humeral head that may result from anterior dislocation of the shoulder. The glenoid labrum (cartilage) or bone may also be injured, resulting in a *Bankart lesion.*

A Barton fracture, like a Colles fracture, usually results from a fall on an outstretched hand. The dorsal rim of the radius is fractured, and the fracture line extends to the articular surface.

214–216. The answers are: 214-B, 215-D, 216-A.   *(Resnick, ed. 2, pp 2469–2473, 3645-3648, 3697-3701, 3842-3845, 4057-4070.)*   Osteofibrous dysplasia (formerly called ossifying fibroma) differs from classical fibrous dysplasia in that the former has bone spicules that are rimmed by osteoblasts. In osteofibrous dysplasia, the lesions are nearly always limited to the tibia and/or fibula. Most cases occur by the age of 10 years, and the younger the age of occurrence, the more likely the chance of recurrence without massive resection. The lesion usually starts within the anterior diaphyseal cortex and expands longitudinally and may appear to have a rim of sclerosis. Anterior bowing of the involved bone is also a common feature.

Adamantinoma is a poorly understood low-grade neoplasm that occurs at an average age of 35. Most cases affect the tibia and involve the anterior middle or distal diaphysis. The lesion often appears expansile or multiloculated, with a lytic matrix which may have regions of bone sclerosis. It is distinguished from osteofibrous dysplasia mainly on the basis of age, because histologic differentiation is difficult. Adamantinoma has many features of an epithelial neoplasm.

Monostotic fibrous dysplasia accounts for 70–80% of cases of fibrous dysplasia, the remainder being of the polyostotic type. A classic smoked-filled, or ground-glass, matrix results from spicules of woven bone within the lesion. The McCune-Albright syndrome, occurring predominantly in females, is the constellation of polyostotic fibrous dysplasia, irregular cutaneous café-au-lait spots, and precocious puberty. It is associated with a variety of endocrine abnormalities that include hyperthyroidism, goiter, gigantism/acromegaly, and hypophosphatemic rickets/osteomalacia.

Chondromyxoid fibroma (CMF) is a lesion that occurs most often between the ages of 10 and 20 with 75% of cases younger than 30. Seventy-five percent of cases affect the pelvis and lower extremity, and most are metaphyseal, though occasionally some are diaphyseal. They are lytic, with trabeculations within the lesion. They are typically "bubbly," and have a sclerotic rim with a narrow zone of transition. A means of differentiating CMF from osteofibrous dysplasia and adamantinoma is the appearance of the "cortical bubbling" sign, in which a lesion that has eroded the cortex has a thin covering of periosteal new bone, resembling a bubble. This sign is nonspecific, however, and slow-growing lesions, such as aneurysmal bone cysts, may be associated with it. It may sometimes be detected only by CT scanning.

Primary lymphoma of bone is most common in the older population. It is in the class of round cell tumors, and in the past was called reticulum cell sarcoma. Nearly half occur around the knee, but the spine, pelvis, scapulae, and ribs also are common sites.

217–219. The answers are: 217-C, 218-B, 219-A. *(Resnick, ed. 2, pp 1118–1119, 1131, 1500, 3478–3482, 4089–4096.)* Melorrheostosis is a disease of unknown etiology that has a distinctive appearance which is likened to dripping candle wax. It may involve the soft tissues as well as the bones and typically maintains a dermatomal distribution.

Osteopetrosis, also known as *Albers-Schönberg disease,* or marble bone disease, is characterized by dense and lucent alternating bands in the long bones and a bone-within-bone appearance in the flat bones and spine. It is a progressive disease, and bone marrow transplant has been used successfully to treat it.

Anklyosing spondylitis, one of the seronegative spondyloarthropathies that are related to HLA-B27, is characterized by progressive syndesmophyte formation. Affected joints are painful and stiff, which is characteristically aggravated by rest. Bone erosion at the anterior surface of the vertebral bodies, along the superior and inferior edges, causes the vertebral bodies to assume a square configuration on the lateral view, which is especially prominent in the lumbar spine. "Squaring" of the vertebral bodies may be one of the first radiographic signs of ankylosing spondylitis. Healing of this region of erosion and osteitis causes the "shiny corner" sign.

Ultimately the syndesmophytes in the spine, which represent ossification of the annulus fibrosis, progress to give the "bamboo spine" appearance. Often, the ankylosis begins symmetrically in the sacroiliac joints and proceeds up the spine. The hips, shoulders, and knees may also be involved. However, progression of the disease is variable, and fewer than 20% will be significantly disabled by it.

220–222. The answers are: 220-A, 221-C, 222-A. *(Resnick, ed. 2, pp 1079–1080.)* Overtubulation of bones whether metabolic, neurologic, or arthritic in etiology, affects growing bones most prominently. Both overtubulation of the shafts of long bones and enlargement of the epiphysis are features of juvenile chronic arthritis (formerly *JRA*) and not the typical adult-onset rheumatoid arthritis. Osteoporosis is a feature of both disorders, whereas periostitis is also more commonly seen only in juvenile chronic arthritis.

223–225. The answers are: 223-B, 224-A, 225-A. *(Resnick, ed. 2, pp 3621–3645.)* Osteoid osteoma occurs most commonly between the ages of 7 and 25 years. The nidus is composed of osteoid and woven bone, and it entraps nerve fibers, which accounts for the classic symptom of pain at night, relieved by aspirin. The common sites of involvement are the femoral neck and proximal femur, distal femur, tibia, neck of the talus, posterior arch of the spine (especially near a pedicle), and the bones of the hands and feet.

In the spine, scoliosis may be triggered by the presence of osteoid osteoma and is due to muscle spasm. The lesions are usually smaller than 2 cm, with most being between 1.0 and 1.5 cm. Reactive sclerosis occurs with the intracortical type of osteoid osteoma, and treatment requires only that the nidus be removed. The sclerotic bone is not removed, except when necessary to ensure complete excision. With the intramedullary and rare intracapsular locations, no sclerosis may be present, and indeed, osteoporosis often surrounds the lesion.

Osteoblastoma is a much less common lesion than osteoid osteoma. The age range is similar. However, 40% of osteoblastomas involve the spine and sacrum, as compared to only 7% of osteoid osteomas. Long-bone involvement is 75% diaphyseal, and the rest occur in the metaphyses. They are usually larger than 2 cm. No distinctive radiographic features aid in diagnosis, since the lesion may be lytic, sclerotic, mixed, and occasionally even have an associated soft-tissue mass. Care must be taken during histologic evaluation, as the malignant variant, termed *aggressive* osteoblastoma, may be difficult to differentiate from osteosarcoma.

226–228. The answers are: 226-C, 227-A, 228-C. *(Resnick, ed. 2, pp 895–904, 925–927, 2530–2540.)* Sinus tracts do occur in patients with rheumatoid arthritis (RA). The etiologies that have been proposed include increased intraarticular pressure and a superimposed septic arthritis. Both the formation of synovial cysts (Baker cysts) and sinus tracts help reduce the elevated intraarticular pressure. Percutaneous aspiration has been cited as the most common cause of the formation of sinus tracts in joints with synovial cysts.

Juxtaarticular osteoporosis reflects a decrease in mineralization that results from hyperemia. Any inflammatory process, therefore, can cause it. It is a typical feature that accompanies the soft-tissue swelling and inflammatory synovitis of RA. In children, osteomyelitis most often involves the metaphysis because the vessels turn sharply in the metaphyses, and bacteria have a tendency to become lodged there.

229. The answers are: A-N, B-Y, C-N, D-Y, E-N. *(Resnick, ed. 2, pp 3757–3776.)* Giant cell tumor (GCT) of bone occurs between ages 20 and 40, with an average age of 32. Favored sites include the knee, distal radius, proximal humerus, sacrum, proximal femur, and distal tibia. The lesion typically contains a purely lytic matrix and has no sclerotic rim. Although, GCT characteristically involves the end of a bone, it may preferentially extend toward the diametaphysis. Histologically and radiographically, GCT may be indistinguishable from the brown tumor of hyperparathyroidism. It is a tumor which is often aggressive and unpredictable, with frequent local recurrence following excision, and even distant metastasis.

Regarding other end-of-bone lesions, an intraosseous ganglion may appear quite similar. Common locations of the latter include the medial malleolus, carpus, and hip, and it also frequently has a sclerotic rim. In young patients, especially in whom the growth plate has not fused, chondroblastoma should be considered, particularly if there is any mineralization within the matrix.

230. The answers are: A-Y, B-Y, C-N, D-Y, E-Y. *(Resnick, ed. 2, pp 965–967, 971–978.)* The boutonniere deformity and the swan neck deformity (described correctly in question 230) are common in rheumatoid arthritis (RA). Capsular distension and synovial inflammation and hyperplasia deform the normal support structures, both ligamentous and osseous, resulting in an alteration of the forces on the joint and subsequent slippage. Ulnar deviation is common in RA, but is by no means pathognomonic. Other inflammatory arthritides may cause similar joint disturbances.

The mallet (baseball) finger results from traumatic avulsion of the insertion of the extensor digitorum tendon at the dorsum of the base of the distal phalynx. This type of injury can also cause a swan neck deformity.

Erosion of the ulnar styloid in RA occurs because of synovial proliferation in the prestyloid recess (primarily at the tip of the ulnar styloid), involvement of the extensor carpi ulnaris (medial surface of distal ulna), or synovial proliferation in the distal radioulnar joint. Soft-tissue swelling is an early sign of disease.

231. The answers are: A-Y, B-Y, C-Y, D-Y, E-Y. *(Resnick, ed. 2, pp 2429–2439.)* Eosinophilic granuloma is a subtype of Langerhans cell histiocytosis (histiocytosis X). About 90% of patients present by age 15, with a mean age of 11. The flat bones are affected in 70% of cases, especially the skull, mandible and maxilla, spine, pelvis, and ribs. When the spine is affected, the vertebral body is involved most frequently, with sparing of the posterior elements and intervertebral disk space.

The radiographic appearance is variable, ranging from a simple skull lesion (soft-tissue density by CT) that has a *"beveled-edge"* appearance to a markedly destructive lesion. Sometimes the degree of periosteal reaction and soft-tissue extension is so great that it is difficult to differentiate from osteomyelitis or a Ewing tumor. In cases of solitary involvement of either the skull or the pelvis/proximal femur, the other typical locations should be carefully examined for further evidence of disease. Although, many lesions are satisfactorily treated with simple curettage or steroid injection, large, recurrent, or sensitively located lesions may require low-dose radiation and/or chemotherapy, in addition to steroids.

232. The answers are: A-Y, B-Y, C-Y, D-Y, E-Y. *(Resnick, ed. 2, pp 2219–2247.)* Among the osseous manifestations of hyperparathyroidism, subperiosteal resorption occurs commonly in the hand as well as the medial proximal tibia, humerus, the ribs (both superior and inferior edges), and the undersurface of the distal clavicle. Subperiosteal resorption may also be manifest along the rims of articulations and cause marginal erosions. When the bones are demineralized, these features may be mistaken for rheumatoid arthritis (RA). Recall in trying to differentiate between the two that RA has a propensity for the proximal interphalangeal joints and that it causes bone proliferation at entheses and narrows joint spaces.

In the knee, as well as other joints, joint space narrowing may occur following subchondral bone resorption, with collapse of the articular surface and the development of a secondary type of crystal deposition disease which complicates the radiographic appearance.

Less specific findings are intracortical, endosteal, or subchondral bone resorption. Subchondral bone loss most often occurs centrally, involving the vertebral endplates, pubic symphysis, and sacroiliac, sternoclavicular, acromioclavicular joints. The peripheral skeleton may also be affected.

233. The answers are: A-Y, B-Y, C-Y, D-Y, E-Y. *(Resnick, ed. 2, pp 2022–2081.)* Osteoporosis, along with its increased risk for fractures and their complications, is one of the most prevalent and costly diseases of bone in the modern world. The problem is a lack of normal bone mass, but otherwise normal bone architecture and composition. Osteoporosis may be focal or generalized. Senescent and postmenopausal osteoporosis are the most common forms and are still poorly understood. Other known causes include catabolic steroids, hyperthyroidism, alcoholism, plasma cell myeloma, and, less often, pregnancy, heparin therapy (greater than 15,000 units per day), hyperparathyroidism, and acromegaly.

Osteomalacia, on the other hand, is a lack of mineralization of well-developed bone. Rickets is osteomalacia prior to growth plate fusion. The etiologies of rickets and osteomalacia are varied and include dietary deficiencies; abnormalities in the absorption, metabolism, or action of vitamin D; and abnormal renal handling of phosphorus and calcium, among many others. Osteoporosis is often difficult to differentiate radiographically from osteomalacia, and a bone biopsy may be necessary. Osteopenia, the x-ray appearance of reduced bone mineral, is a nonspecific finding that occurs with a large number of disorders. A variety of noninvasive means to measure bone density is available.

234. The answers are: A-N, B-Y, C-N, D-Y, E-N. *(Resnick, ed. 2, pp 3831–3842.)* Aneurysmal bone cyst (ABC) is a nonneoplastic vascular disorder of bone that some have considered an intraosseous or periosteal vascular malformation. It is thought to arise in response to trauma or an underlying lesion within the bone. Among the bone lesions that are frequently associated with ABC are giant cell tumor, chondroblastoma, osteoblastoma, fibrous dysplasia, and telangiectatic osteosarcoma. In 50% of cases, no underlying lesion is found, and it may be because the ABC has completely replaced the underlying lesion. Eighty-five percent of patients are less than 20 years old, with cases rarely found below age 5 or above 50.

ABC occurs in both the axial and appendicular skeletons. In the long bones, 75% are metaphyseal, and when found in an end-of-bone location, a giant cell tumor or chondroblastoma is often associated. In the spine, the posterior elements are usually the primary site of involvement, though ABC may extend into the vertebral body. The lesions are expansile, eccentric, and have a lytic matrix, which gives them a blown-out appearance.

235. The answers are: A-N, B-Y, C-N, D-Y, E-N. *(Resnick, ed. 2, pp 2332, 2415.)* The H-shaped vertebra is most typical of sickle cell anemia, but may also occur in Gaucher disease and thalassemia. It is thought to be caused by ischemic necrosis and partial collapse of the central portion of the vertebral end plates. Sickle cell patients may have smoothly biconcave vertebra, which may also be seen in osteoporosis and osteomalacia. All the choices given may also produce a modeling deformity of undertubulation, termed the *Erlenmeyer flask* deformity, which is best appreciated in the distal femoral metaphyses.

236. The answers are: A-Y, B-N, C-Y, D-N, E-Y. *(Resnick, ed. 2, pp 2037–2043.)* Reflex sympathetic dystrophy syndrome (RSDS), also called *Sudeck atrophy,* has three clinical stages. *Stage 1:* Lasts 3 to 6 months and is characterized by stiffness, pain, vasomotor changes, tenderness, weakness, swelling, and hyperesthesia. *Stage 2:* The swelling and vasospasm or vasodilatation improve, but the skin atrophies and contractures appear. *Stage 3:* Tenderness and vasomotor changes resolve, but skin atrophy, hypertrichosis, hyperhidrosis, and nail changes are prominent.

Reflex sympathetic dystrophy syndrome may resolve over the course of years, but it is sometimes irreversible. It is a bilateral process, although involvement of one side is often more prominent. The above stages are not always distinct. The entire extremity distal to the region of injury is usually involved, though the radiographic changes on the contralateral side may be patchy. Rapid, severe bone demineralization occurs most markedly at the juxtacortical areas, along with swelling of the soft tissues. Joint space narrowing and intraarticular erosions, however, are not a feature of this disorder.

237. The answers are: A-Y, B-N, C-N, D-Y, E-N. *(Resnick, ed. 2, pp 2962–2965.)* Slipped capital femoral epiphysis is an entity that affects males more often than females and blacks more often than whites. The mean age is 13 to 14 years of age in males and 11 to 12 years of age in females, with a range of 10 to 17 in males and 8 to 15 in females.

Overweight and physically active adolescents are at increased risk. The adolescent growth spurt has been identified as the period of greatest risk, hence the coincidence in the age ranges with puberty. Approximately 20–25% of patients, mostly girls, have bilateral involvement. An underlying disorder or traumatic cause should be sought when the diagnosis is made in an infant or young child. The most common direction of slippage is for the femoral head to slip posteriorly, medially, and inferiorly with respect to the femoral shaft. Complications include severe deformity of the femoral neck and varus angulation, with osteonecrosis and osteoarthritis occurring as longer-term complications.

238. **The answers are: A-N, B-Y, C-Y, D-Y, E-N.** *(Resnick, ed. 2, pp 3203–3234.)* The natural history of osteonecrosis at an articular surface of bone (avascular necrosis) is similar to an intramedullary bone infarction. Initially, hyperemia of the surrounding viable tissues causes local demineralization which spares the dead bone. This results in the misleading radiographic appearance of increased density in the infarcted area ("snow cap" sign). In fact, the bone mineral density at the center of the infarcted area has not changed.

Surrounding the region of infarct, a rim of osteoclasts forms that begin to resorb the dead bone, and areas of new bone begin to form peripherally. By this mechanism, the body tries to recover the region of dead bone by slowly resorbing the dead bone and introducing a vascular supply by depositing new viable bone, which may later be remodeled along lines of stress. This reparative process, known as *creeping substitution* or *creeping apposition,* occurs at a variable rate in different individuals.

Following an infarct, the dead bone loses none of its mechanical strength. However, during the process of remodeling, the bone is weaker and fracture may occur, which produces the "crescent" sign. This loss of support for the cartilage surface may then lead to buckling and collapse of the articular surface and the development of osteoarthritis.

239. **The answers are: A-Y, B-N, C-Y, D-N, E-Y.** *(Resnick, ed. 2, p 2172–2195.)* Acromegaly is caused by an increased level of growth hormone which causes chondrocyte proliferation and hypertrophy of hyaline cartilage and fibrocartilage. As a result, the joint spaces appear widened radiographically. The hyaline cartilage may fissure and denude, with degenerative joint disease following in some cases.

The enthesis is the site of muscular and ligamentous attachment to bone. In acromegaly, the fibrocartilage there similarly hypertrophies. It then undergoes calcification and ossification, producing osteophytes and calcinosis. The soft tissues are also affected. The facial features become coarsened and the heel-pad thickens. Neuropathic joint changes are not a feature of acromegaly.

240. **The answers are: A-Y, B-Y, C-Y, D-Y, E-N.** *(Resnick, ed. 2, pp 1593, 1603–1611.)* Ossification of the posterior longitudinal ligament (OPLL) usually presents in patients between the ages of 50 and 60. The cervical spine is the most commonly affected region, with C3 to C5 being the usual site. People with OPLL may be asymptomatic, or may have a variety of motor and/or sensory symptoms. The thickness of the ossified posterior longitudinal ligament seen on radiographic exams is significant, and spinal cord signs arise once the ossification fills 60% of the sagittal diameter of the spinal canal. OPLL occurs in 50% of patients with diffuse idiopathic skeletal hyperostosis (DISH), and 20% of people with OPLL also have DISH.

Neuroradiology

DIRECTIONS: Each question below contains five suggested responses. Select the **one best** response to each question.

241. The 5-year-old boy whose MR scan is shown in the figure, was first seen by a dermatologist for evaluation of skin lesions. The MOST likely diagnosis is

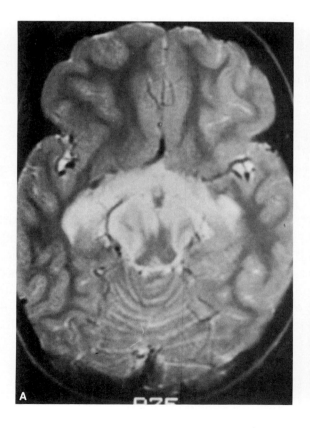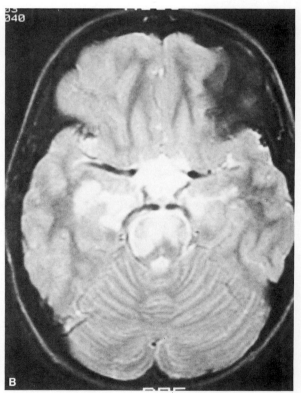

(reprinted with permission AJR, 1992)

    (A)   von Hippel-Lindau disease
    (B)   neurofibromatosis type 1
    (C)   neurofibromatosis type 2
    (D)   Sturge-Weber disease
    (E)   tuberous sclerosis

242. A 47-year-old man spontaneously developed dissociated sensory loss and vomiting. An emergent MR was obtained and is shown in the figure. The abnormality is in the territory supplied by the

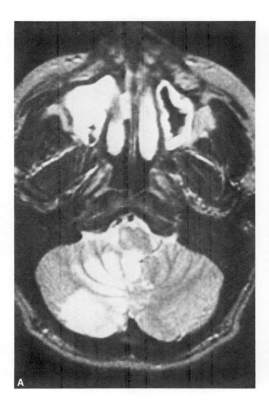 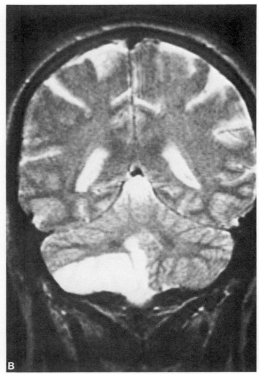

(reprinted with permission AJR, 1992)

(A)   occipital artery
(B)   basilar artery
(C)   anterior inferior cerebellar artery
(D)   posterior inferior cerebellar artery
(E)   superior cerebellar artery

---

243. All the following have a short T1 relaxation time EXCEPT

(A)   posterior pituitary gland
(B)   lipoma of corpus callosum
(C)   melanotic melanoma metastasis
(D)   arachnoid cyst
(E)   craniopharyngioma cyst

244. MR is usually superior to myelography in the detection of all the following EXCEPT

(A)   arachnoiditis
(B)   astrocytoma
(C)   tonsillar ectopia
(D)   herpes myelitis
(E)   multiple sclerosis

245. Herpes encephalitis is typically associated with all the following EXCEPT

(A)   involvement of the globus pallidus
(B)   gyral enhancement
(C)   prolonged T1 and T2 relaxation times in the medial temporal lobes
(D)   involvement of the insular cortex
(E)   small foci of hemorrhage

246. A 30-year-old man presented to the emergency room with a seizure. After stabilization, the contrast-enhanced CT scan shown in the figure was obtained. The MOST likely diagnosis is

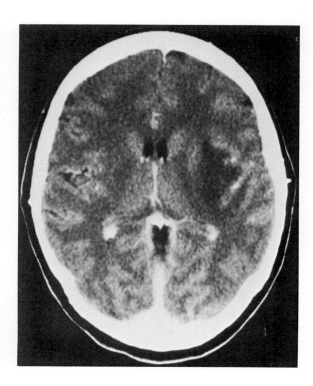

(A) astrocytoma
(B) infarction
(C) herpes encephalitis
(D) toxoplasmosis
(E) lymphoma

247. All the following statements regarding thyroglossal duct cysts are true EXCEPT

(A) the cyst wall is lined by squamous epithelium
(B) 80% of cysts occur in a suprahyoid location
(C) they occur along the midline or just off the midline
(D) the majority arise in patients under 30 years of age
(E) they lie adjacent to strap muscles

248. Based on the T1-weighted sagittal MR scan in the figure, the MOST likely diagnosis is

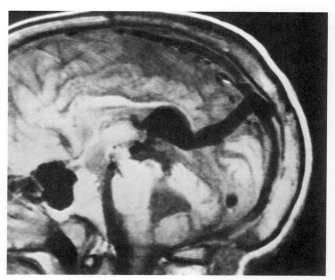

(reprinted with permission AJR, 1992)

(A) corpus callosum lipoma
(B) giant posterior inferior cerebellar artery (PICA) aneurysm
(C) cavernous angioma
(D) sagittal sinus thrombosis
(E) vein of Galen malformation

249. All the following are associated with Chiari II malformations EXCEPT

(A) stenogyria
(B) tectal beaking
(C) interdigitating gyri
(D) lückenschädel skull
(E) heterotopic gray matter

250. All the following neoplasms are associated with subarachnoid metastases in the lumbar subarachnoid space EXCEPT

(A) germinoma
(B) acoustic schwannoma
(C) glioblastoma multiforme
(D) medulloblastoma
(E) choroid plexus papilloma

251. The 6-year-old boy in the figure complained of headaches for 3 weeks. A physical examination revealed papilledema. The MOST likely diagnosis is

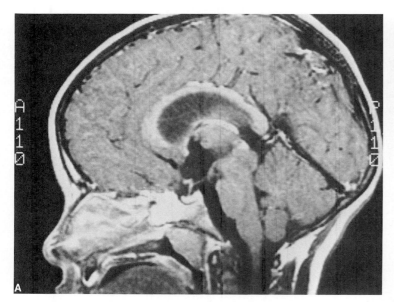

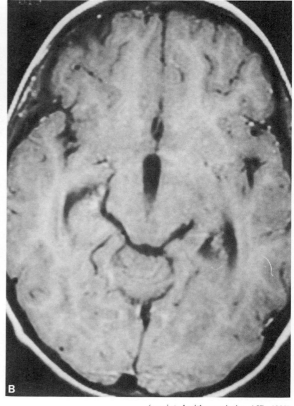

(reprinted with permission AJR, 1992)

(A) incisural meningioma
(B) germinoma
(C) hemangioblastoma
(D) brainstem glioma
(E) ependymoma

252. Important components of the ostiomeatal unit include all the following EXCEPT

(A) infundibulum
(B) uncinate process
(C) inferior turbinate
(D) hiatus semilunaris
(E) ethmoid bulla

253. A 30-year-old man develops a parenchymal hematoma in the left parietal lobe. The LEAST likely cause is

(A) amyloid angiopathy
(B) arteriovenous malformation
(C) cocaine use
(D) metastatic melanoma
(E) mycotic aneurysm

254. Judging from the contrast-enhanced CT scan in the figure, what would you say is the MOST likely diagnosis?

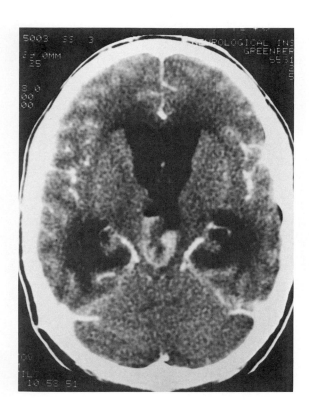

    (A)   Pineoblastoma
    (B)   Colloid cyst
    (C)   Giant cell astrocytoma
    (D)   Epidermoid
    (E)   Hemangioblastoma

255. All the following statements regarding the great vessels and their branches are true EXCEPT

    (A)   the right vertebral artery is usually dominant
    (B)   the left vertebral artery arises directly from the aorta approximately 5% of the time
    (C)   a "bovine arch" is encountered in approximately 10% of cases
    (D)   as it ascends, the vertebral artery enters the foramen transversarium of C6 in over 90% of cases
    (E)   the incidence of aberrant right subclavian artery is approximately 1%

256. A prenatal ultrasound performed on the neonate in this case revealed a cystic intracranial lesion. The T1-weighted MR image shown in the figure was obtained shortly after birth. The MOST likely diagnosis is

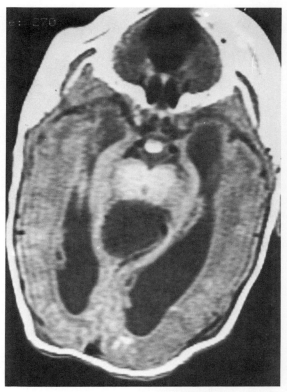

(reprinted with permission AJR, 1992)

    (A)   Dandy-Walker cyst
    (B)   mega cisterna magna
    (C)   arachnoid cyst
    (D)   cystic craniopharyngioma
    (E)   Rathke cleft cyst

257. The signal-to-noise ratio (SNR) of an MR scan is increased by all the following EXCEPT

    (A)   an increase in the number of averages
    (B)   an increase in the slice thickness
    (C)   an increase in the matrix size
    (D)   a decrease in the TE
    (E)   an increase in the field-of-view

253. A 62-year-old man had a long history of a draining left ear. He recently noticed pain and swelling behind the left ear, and the CT and MR scans shown at left and right, respectively, in the figure were obtained. The MOST likely diagnosis is

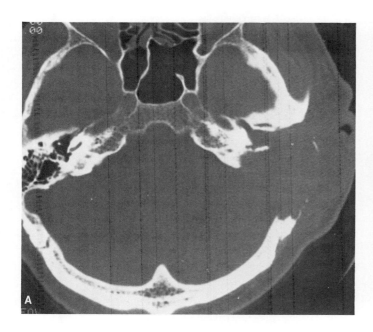
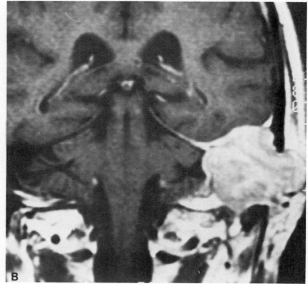

(reprinted with permission AJR, 1992)

(A) cholesteatoma
(B) cholesterol granuloma
(C) glomus jugulare
(D) squamous cell carcinoma
(E) chordoma

259. All the following statements concerning magnetic resonance angiography are true EXCEPT

(A) a significant drawback to phase contrast imaging is the long acquisition time
(B) time-of-flight imaging exploits the inflow of fully magnetized blood into saturated stationary tissue
(C) materials with short T1 relaxation times, such as methemoglobin, may simulate flow on phase contrast studies
(D) phase contrast techniques employ bipolar pulse sequences to detect the phase shift caused by moving blood through a magnetic field gradient
(E) aliasing is an artifact that is encountered only with phase contrast imaging and does not affect time-of-flight phenomena

260. Judging from the spinal MR scans in the figure, which ONE of the following would you say is the MOST likely diagnosis?

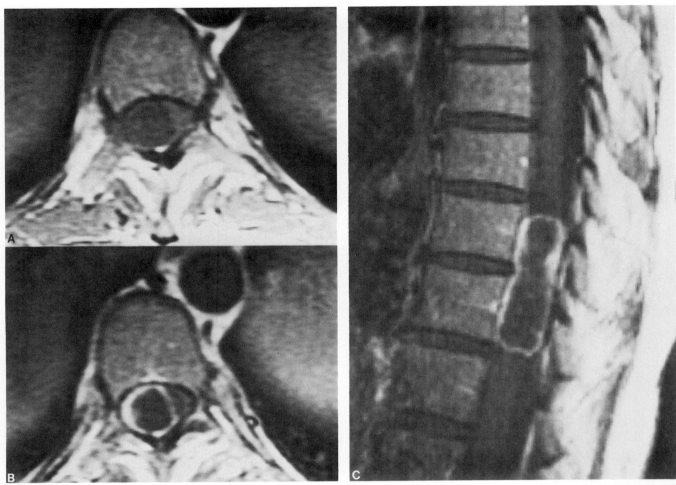

(reprinted with permission AJR, 1992)

(A)   Astrocytoma
(B)   Ependymoma
(C)   Arachnoid cyst
(D)   Schwannoma
(E)   Epidural abscess

261. Based on the pre- and post-contrast T1-weighted MR images of the lumbar spine shown in the figure, the LEAST likely diagnosis is

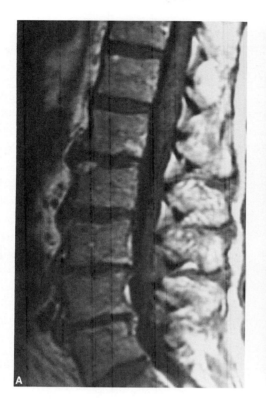 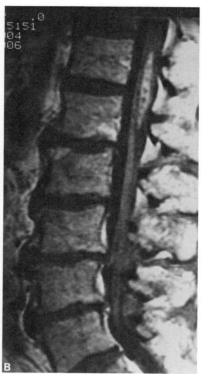

(reprinted with permission AJNR, 1992)

(A) spinal cord infarction
(B) transverse myelitis
(C) myxopapillary ependymoma
(D) meningioma
(E) metastatic melanoma

DIRECTIONS: Each question below contains five suggested answers. For **each** of the **five** alternatives listed, you are to respond either YES or NO. In a given item, **all, some,** or **none of the alternatives may be correct.**

262. True statements about truncation artifacts include which of the following?

(A) Images of the cervical spine are commonly affected
(B) The artifacts appear in the phase-encoded direction
(C) They can be minimized by decreasing pixel size
(D) They are a form of aliasing
(E) High-contrast tissue interfaces become difficult to evaluate

263. Branches of the supraclinoid internal carotid artery include which of the following?

(A) Posterior choroidal artery
(B) Inferolateral trunk
(C) Ophthalmic artery
(D) Anterior communicating artery
(E) Medial tentorial artery

264. Persistent embryonic anastomoses between the carotid and vertebrobasilar circulations which may be seen in the adult include the

(A) artery of Huebner
(B) hypoglossal artery
(C) otic artery
(D) occipital artery
(E) trigeminal artery

265. TRUE statements regarding congenital (berry) aneurysms include which of the following?

(A) Approximately 25% arise in the posterior fossa
(B) There is an associated increased incidence in patients with autosomal dominant polycystic kidney disease
(C) A giant aneurysm is defined as having a size which exceeds 2.5 cm
(D) Twenty percent or more are multiple
(E) Aneurysms of the posterior communicating artery typically cause a pupillary-sparing third-nerve palsy

266. True statements about white matter disease include which of the following?

(A) The brachium pontis is commonly involved in multiple sclerosis
(B) Central pontine myelinolysis occurs most commonly because of rapid correction of hyperkalemia
(C) Chronic multiple sclerosis plaques have a long T1 relaxation time
(D) Acute disseminated encephalomyelitis is most commonly associated with the measles
(E) Periventricular multiple sclerosis plaques are best detected on proton density images

267. Regarding brain lesions in HIV-infected patients,

(A) progressive multifocal leukoencephalopathy (PML) is typically symmetrical and periventricular
(B) tuberculosis is associated with the formation of gelatinous pseudocysts
(C) cryptococcal infection follows the path of the Virchow-Robin spaces
(D) metastatic deposits of Kaposi sarcoma in the brain occur more commonly than primary CNS lymphoma
(E) the causative agent in PML is thought to be a virus of the herpes family

268. True statements about pituitary tumors include which of the following?

(A) Prolactinoma is the most common hormonally active adenoma
(B) T2-weighted scans are best for detecting microadenomas
(C) Microadenomas are, by definition, less than 5 mm in diameter
(D) Lateral displacement of the carotid artery is diagnostic of invasion of the cavernous sinus
(E) Some adenomas have hyperintense foci which represent cystic collections of old hemorrhage

269. True statements regarding cerebrovascular disease include which of the following?

   (A) Septum pellucidum hemorrhage is typically associated with basilar tip aneurysms
   (B) The moya-moya vascular pattern develops in the setting of common carotid artery occlusion
   (C) Asparaginase treatments can precipitate intracranial hemorrhage
   (D) Amphetamine use is associated with cerebral vasculitis
   (E) The superior ophthalmic vein becomes dilated in cases of carotid-cavernous fistula

270. Correct statements regarding the characteristics of supratentorial intraaxial tumors include which of the following?

   (A) Ring enhancement is common in AIDS-related lymphoma
   (B) Glioblastoma multiforme often has areas of hemorrhage
   (C) Calcification is common in lymphoma
   (D) Gangliogliomas frequently have cystic components
   (E) Oligodendrogliomas usually have areas of calcification

271. Structures which normally enhance on T1-weighted MR scans following gadolinium administration include the

   (A) anterior commissure
   (B) infundibulum
   (C) choroid plexus
   (D) pineal gland
   (E) filum terminale

272. True statements about traumatic injury to the brain include which of the following?

   (A) T1-weighted MR scanning is the imaging method of choice for detecting subarachnoid hemorrhage
   (B) Shear injuries frequently affect the corpus callosum and gray-white junction
   (C) Longitudinal fractures of the temporal bone most often cause a sensorineural hearing loss
   (D) Epidural hematomas have a convex medial border
   (E) Traumatic subdural hematomas in infants are bilateral in approximately 80% of cases

273. TRUE statements concerning cerebellopontine (CP) angle lesions include which of the following?

   (A) Epidermoids show homogeneous enhancement
   (B) Meningiomas calcify more frequently than acoustic schwannomas
   (C) The cerebellar nodulus may mimic a CP angle mass
   (D) Acoustic schwannomas typically form an acute angle at the interface with the adjacent temporal bone
   (E) Bilateral acoustic schwannomas are diagnostic of neurofibromatosis type 1 (NF1)

274. Regarding diseases of the white matter,

   (A) in Leigh disease, the temporal lobes are most severely affected
   (B) the frontal areas are involved first in Alexander disease
   (C) microcephaly is a feature of Canavan disease
   (D) the occipital white matter is affected first in X-linked adrenal leukodystrophy
   (E) periventricular leukomalacia (PVL) most severely affects the periatrial white matter

275. Regarding congenital anomalies, which of the following are TRUE statements?

(A) The cortical layer is thickened in agyria

(B) Schizencephaly features white-matter-lined clefts which extend from the lateral ventricles to the inner table of the skull

(C) In alobar holoprosencephaly, the thalami are fused

(D) The falx cerebri is present in hydranencephaly

(E) Dysgenesis of the corpus callosum occurs in 60% of patients with the Dandy-Walker malformation.

276. TRUE statements regarding the phakomatoses include which of the following?

(A) Supratentorial hemangioblastoma is the most common brain tumor in patients with von Hippel-Lindau disease

(B) The most common CNS manifestation of Sturge-Weber disease is periventricular calcification around the occipital horns

(C) The giant cell astrocytomas which arise in patients with tuberous sclerosis occur most commonly at the foramen of Monro

(D) Eighty percent of patients with lateral thoracic meningoceles have neurofibromatosis

(E) Antoni type A histology is typical of the plexiform neurofibromas found in neurofibromatosis

277. TRUE statements about brain tumors in children include which of the following?

(A) Calcification is more frequent in ependymoma than in medulloblastoma

(B) The classic presentation of brainstem glioma is hydrocephalus

(C) Thirty percent of craniopharyngiomas have calcification visible on CT

(D) Choroid plexus papilloma most frequently occurs in the fourth ventricle

(E) Extension through the foramen of Magendie is typical of pilocytic cerebellar astrocytoma

278. Regarding degenerative spine disease,

(A) far lateral disk herniations are best detected with myelography

(B) degenerated intervertebral disks have a long T2

(C) an L4-L5 far lateral disk herniation causes an L5 radiculopathy

(D) type 1 endplate changes have a short T1 and a short T2

(E) synovial cysts are most common in the cervical spine

279. Regarding infections of the spine,

(A) the most common pathogen in epidural abscesses is *Staphylococcus aureus*

(B) tuberculosis typically spreads along the anterior longitudinal ligament

(C) in diskitis, the disk becomes hypointense on T2-weighted MR images

(D) the arterial route is the most common path of infection in osteomyelitis

(E) diskitis more commonly occurs in the lumbar spine

280. Regarding primary tumors of the spinal column, which of the following is (are) TRUE?

(A) Osteoid osteomas occur most frequently in the lumbar spine

(B) Osteoblastoma most frequently involves the posterior elements

(C) Giant cell tumors arise most commonly in the sacrum

(D) The clivus is the most common location of chordomas

(E) Aneurysmal bone cysts favor the posterior elements

281. TRUE statements about orbital lesions include which of the following?

(A) Grave disease is more likely to involve the tendinous extraocular muscle insertions than is orbital pseudotumor

(B) Dacrocystitis refers to inflammation of the lacrimal glands

(C) Tram-track calcification is characteristic of optic nerve gliomas

(D) Dermoids most often occur in the intraconal space

(E) Retinoblastoma is bilateral in about 30% of cases

282. TRUE statements regarding the masticator space include which of the following?

(A) Chondrosarcomas arise typically from the temporomandibular joint

(B) The superior alveolar nerve is the principal sensory branch of the masticator space

(C) Masses displace the parapharyngeal space posteriorly

(D) The temporalis muscle inserts on the coronoid process of the mandible

(E) Injury or involvement by malignant tumor of CN V_2 results in motor atrophy and diminished masticator space volume

283. Regarding temporal bone lesions,

(A) pars flaccida cholesteatomas involve Prussak's space

(B) cholesterol granuloma is hyperintense on T1- and T2-weighted MR images

(C) the principal organism involved in malignant otitis externa is *Pseudomonas aeruginosa*

(D) primary cholesteatoma of the middle ear arises most commonly in the epitympanum

(E) pulsatile tinnitus is best evaluated by MR imaging

284. Regarding lesions of the salivary glands,

(A) Warthin tumors are bilateral in 60% of cases

(B) mucoepidermoid carcinomas are most likely to show perineural spread

(C) pleomorphic adenomas are hyperintense on T2-weighted MR images

(D) lymphangiomas are the most common salivary gland tumors in children

(E) ranulas most commonly involve the sublingual salivary glands

285. The pterygopalatine fossa communicates with the

(A) infratemporal fossa via the pterygomaxillary fissure

(B) oral cavity via the pterygopalatine canal

(C) orbit via the superior orbital fissure

(D) middle cranial fossa via the foramen ovale

(E) inferior meatus of the nasal cavity via the sphenopalatine foramen

DIRECTIONS: Each group of questions below consists of lettered headings followed by a set of numbered items. For each numbered item select the **one** lettered heading with which it is **most** closely associated. Each lettered heading may be used **once, more than once,** or **not at all.**

Questions 286–288

Match the following clinical findings with the disease with which they are most closely associated.

  (A) Chordoma
  (B) Acoustic schwannoma
  (C) Cholesteatoma
  (D) Petrous apicitis
  (E) Glomus tympanicum

286.   Pulsatile tinnitus

287.   Retrocochlear hearing loss

288.   Gradenigo syndrome

DIRECTIONS: Each group of questions below consists of four lettered headings followed by a set of numbered items. For each numbered item select

A	if the item is associated with	(A) **only**
B	if the item is associated with	(B) **only**
C	if the item is associated with	**both** (A) and (B)
D	if the item is associated with	**neither** (A) nor (B)

Each lettered heading may be used **once, more than once,** or **not at all.**

Questions 289, 290

(A) Myxopapillary ependymoma
(B) Fibrolipoma
(C) Both
(D) Neither

289. Filum terminale

290. Aqueduct of Sylvius

Questions 291, 292

(A) Hemangioblastoma
(B) Glomus tympanicum
(C) Both
(D) Neither

291. Flow voids on MR

292. Enlarged ascending pharnygeal artery

Questions 293, 294

(A) Neurofibromatosis
(B) Marfan syndrome
(C) Both
(D) Neither

293. Dural ectasia

294. Optic nerve glioma

Questions 295, 296

(A) Cervical hemangioblastoma
(B) Chiari I malformation
(C) Both
(D) Neither

295. Holocord syrinx or cyst

296. Tectal "beaking"

Questions 297, 298

(A) Dentate gyrus
(B) Choroid fissure
(C) Both
(D) Neither

297. Temporal lobe

298. Cerebellum

Questions 299, 300

(A) Pineal region
(B) Suprasellar region
(C) Both
(D) Neither

299. Germinoma

300. Craniopharyngioma

Neuroradiology

Answers

241. The answer is B. *(Atlas, pp 539–566.)* The axial T2-weighted MR images in the figure show extensive, abnormal hyperintensity in the optic chiasm, optic tracts, and optic radiations bilaterally, which is virtually diagnostic of neurofibromatosis type 1. This appearance usually represents a very low grade neoplastic (astrocytic) process. Enhancement following gadolinium administration does not typically occur. This patient also has abnormal hyperintensity in the brainstem, demonstrating that individuals with neurofibromatosis type 1 often have other areas of involvement in the brain parenchyma. The precise histologic correlate of the lesions outside the optic pathways is not always certain.

242. The answer is D. *(Atlas, pp 411–437.)* The axial and coronal T2-weighted images in the figure show a typical posterior inferior cerebellar artery (PICA) territory infarction. There is a large, well-demarcated area of high signal in the cerebellum inferiorly, indicating cytotoxic edema, as well as involvement of the right lateral medulla. Occlusion of the PICA may result in the lateral medullary syndrome of Wallenberg, which includes ipsilateral facial analgesia, ipsilateral Horner syndrome, contralateral analgesia, and contralateral hemiparesis.

The signal voids in both vertebral arteries attest to their patency. The occipital artery is an extracranial branch of the external carotid artery, and its occlusion would not ordinarily affect intracranial structures.

243. The answer is D. *(Atlas, pp 23–38, 626–627.)* Fatty tissue (corpus callosum lipoma), proteinaceous fluid (craniopharyngioma cyst), melanin (melanotic melanoma metastasis), and methemoglobin are bright on T1-weighted MR images by virtue of their short T1 relaxation times. The cause of the posterior pituitary "bright spot" remains a controversial topic. The phospholipid vesicles which transport the releasing factors from the hypothalamus to the posterior pituitary gland may play a role.

Arachnoid cysts usually behave similarly to cerebrospinal fluid (CSF) on all pulse sequences. Their T1 and T2 relaxation times are long, making them dark on T1-weighted images and bright on T2-weighted images.

244. The answer is A. *(Atlas, pp 980–982. Banna, pp 277–278.)* MR imaging provides unparalleled sensitivity in the detection of intramedullary spinal cord abnormalities such as neoplasm (astrocytoma), infection (herpes myelitis), and demyelination (multiple sclerosis). Nonexpanding intramedullary spinal cord lesions may be difficult or impossible to detect with myelography, even if combined with CT scanning directly following intrathecal injection of contrast. Tonsillar ectopia, the caudal extension of the cerebellar tonsils beneath the foramen magnum, is best evaluated with sagittal MR imaging, where the precise margins of the foramen magnum are readily visible. Not only is the slightest degree of tonsillar ectopia recognizable, but the morphology of the cerebellar tonsils and the inferior fourth ventricle is also detailed.

Although arachnoiditis may sometimes be diagnosed by MR imaging, myelography, especially in combination with postmyelography CT scanning, remains the best means of identifying and characterizing the extent of disease. This is particularly true of mild arachnoiditis, when subtle root thickening or a "sleeveless" nerve root is the only clue to the presence of disease.

245. The answer is A. *(Atlas, pp 502–504.)* The herpes simplex virus is the most common cause of nonepidemic fatal encephalitis in the United States. The illness is characterized by extensive and asymmetrical hemorrhagic necrosis of the temporal and frontal lobes. The insular cortex is also frequently involved.

Because the basal ganglia (caudate, putamen, and globus pallidus) are usually spared, cross-sectional images typically reveal a sharply defined medial border between the involved insula and the uninvolved putamen. By CT, the involved area is usually edematous and appears relatively lucent. On MR images, the prolongation of T1 and T2 relaxation times of the diseased temporal lobes produces hypointensity on T1-weighted images and hyperintensity on T2-weighted images. Enhancement may be patchy or gyriform.

246. The answer is A. *(Williams & Haughton, pp 150–167.)* The figure shows a hypodense, nonenhancing lesion in the left subinsular white matter. There is mild mass effect on the adjacent putamen medially and on the sylvian fissure laterally. The insular cortex is uninvolved. These features are most typical of a low-grade astrocytoma.

An infarction of this size should not spare the adjacent gray matter structures (basal ganglia and insular cortex). Herpes encephalitis frequently involves the insular and temporal lobe cortices and often enhances. Focal hemorrhage may also be present. Toxoplasmosis and lymphoma typically enhance; moreover, non-AIDS CNS-related lymphoma is characteristically hyperdense on precontrast CT scans.

247. The answer is B. *(Harnsberger, pp 212–215.)* Thyroglossal duct cysts arise from rests that may persist anywhere along the thyroglossal duct remnant, which is a midline structure extending from the foramen cecum at the base of the tongue to the thyroid gland. Some cysts enlarge asymmetrically and so appear just off the midline. They usually occur at (15%) or just below (65%) the hyoid bone. Only 20% are found in a suprahyoid location.

Most cases involve patients under the age of 30, and half are younger than 10 years old. The cysts are lined by squamous epithelium, with a reported incidence of carcinoma of less than 1%. By CT, they are characteristically less dense than the surrounding strap muscles, which lie in close association. Treatment involves surgical removal of the cyst and its entire lining, to prevent regrowth.

248. The answer is E. *(Barkovich, p 327–332.)* The figure shows a classic vein of Galen "aneurysm," or AVM. An abnormal collection of small vessels (the nidus) is located in the upper brainstem. The vein of Galen is enormous due to the high-volume shunt which results. There is also high flow into an accessory falcine vein and away from the straight sinus, which is atretic and not visible on the image.

A corpus callosum lipoma is hyperintense on T1-weighted images. A giant PICA aneurysm would be located more inferiorly; moreover, there would not be a nidus or any abnormal veins. Cavernous angiomas are typically hyperintense on T1-weighted images due to methemoglobin; there is also a hypointense periphery (hemosiderin). Sagittal sinus thrombosis would result in abnormal signal in the sagittal sinus without the features seen in this case.

249. The answer is E. *(Barkovich, pp 109–113.)*   The Chiari II malformation is a complex congenital disorder involving the hindbrain, spine, and mesoderm. Almost all these patients have a myelomeningocele. Although multiple abnormalities are found in the brains of these patients, it is unusual to encounter all of them in a single individual.

Gray matter heterotopias are collections of neurons in abnormal locations, which occur as an arrest of the normal radial migration of neurons from the germinal matrix. They do not occur in specific association with the Chiari II malformation.

The other choices *are* associated with Chiari II malformations. Stenogyria refers to an abnormal gyral pattern in the medial aspect of the parietal and occipital lobes and is best appreciated on sagittal MR scans. The tectal plate is invariably abnormal, with varying degrees of fusion of the colliculi. Moreover, the tectum may be compressed by the temporal lobes and the cerebellum, contributing to the characteristic "beaking." The falx cerebri is usually deficient in areas, resulting in protrusion of gyri from both hemispheres across the interhemispheric fissure and "interdigitation." Lückenschädel (lacunar) skull is the result of a mesodermal dysplasia, producing thinned areas which give the skull radiographs of newborn patients a scalloped appearance.

250. The answer is B. *(Banna, pp 263–265.)*   Most of the primary CNS tumors which metastasize through CSF pathways are either aggressive, such as glioblastomas, retinoblastomas, medulloblastomas, or germinomas; and/or have direct access to the ventricular system, as in the case of ependymomas and choroid plexus papillomas. Acoustic schwannomas are benign neoplasms which virtually never metastasize along CSF pathways. Tumors arising outside the CNS can also invade and spread along the spinal subarachnoid space.

In the spine, subarachnoid metastases most often occur in the lumbar region, probably due to the effect of gravity. Gadolinium-enhanced MR imaging and myelography are both sensitive in detecting leptomeningeal tumor spread.

251. The answer is D. *(Barkovich, p 124.)*   The midline sagittal T1-weighted MR scan in the figure at left shows obliteration of the aqueduct of Sylvius by the abnormal tectum and resultant mild hydrocephalus. The normally enhancing pineal gland is the high-signal structure located just rostral to the tectum. The axial image in the figure at right shows diffuse thickening of the tectum (quadrigeminal plate), without any enhancement. There is mild dilatation of the third ventricle and the atria of the lateral ventricles. These findings are typical for a tectal (upper brainstem) glioma. In contrast to those gliomas which occur in this location, lower brainstem gliomas generally present with cranial nerve palsies, rather than hydrocephalus.

Regarding the other choices, an incisural meningioma is an extraaxial tumor, whereas the lesion in this case is clearly an infiltrative, intraaxial process. Germinomas typically involve the pineal or suprasellar region. Most hemangioblastomas occur in the cerebellum or spinal cord, and they characteristically show intense enhancement on both CT and MR scans. Infratentorial ependymomas typically arise in the fourth ventricle, and are usually inhomogeneous and enhance following contrast administration.

252. The answer is C. *(Harnsberger, pp 382–389.)*   The ostiomeatal unit is defined as the area of the superomedial maxillary sinus and the middle meatus that conveys the mucociliary drainages of the maxillary, frontal, and anterior and middle ethmoid sinuses into the nose. Because of its strategic location and the emergence of transnasal endoscopic surgery, the ostiomeatal unit has become very important. It must be fully evaluated on all screening CT scans of the sinuses; this is best accomplished in the coronal plane.

The infundibulum, uncinate process, hiatus semilunaris, and ethmoid bulla are all part of the ostiomeatal unit and are associated with the *middle* turbinate of the nose.

253. The answer is A. *(Atlas, pp 578–580.)* Amyloid angiopathy, arteriovenous malformation, cocaine use, metastatic melanoma, and mycotic aneurysm are all important causes of parenchymal cerebral hemorrhage. However, amyloid (congophilic) angiopathy is a disease of the elderly, and should not be included in the differential diagnosis for a young adult.

Amyloid angiopathy is an important cause of atraumatic lobar hemorrhage in the elderly, and occurs frequently in the setting of Alzheimer disease. The amyloid infiltrates the walls of the cerebral vessels, gradually replacing the entire thickness and producing vascular fragility. Small- and medium-sized cortical and leptomeningeal vessels are affected and therefore are the most prone to rupture.

254. The answer is A. *(Williams & Haughton, pp 183–190.)* The figure shows a dense and/or enhancing posterior third-ventricular region lesion. There is associated obstructive hydrocephalus and transependymal interstitial edema. The appearance is that of an aggressive process arising in the pineal region and, of the choices given, is most consistent with a pineoblastoma.

Colloid cysts typically arise near the foramina of Monro, and obstruct only the lateral ventricles, as do giant cell astrocytomas, which occur most commonly in patients with tuberous sclerosis.

Epidermoids tend to occur off the midline, commonly in the cerebellopontine angles. Moreover, they are typically hypodense and do not enhance. Hemangioblastomas also do not occur in the pineal region. They are the most common primary posterior fossa tumor in adults and are frequently seen in patients with von Hippel-Lindau disease.

255. The answer is A. *(Osborn, pp 33–48.)* The left vertebral artery is the same size or larger than the right vertebral artery in 75–80% of cases. This anatomic fact is important when performing selective vertebral arterial angiography, as the larger size of the left vertebral artery makes it safer to catheterize. In addition, when injecting the dominant vessel, one has a greater chance of refluxing down the contralateral side, so that both distal vertebral arteries may be visualized with one injection. However, both may have to be studied individually if the posterior inferior cerebellar arteries (PICAs) need to be evaluated closely.

A "bovine arch," a nonpathologic anatomic variant in which the left common carotid artery arises from the innominate artery, is found in 10–15% of cases.

256. The answer is C. *(Atlas, pp 364–365.)* The infant shown in the figure has a round, low-intensity lesion involving the quadrigeminal plate. The lesion has the same signal characteristic as the cerebrospinal fluid (CSF) in the dilated lateral ventricles. This appearance is typical of an arachnoid cyst arising in the quadrigeminal plate cistern.

Arachnoid cysts either may arise from a congenital defect in the development of the arachnoid membrane or may occur as the sequela of inflammation. They may trap or secrete CSF, causing them to expand. Though they are often asymptomatic, some may come to attention because of ventricular obstruction. Other common locations of arachnoid cysts include the anterior temporal lobe, suprasellar cistern, cerebellopontine angle, and retrocerebellar region.

Rathke cleft cysts and craniopharyngiomas arise in a suprasellar or intrasellar location; Dandy-Walker cysts and mega cisterna magna are situated posterior to the cerebellum.

257. The answer is C. *(Brant-Zawadzki, p 44.)* Signal strength is improved by maneuvers that increase the number of protons which are excited in the imaging volume. Increasing the slice thickness and field-of-view will accomplish this directly. An increase in the number of signal averages increases the SNR by a square root factor. Decreasing the TE will also boost SNR because there is less time for signal decay, but this is achieved at the expense of less tissue contrast. The cost of increasing slice thickness and field-of-view is reduced resolution; increasing the number of signal averages increases scan time.

Increasing the matrix size causes a decrease in the SNR, because each pixel in the matrix will have fewer excited protons. Theoretically, this should improve resolution, but the resultant low SNR makes this trade-off undesirable.

258. The answer is D. *(Friedman, AJNR, vol 12; pp 872–874.)* The figure at left is a CT scan of the posterior fossa windowed for bone. It shows a highly destructive process involving the left temporal bone, with extension into the middle ear and destruction of the ossicles. The adjacent temporal squamosa is thickened and sclerotic. The figure at right, a coronal T1-weighted gadolinium-enhanced MR scan, reveals the aggressive mass which is responsible. It also shows thickening and enhancement of the adjacent dura. This appearance is most consistent with carcinoma arising in the temporal bone, in this case a primary squamous cell neoplasm that has originated in the middle ear or external auditory canal. Metastatic squamous cell carcinoma may also have a similar appearance.

Cholesteatomas may erode bone, but they are rarely this aggressive. Cholesterol granulomas typically arise at the petrous apex. The glomus jugulare, one of a group of vascular "glomus" tumors (also known as *chemodectomas*), originates in the jugular fossa, which is situated caudally to the mass. Intracranial chordoma, a neoplasm which arises from notochordal rests, generally arises in the midline, usually from the clivus. Though they can cause marked bony destruction, a tumor which originates so far laterally would be extraordinary.

259. The answer is C. *(Huston et al, Radiology 1991, 181:3, 721–730.)* Recently, time-of-flight and phase contrast MR angiography (MRA) techniques have been successfully applied to the study of intracranial cerebrovascular disease. Statements (B) and (D) accurately describe the principles which underlie each.

Limitations of 3D time-of-flight imaging include susceptibility to saturation effects, artifacts from air-bone susceptibility gradients, and simulation of flow (bright signal) by materials with short T1 relaxation times. However, a major advantage is the reduced acquisition time when compared to phase contrast imaging.

One drawback of phase contrast MRA is aliasing. Normal flow images display a smooth transition between adjacent pixels, as one would expect with laminar flow. Aliasing appears as a sharp transition between black and white within vascular lumina which results in a mottled-appearing vessel. Advantages of phase contrast include superior background suppression, low sensitivity to saturation effects, variable velocity detection, and greater functional flow information.

260. The answer is D. *(Atlas, pp 946–952.)* The figures at left are pre- and post-gadolinium T1-weighted axial MR scans of the thoracic spine, respectively. The figure at right is a sagittal contrast-enhanced T1-weighted image. They show a hypointense, peripherally enhancing lesion whose location is intradural, but extramedullary. The most common lesions in this compartment include meningioma and schwannoma, the latter being the diagnosis in this case. As a rule, meningiomas tend to occur more frequently in the thoracic spine, whereas schwannomas are more common in the cervical and lumbosacral spine. Additionally, the pattern of peripheral enhancement helps distinguish the two, as meningiomas tend to enhance uniformly, and schwannomas heterogeneously.

Less commonly, "drop" metastases and arachnoid cysts occur in this location. Astrocytomas and ependymomas, while arising in the intradural compartment, are *intra*medullary neoplasms.

Epidural abscesses, like spinal metastases, may produce devastating cord and nerve root symptoms, but do so by extrinsic compression of the thecal sac. The dural outline is clearly preserved in this case.

261. **The answer is D.** *(Atlas, pp 952–961, 987–1001.)* The figures reveal enlargement of the conus medullaris and central enhancement after gadolinium. The patient in this case had severe atherosclerotic vascular disease. He suffered an infarction of his distal spinal cord when its tenuous blood supply was further compromised during a hypotensive episode. The differential diagnosis of lesions in the intramedullary compartment includes astrocytoma, ependymoma, syrinx, myelitis, infarction, and metastases.

   Of the choice given, meningioma is the only lesion which is not intramedullary. Meningiomas arise from the meninges and are therefore intradural, but also extramedullary in location.

262. **The answers are: A-Y, B-Y, C-Y, D-N, E-Y.** *(Atlas, pp 117–120.)* The profile of signal strength across high-contrast interfaces is characterized by abrupt changes in signal magnitude. The Fourier transformation used to construct the images cannot precisely reproduce this rapid a transition of spatial frequencies and therefore undershoots or overshoots slightly near the border between the two tissues. The result is a series of ripples on either side of the tissue interface.

   Truncation artifacts are common in the cervical spine, where there is a sharp difference between the signal of the spinal cord and adjacent subarachnoid space. The larger the pixels, the more likely it is that a signal will vary across the width of one pixel. Therefore, decreasing pixel size will minimize the truncation effect.

   Since scan time is proportional to the number of pixels in the phase-encoded direction, the matrix is usually set up with fewer pixels in that direction (e.g., 256 × 128). As a result of the larger pixel size along the phase-encoded dimension, the truncation artifacts are relatively worse along that axis. Changing the matrix size to 256 × 256 would reduce the artifact, but at the expense of greater scan time.

   Aliasing or "wraparound" artifacts are created by the anatomy of the patient which extends beyond the designated field of view but which is magnetized and emits signal. The computer incorrectly assigns a location to those structures to *within* the image.

263. **The answers are: A-N, B-N, C-Y, D-N, E-N.** *(Osborn, pp 109–184.)* Prior to its terminal bifurcation into the anterior and middle cerebral arteries, the intracranial extracavernous internal carotid artery (ICA) gives rise to several important branches. These include the superior hypophyseal, ophthalmic, posterior communicating, and anterior choroidal arteries. The latter three are important both in radiography, as angiographic landmarks, and in clinical practice. The supraclinoid ICA also sends small unnamed branches to the hypothalamus, optic tract, and optic chiasm.

   The ophthalmic artery, which is the only correct choice among those given, supplies the globe and orbital contents. It is also an important source of collateral flow in cases of cervical ICA occlusion. The anterior falx artery and, occasionally, the middle meningeal artery arise from it.

   The posterior communicating (PCOM) artery arises from the posteromedial surface of the ICA and sweeps backward, above the third cranial nerve, to join the posterior cerebral artery (PCA), thereby linking the anterior and posterior cerebral circulations. It also gives rise to important thalamoperforating branches. One or both PCOMs are hypoplastic in 20% of cases.

   The *anterior* choroidal artery normally arises from the posteromedial aspect of the ICA above the PCOM. It is divided into proximal (cisternal) and distal (plexal) segments. It is an important supply to the choroid plexus of the temporal horn of the lateral ventricle and also to portions of the optic tract, thalamus, and internal capsule.

   The posterior choroidal artery arises from the posterior cerebral artery (PCA). The anterior communicating (ACOM) artery connects the two anterior cerebral arteries (ACAs) at their A1-A2 junctions. The medial tentorial artery is a branch of the meningohypophyseal trunk which, along with the inferolateral trunk, arises from the cavernous ICA.

264. The answers are: A-N, B-Y, C-Y, D-N, E-Y. *(Osborn, pp 153–154.)* The primitive trigeminal, otic, and hypoglossal arteries are transient anastomoses between the internal carotid arteries (ICAs) and the precursors of the basilar artery system. If these vessels fail to regress during development, a persistent carotid-basilar connection results. These may be more than just angiographic curiosities, however, since aneurysms, AVMs, and other vascular abnormalities have occurred in conjunction with them. Additionally, they serve as potential conduits through which atheromatous emboli can pass from the internal carotid artery into the posterior circulation.

The most frequent of these vessels is the persistent trigeminal artery, which is discovered in 0.1–0.2% of cerebral angiograms. It arises just before the cavernous segment of the ICA and joins the basilar artery between the origins of the superior cerebellar artery and the anterior inferior cerebellar artery (AICA). The basilar artery proximal to the junction is usually hypoplastic and the posterior communicating artery is usually absent.

The persistent hypoglossal artery originates more caudally, in the cervical segment of the ICA. It then enters the hypoglossal canal and joins the proximal basilar artery. The rare persistent otic artery arises from the petrous portion of the ICA and anastomoses to the AICA.

The occipital artery is a normal branch of the external carotid artery. The recurrent artery of Huebner is one of the important medial lenticulostriate branches.

265. The answers are: A-N, B-Y, C-Y, D-Y, E-N. *(Newton & Potts, pp 2448–2449. Atlas, pp 396–408.)* Intracranial aneurysms are the most common atraumatic cause of subarachnoid hemorrhage. Only about 10% occur in the posterior fossa, the majority of these arising at the basilar tip, the remainder being in the anterior circulation. At least 20% are multiple; therefore, anyone being evaluated for aneurysmal rupture needs to have the entire cerebral circulation thoroughly scrutinized.

The distribution of subarachnoid blood may be helpful in localizing the source of bleeding. For example, sylvian fissure hemorrhage usually indicates a middle cerebral artery bifurcation aneurysm, whereas blood in the septum pellucidum usually indicates an aneurysm of the anterior communicating artery.

By definition, aneurysms larger than 2.5 cm are termed *giant*. They may present because of mass effect or subarachnoid hemorrhage. Common locations include the cavernous internal carotid artery, middle cerebral artery bifurcation, and basilar tip.

An isolated and complete third-nerve palsy, with a dilated pupil, is a classic presentation of an unruptured posterior communicating artery aneurysm. A pupillary-sparing third-nerve palsy is characteristic of diabetic microvascular disease. This is because the parasympathetic fibers which control pupillary constriction course along the periphery of the optic nerve, and microvascular infarction occurs centrally.

Although the vast majority of berry aneurysms occur in isolation, certain diseases predispose to their formation. These include autosomal dominant polycystic kidney disease (6% incidence of aneurysm), arteriovenous malformation, fibromuscular dysplasia, coarctation of the aorta, and collagen vascular disease.

266. The answers are: A-Y, B-N, C-Y, D-Y, E-Y. *(Atlas, pp 467–500.)* Multiple sclerosis is a demyelinating disease of unknown etiology which most frequently affects young adults. The classic lesions seen on MR scans are plaques, which occur commonly in the periventricular white matter, internal capsule, corpus callosum, pons, and brachium pontis. They are best seen on long TR sequences, appearing as hyperintense foci due to a prolonged T2 relaxation time. When the plaques are periventricular in location, they may not be apparent on T2-weighted scans due to the similar signal of cerebrospinal fluid; rather, proton density–weighted scans will better reveal them as hyperintense foci adjacent to darker cerebrospinal fluid.

Acute disseminated encephalomyelitis (ADEM) is a virally-induced, immune-mediated white matter disease. It is most commonly encountered following measles infection. Rubella is the next most common, followed by varicella, and Epstein-Barr virus. The majority of patients recover completely.

Central pontine myelinolysis occurs most commonly in association with certain electrolyte abnormalities; classically, it is associated with the rapid correction of profound hyponatremia. It may occur in alcoholics, who often have multiple electrolyte disturbances. Typically, T2-weighted MR scans reveal a central area of hyperintensity in the pons, with sparing of a peripheral rim of tissue, although other portions of the brainstem may be affected.

267. The answers are: A-N, B-N, C-Y, D-N, E-N. *(Atlas, pp 302–307, 477–478, 523–524.)* The most common brain lesions in HIV-infected patients include HIV encephalitis, progressive multifocal leukoencephalopathy (PML), opportunistic infection (especially toxoplasmosis and cryptococcus), and primary lymphoma. The first two diseases typically do not enhance following contrast administration (CT or MR), whereas the latter two do. HIV encephalitis is characteristically periventricular and symmetrical, in contrast to PML, which is more often subcortically located and symmetrically distributed. In the latter stages of PML, the lesions may become confluent. PML is not caused by herpetic infection, but rather by the reactivation of a dormant papovavirus.

Cryptococcal infection involves the meninges, particularly in the basal cisterns. The organisms penetrate the Virchow-Robin spaces, especially in the region of the basal ganglia. Gelatinous pseudocysts, which contain masses of encapsulated organisms, are found frequently and usually show little or no enhancement.

The most common CNS neoplasm in HIV-infected patients is primary lymphoma. It is a highly aggressive tumor, with few patients surviving beyond one year. Kaposi sarcoma rarely metastasizes to the brain.

268. The answers are: A-Y, B-N, C-N, D-N, E-Y. *(Atlas, pp 632–640.)* Pituitary adenomas are the most common intrasellar tumor, representing 10–15% of all intracranial neoplasms. Prolactinomas account for 40–50% of hormonally active adenomas; less commonly, adenomas may produce growth hormone (20%) and ACTH (20%). Adenomas are classified as *micro-* or *macro-*, depending on size, with a diameter of 10 mm being the point of division.

The coronal plane is the best for evaluating the sella and its contents. T1-weighted MR scans are better for visualizing the pituitary because the bright signal of the surrounding CSF on T2-weighted images often obscures the gland. Gadolinium enhances the ability to detect microadenomas, particularly the very small ACTH-producing tumors.

Hemorrhage into macroadenomas is not uncommon and extracellular methemoglobin will produce bright signal on both T1- and T2-weighted images.

Lateral displacement of the cavernous carotid artery by a macroadenoma is not an uncommon occurrence, but the finding is not specific for invasion of the cavernous sinus. Studies have shown that lateral extension and interposition of abnormal tissue between the lateral wall of the cavernous sinus and the carotid artery is the most reliable indicator of invasion.

269. The answers are: A-N, B-N, C-Y, D-Y, E-Y. *(Williams & Haughton, pp 84, 111, 144. Barkovich, p. 345.)* The pattern of blood in the subarachnoid space is useful in predicting the location of a ruptured berry aneurysm. Hemorrhage in the septum pellucidum is almost specific for an anterior communicating artery aneurysm. *Moya-moya,* or "puff of smoke," is the description of the pattern of small collateral vessels which develop in response to a slowly progressive occlusion of the proximal intracranial arteries; the *common* carotid arteries are not involved.

Asparaginase is an important chemotherapeutic agent used in the treatment of some childhood leukemias. It can cause multiple clotting problems, and intracranial hemorrhage is a well-recognized complication in this patient population.

Amphetamine use may result in a classic drug-induced vasculitis. Angiography shows multiple irregular areas of arterial narrowing. However, these findings are not specific and the diagnosis rests upon the clinical picture and the history. Carotid-cavernous fistulae occur most commonly in the setting of trauma, but may result from the rupture of a cavernous carotid aneurysm. In a patient with pulsatile exophthalmos, the CT findings of proptosis and ipsilateral cavernous sinus and ophthalmic vein distension are virtually diagnostic.

270. The answers are: A-Y, B-Y, C-N, D-Y, E-Y.   *(Atlas, pp 223–326.)*   Primary CNS lymphoma occurring in AIDS patients is a highly aggressive malignancy which is frequently necrotic and surrounded by vasogenic edema. The central necrotic portion is hypodense on CT, and the periphery often enhances with contrast. In contrast, lymphoma occurring in patients who do not have AIDS is more typically a solid, hypercellular tumor and is therefore often hyperdense on noncontrast CT scans. Following gadolinium or iodinated contrast, enhancement is typically uniform. Primary CNS lymphoma virtually never calcifies.

Glioblastoma multiforme is a devastating neoplasm which has such malignant vascular endothelial proliferation that hemorrhage and necrosis are frequently found not only in the tumor, but also in the brain tissue which is being invaded.

Gangliogliomas are indolent tumors composed of both neural and glial elements. They occur in children and young adults, most commonly in the temporal lobes. Since cystic areas are present in at least 40% of cases, the presence of a partially cystic mass in the temporal lobe of a child should suggest the diagnosis.

Oligodendrogliomas are the most common intracranial tumor to calcify. Linear or nodular calcific deposits appear in 50–90% of lesions. These neoplasms occur most frequently in the frontal and frontotemporal regions.

271. The answers are: A-N, B-Y, C-Y, D-Y, E-N.   *(Atlas, pp 245–249.)*   Normally, intravascular contrast media are prevented from reaching the cerebral extravascular space by the unique capillary structure which constitutes the blood-brain barrier. There are special tight junctions in the foot processes of the pericytes which prevent the passage of large molecules across the basement membrane. Lipid soluble compounds and ethanol, however, pass unhindered. Additionally, any process which alters the permeability of the endothelium, such as infection and neoplasia, will disrupt the blood-brain barrier.

Many normal intracranial structures are "outside" the blood-brain barrier, often as a means to allow them to monitor blood levels of chemical mediators or neurohormones. These include the pituitary stalk (infundibulum), pituitary gland, and pineal gland. The choroid plexus does not have a blood-brain barrier.

The anterior commissure, a white matter tract, and the filum terminale of the spinal cord do not ordinarily enhance with gadolinium.

272. The answers are: A-N, B-Y, C-N, D-Y, E-Y.   *(Latchaw, 2d ed., 1991, pp 178–179, 203–265. Harnsberger, pp 325–326. Barkovich, pp 68–71.)*   CT scanning remains the best imaging modality for the detection of subarachnoid hemorrhage (SAH). MR imaging often fails to display SAH, probably due to the relatively high Po_2 in the cerebrospinal fluid (CSF) preventing the formation of paramagnetic deoxyhemoglobin.

Shear (diffuse axonal) injuries are common with severe, blunt head trauma. They develop secondary to differential movements of one portion of the brain with respect to another and occur most commonly at the gray-white junction in the cerebral hemispheres, followed by the corpus callosum and the upper brainstem.

Longitudinal temporal bone fractures occur along the petrous ridge. Because the ossicles are disrupted but the eighth nerve remains intact, a conductive hearing loss results. Hemorrhagic CSF otorrhea commonly occurs and the internal carotid artery may also suffer injury. In contrast, transverse temporal bone fractures, which are less common, may result in sensorineural hearing loss and facial nerve injury.

Acute epidural hematomas are sharply defined, biconvex collections which have a higher density than adjacent gray matter. Linear skull fractures are present in 60–90% of cases, but their absence does not preclude significant hemorrhage. Epidural hematomas do not cross suture lines. Acute subdural hematomas are typically crescentic: they conform to the inner table of the skull and can cross sutures. Skull fractures are seen in about 40% of cases.

Whereas traumatic subdurals are more commonly unilateral in adults, they are bilateral in 80% of infants. The possibility of child abuse should be raised in the appropriate clinical setting.

273. **The answers are: A-N, B-Y, C-N, D-Y, E-N.** *(Atlas, pp 327–378.)* Epidermoid cysts are congenital lesions of ectodermal origin. They are characteristically lobular and hypodense on CT, and do not enhance. Although they may appear similar in intensity to CSF on MR scans, proton density images can usually help distinguish them from arachnoid cysts, since epidermoids usually have a higher signal. In addition to the cerebellopontine (CP) angle, epidermoids also occur commonly in a parasellar location.

Acoustic schwannomas are the most common nerve sheath tumor in the CNS and usually arise from the superior division of the vestibular nerve (CN VIII). Unlike meningiomas, they typically form an acute angle with the adjacent temporal bone. Meningiomas are broader-based and form obtuse angles with the petrous ridge. Meningiomas calcify far more frequently than schwannomas.

When acoustic schwannomas occur bilaterally, a diagnosis of neurofibromatosis type 2 (NF2) can be made. It is a distinct entity from NF1 and has a different set of associated abnormalities in the CNS.

The flocculus is a normal cerebellar structure which may protrude anterolaterally into the CP angle and mimic a mass. The nodulus is another normal cerebellar structure which lies in the midline, posterior to the fourth ventricle. It, too, can be mistaken for a mass.

274. **The answers are: A-N, B-Y, C-N, D-Y, E-Y.** *(Barkovich, pp 35–75.)* Leigh disease (subacute necrotizing encephalopathy) is an autosomal recessive disease characterized by abnormalities in both basal ganglia (particularly the putamen), as well as lesions in the brainstem and white matter. Affected individuals are usually in the pediatric age group. Alexander disease (fibrinoid leukodystrophy) is a dysmyelinating disorder which is characterized first by abnormalities in the frontal white matter. The lesions progress posteriorly and inferiorly with time. Both Alexander disease and Canavan disease present with macrocephaly; this is very important in the clinical evaluation of these patients. Death usually occurs in early childhood. Canavan disease (spongiform leukodystrophy) is an autosomal recessive disorder that manifests as diffuse, symmetrical abnormalities of the cerebral white matter. Classic X-linked adrenal leukodystrophy is seen exclusively in males; it usually presents in childhood between the ages of 5 and 10. Abnormal white matter appears first in the occipital region, and progresses anteriorly with time. The anterior edge of the abnormal white matter frequently enhances after contrast administration.

Periventricular leukomalacia is most often seen in premature infants. MR findings include attenuation of the periventricular white matter (especially around the atria), enlargement and irregularity of the body and atrium of the lateral ventricles, thinning of the posterior body and splenium of the corpus callosum, and hyperintensity of the periventricular white matter (especially around the atria).

275. The answers are: A-Y, B-N, C-Y, D-Y, E-N. *(Barkovich, pp 60–61, 77–121.)* Agyria (complete lissencephaly) is a migrational disorder characterized by absence of gyri on the surface of the brain. The areas most frequently affected are the parietal and occipital lobes. The cortex is smooth and thickened, with decreased white matter and shallow sylvian fissures. Schizencephaly is also a migrational disorder, in which gray-matter-lined clefts extend from the lateral ventricles to the inner table of the skull. Cerebrospinal fluid may fill the cleft ("open lip"), or the cleft may be fused ("closed lip"). The clefts are most commonly near the pre- and postcentral gyri. Seizures are the most common clinical manifestation.

In hydranencephaly, the cerebral hemispheres (in the distribution of the anterior circulation) are replaced by sacs containing cerebrospinal fluid. In utero occlusion of the internal carotid arteries (by a variety of possible insults) is felt to be the underlying etiology. The falx cerebri is present, as compared to alobar holoprosencephaly (the most severe form of holoprosencephaly), which is a group of disorders characterized by a failure of differentiation and cleavage of the prosencephalon. In the alobar type, the thalami are fused, the falx is absent, and a crescent-shaped monoventricle is present. Severe midline facial anomalies usually coexist with the intracranial defects.

The Dandy-Walker malformation consists of cystic dilatation of the fourth ventricle, agenesis of the cerebellar vermis, and marked enlargement of the posterior fossa. Hydrocephalus develops in 75% of patients; dysgenesis of the corpus callosum occurs in 20–25% of patients.

Incidentally, T1-weighted MR scanning, with its superb anatomic detail, is ideally suited for the evaluation of these and other congenital malformations.

276. The answers are: A-N, B-N, C-Y, D-Y, E-N. *(Barkovich, pp 123–147.)* Von Hippel-Lindau disease is an autosomal dominant disorder characterized by retinal angiomas, cerebellar and spinal cord hemangioblastomas, angiomas of the liver and kidney, and cysts of the pancreas, kidney, and liver. Renal cell carcinomas also arise more frequently in these patients. Supratentorial hemangioblastomas may occur, but they are rare and far less common than the cerebellar lesions.

Sturge-Weber disease is a congenital disorder characterized by angiomatosis involving the face, the choroid of the eye, and the leptomeninges. Calcifications occur in the cerebral cortex underlying the meningeal angiomatosis and are the most frequent CT finding. The calcifications are gyriform in shape, and are most frequently seen in the temporoparietooccipital regions.

Tuberous sclerosis is characterized by multiple subependymal hamartomas. Giant cell astrocytoma refers to enlarging subependymal nodules that tend to be situated near the foramina of Monro; they are seen in 5–10% of patients with tuberous sclerosis.

Lateral thoracic meningoceles are a common manifestation of spinal neurofibromatosis; most authors believe that they are secondary to meningeal dysplasia. Eighty percent of patients with lateral thoracic meningoceles have neurofibromatosis. The plexiform type of neurofibroma is virtually pathognomonic of neurofibromatosis. Antoni type A and type B histology refer to schwannomas; the former has a cellular pattern, whereas the latter is hypocellular and prone to cystic and myxoid degeneration. The presence of the type B pattern accounts for the more inhomogeneous appearance of schwannomas as compared to neurofibromas.

277. The answers are: A-Y, B-N, C-N, D-N, E-N. *(Barkovich, pp 149–203.)* The most typical appearance of a posterior fossa ependymoma on CT is that of an iso- to hyperdense fourth ventricular mass with punctate calcifications, small cysts, and moderate contrast enhancement. Nearly 50% will show multifocal, small calcifications; larger calcifications are occasionally seen. Calcification is much less common in medulloblastoma, occurring in up to 20% of cases.

Brainstem glioma most commonly occurs in the pons; the classic presentation is multiple cranial nerve palsies. Hydrocephalus is unusual in brainstem glioma; however, it can be seen with tectal gliomas. Regarding the CT appearance of craniopharyngiomas, 90% will have a cystic component and the same percentage will be at least partly calcified. The calcification may be peripheral or chunky. In addition, over 90% enhance with contrast.

In the pediatric age group, choroid plexus papilloma most commonly arises in the lateral ventricles; in adults, the fourth ventricle is the most common site. Extension through the foramina of Luschka occurs in up to 15% of fourth ventricular ependymomas. Up to 60% of these ependymomas grow through the foramen of Magendie into the cisterna magna, through the foramen magnum, and into the cervical spinal canal. Extension through fourth ventricular outlets is not typical of pilocytic cerebellar astrocytoma.

278. **The answers are: A-N, B-N, C-N, D-N, E-N.** *(Atlas, pp 795–864.)* Far lateral disk herniations affect the root exiting *above* the disk space; that is, a far lateral L4-L5 disk herniation will impinge upon the L4 root which has exited under the L4 pedicle. The more frequent paracentral disk herniation will affect the lower root as it exits the thecal sac; that is, an L4-L5 paracentral disk herniation will impinge upon the L5 root. Far lateral disk herniations are often missed by myelography, since the root sleeve terminates proximal to the site of herniation. All axial CT/MR spine images should be carefully scrutinized for the presence of lateral herniations.

The normal intervertebral disk contains water; with age and/or degeneration, the disk loses water and becomes dessicated. Therefore, a T2-weighted image of a normal disk reveals high intensity (long T2), whereas a degenerated disk is hypointense (short T2). It is also common to see changes in the endplates of the vertebral bodies around the degenerated disks. Type 1 is a pattern of hypointensity (long T1) on T1-weighted images and hyperintensity (long T2) on T2-weighted images. It most likely represents vascularized marrow with increased water signal. Type 2 (fatty) endplate changes show the opposite signal.

Synovial cysts are most common in the lumbar region, especially at L4-L5 and L5-S1. They are probably related to facet degeneration and/or trauma. Signal on MR is similar, but not identical to CSF, and they may contain hemorrhage.

279. **The answers are: A-Y, B-Y, C-N, D-Y, E-Y.** *(Atlas, pp 1001–1007.)* Infections in the spine may be due to hematogenous (arterial) bacterial spread, direct extension of a soft-tissue infection, penetrating injury, or surgery. The arterial route is believed to be the most common pathway in cases of spinal osteomyelitis. *Staphylococcus aureus* is the most frequent pathogen to cause diskitis, osteomyelitis, and epidural abscess. Gram-negative organisms are also important pathogens. Diskitis and osteomyelitis are most common in the lumbar spine. The classic findings on MR include narrowing of the disk space, hyperintensity of the disk and adjacent bone on T2-weighted images, and loss of the margin between the disk and vertebral endplates. There may be an associated paraspinal mass. Tuberculous osteomyelitis (Pott disease) is characterized by late preservation of the disk space, multilevel involvement, and a tendency to spread along the anterior longitudinal ligament. This latter finding may result in extensive prevertebral soft-tissue swelling.

280. **The answers are: A-Y, B-Y, C-Y, D-N, E-Y.** *(Atlas, pp 926–944.)* Osteoid osteoma is a benign bone lesion with the characteristic presentation of pain at night, which is relieved by aspirin. Plain films show a lucent nidus surrounded by sclerosis. These lesions can occur in virtually any bone; within the spine, the lumbar region (59%) is most common, followed by the cervical spine (27%). Osteoblastoma has a predilection for the spine, and occurs there in 25–50% of cases. These uncommon benign bone tumors usually involve the posterior elements, though occasionally extend to involve the vertebral body.

Giant cell tumors typically affect adults aged 20 to 40; regarding spinal lesions, a significant majority occur in the sacrum. Plain films reveal a lytic, expansile lesion. Chordoma is an aggressive tumor which arises from notochordal remnants and which is capable of metastasis. Because the notochord extends from the skull base (clivus) to the sacrum, chordomas can occur in a wide variety of locations: 50% arise in the sacrum, 35% in the clivus, and the remainder elsewhere along the spine. Aneurysmal bone cysts are benign lesions which occur in the spine in up to 20% of cases; 60% involve the posterior elements and 40% arise in the vertebral body. Plain films typically show an expansile lytic lesion with a very thin cortical margin.

281. The answers are: A-N, B-N, C-N, D-N, E-Y. *(Som, Bergeron, ed. 2, 1991, pp 693–828.)* Grave disease may result in thyroid ophthalmopathy, which is the most common cause of bilateral exophthalmos in an adult. Pathologically, there is deposition of mucopolysaccharides and infiltration by lymphocytes in the muscle bodies and retroorbital fat. Imaging reveals bilateral enlargement of the muscle bodies, with sparing of their tendinous muscle insertions on the globe. This is in contrast to orbital pseudotumor (myositis), wherein the tendinous insertions *are* involved.

Dacrocystitis refers to inflammation of the lacrimal sac, which is usually found to be filled with purulent material. Dacroadenitis is an inflammation of the lacrimal glands, which may occur in viral infections, most notably mumps.

Tram-track calcification is typical of optic nerve meningiomas. It represents calcification in a tumor which surrounds the optic nerve. Calcification is very unusual in optic nerve gliomas and would not have a "tram-track" appearance.

Dermoids are congenital benign tumors that most often arise anteriorly between the globe and the orbital periosteum in the extraconal space. They may cause smooth bony erosion and have fluid or fat density as measured by CT. Retinoblastoma occurs most commonly in children under 3 years of age (98%), and is bilateral in approximately one-third of cases. It is the most common tumor of the globe in children. The presence of bilateral retinoblastoma should prompt a search for a pineal cell neoplasm *(trilateral retinoblastoma)*.

282. The answers are: A-Y, B-N, C-Y, D-Y, E-N. *(Harnsberger, pp 46–60, 34.)* The principal structures of the masticator space are the mandible and muscles of mastication. Hence, primary malignant tumors are most frequently sarcomas. Chondrosarcomas generally arise from the temporomandibular joint. Since the masticator space is anterior to the parapharyngeal space, a mass would displace the parapharyngeal fat posteriorly.

Regarding the normal anatomy of the masticator space, the temporalis muscle inserts on the coronoid process of the mandible. The muscles of mastication are supplied by the masticator nerve, which is a branch of CN V_3. Injury to the nerve will result in atrophy of these muscles. The inferior alveolar nerve, which provides sensation to the mandible and teeth, is the other major nerve in the masticator space.

283. The answers are: A-Y, B-Y, C-Y, D-Y, E-N. *(Harnsberger, pp 310–320.)* Cholesteatomas may be primary (congenital) or secondary (acquired). Primary cholesteatomas arise from epithelial rests and, in the middle ear compartments, most often occur in the epitympanum. The petrous apex is another important location. Secondary cholesteatoma is an acquired, postinflammatory lesion which develops from ingrowth of squamous epithelium through the eardrum. The accumulation of squamous and keratin debris within the middle ear gradually causes erosion of the petrous bone and ossicles. Pars flaccida cholesteatomas are much more common than pars tensa lesions; the former typically herniate into Prussak's space in the lateral attic. Cholesterol granulomas are postinflammatory lesions of the petrous apex that generally occur in pneumatized petrous apices. They cause varying degrees of expansion of the petrous apex, and their signal characteristics (hyperintensity on T1- and T2-weighted MR images) help distinguish them from primary cholesteatomas.

Malignant otitis externa is a highly aggressive infection which most often occurs in diabetic patients; *Pseudomonas aeruginosa* is usually the offending organism. It can result in extensive destruction of the skull base and may mimic a neoplasm.

The differential diagnosis of pulsatile tinnitus includes paraganglioma, dural arteriovenous malformation, aberrant internal carotid artery, and a dehiscent or high jugular bulb. CT and angiography are the best modalities to evaluate these clinical problems, as all these lesions may be missed by MR imaging.

284. The answers are: A-N, B-N, C-Y, D-N, E-Y. *(Som & Bergeron, ed. 2, pp 277–348.)* A wide variety of neoplasms may affect the salivary glands. Pleomorphic adenoma (benign mixed tumor) is the most common benign parotid tumor. It is characteristically very well circumscribed and hyperintense on T2-weighted MR images. Warthin tumor (papillary cystadenoma lymphomatosum) is the second most common. It occurs more frequently in males, and is bilateral in 10–30% of cases. It probably arises in heterotopic salivary gland ductal epithelium that is trapped within intraparotid and periparotid lymph nodes. As a result, cystic spaces are common within the tumor.

Adenoid cystic carcinoma (cylindroma) is an infiltrating salivary gland malignancy with a well-known propensity to spread perineurally, which accounts for the frequent clinical presentation of pain. Lymph node metastases are uncommon. Mucoepidermoid carcinomas, on the other hand, metastasize primarily to lymph nodes, bone, lung, and subcutaneous tissues.

Hemangiomas are the most common salivary gland tumor in children. They may contain phleboliths. Lymphangiomas most frequently arise in the posterior triangle of the neck, although they may spread to salivary glands, muscles, and vessels.

A "simple" ranula is a mucus retention cyst, which most often occurs in the sublingual salivary glands. A "plunging" ranula is a mucocele that develops from rupture of the wall of a simple ranula. It has no epithelial lining and is therefore really a pseudocyst.

285. The answers are: A-Y, B-Y, C-N, D-N, E-N. *(Harnsberger, pp 390–391.)* The pterygopalatine fossa is a small pyramidal space situated below the orbital apex. It is extremely important, as it communicates with multiple fissures, canals, and foramina including (1) the infratemporal fossa, via the pterygomaxillary fissure, (2) the oral cavity, via the pterygopalatine canal, (3) the orbit, via the inferior orbital fissure, (4) the middle cranial fossa, via the foramen rotundum and the vidian canal, and (5) the superior meatus of the nasal cavity, via the sphenopalatine foramen. The pterygopalatine fossa contains the pterygopalatine ganglion and the distal portion of the internal maxillary artery.

It is obvious that once a malignant neoplasm reaches the pterygopalatine fossa, it may easily spread to a wide variety of anatomic locations.

286–288. The answers are: 286-E, 287-B, 288-D. *(Harnsberger, pp 312–321, 468–470.)* Pulsatile tinnitus may be secondary to vascular anomalies (e.g., aberrant internal carotid artery and dehiscent or high jugular bulb), vascular lesions (e.g., AVM and stenosis), or tumor (e.g., paraganglioma). Glomus tympanicum is a paraganglioma arising at the cochlear promontory of the middle ear cavity. It presents with pulsatile tinnitus and/or a vascular tympanic membrane. Since it is a highly vascular tumor, intense enhancement occurs after CT or MR contrast administration.

The acoustic pathway is divided into sensory (cochlear) and neural (retrocochlear) components. Congenital or inflammatory lesions of the cochlea (cochlear otosclerosis) cause a sensory hearing loss. Retrocochlear hearing loss has multiple etiologies; acoustic schwannoma is the classic tumor responsible for a neural hearing loss. Audiometric testing can localize a lesion to either the sensory or neural component of the acoustic pathway.

Gradenigo syndrome refers to inflammation of the petrous apex (petrous apicitis). Patients present with sixth-nerve palsy and pain in the temporal region resulting from involvement of the adjacent fifth cranial nerve. Pneumatization of the petrous apex predisposes to inflammatory lesions in this location. Imaging of patients with Gradenigo syndrome often reveals a destructive lesion involving the petrous apex, often with opacification of the ipsilateral middle ear and mastoid.

Cholesteatomas most commonly result in conductive hearing loss.

289, 290. The answers are: 289-C, 290-D. *(Atlas, pp 894–895, 956–958.)* As the spinal cord approaches its termination, it tapers gradually, forming the conus medullaris. It continues as a filament of fibrous tissue known as the filum terminale, which extends to the second coccygeal segment. Ependymomas are the most common primary tumors to arise in the lower spinal cord, conus medullaris, and filum terminale. One subtype of ependymoma, the myxopapillary form, is particularly common in the conus and filum; it is a mucin-producing tumor, which is prone to bleeding—sometimes presenting as unexplained subarachnoid hemorrhage.

Fibrolipomas frequently occur in the filum terminale, and may be considered a normal variant if not associated with tethering of the spinal cord or neurologic dysfunction. These developmental lesions arise secondary to the persistence of caudally located pleuripotential cells that differentiate into fat. Fibrolipomas of the filum may be intradural or extradural, or both; extradural lesions tend to be diffuse. They do not occur in the region of the aqueduct of Sylvius and are best evaluated by sagittal and axial T1-weighted MR images, because of their high signal (fat).

Ependymomas arising in the aqueduct are extremely unusual. When they occur intracranially, ependymomas tend to have a *cellular* histology. The *myxopapillary* histologic pattern is seen almost exclusively in ependymomas of the conus and filum.

291, 292. The answers are: 291-C, 292-B. *(Atlas, pp 289–292, 700–701. Osborn, pp 69–72.)* Hemangioblastomas are the most common primary neoplasms in the adult posterior fossa and arise most frequently in the cerebellum. Supratentorial hemangioblastomas are rare. The solid portions of these neoplasms are extremely vascular, and the large tumor vessels appear as flow voids on MR images. Glomus tumors, which are typically benign, and are also known as *paragangliomas,* arise from chemoreceptor cells located at several specific sites in the head and neck. The middle ear is the site of glomus tympanicum tumors, whereas glomus jugulare lesions arise in the jugular fossa. Glomus tumors are also extremely vascular, and signal voids secondary to large tumor vessels may be evident on MR scans.

The tympanic branch of the ascending pharyngeal artery is the major source of blood supply to the glomus tympanicum and is therefore often enlarged when a tumor arises there. Cerebellar hemangioblastomas are intraaxial and are therefore usually supplied by the anterior inferior, posterior inferior, or superior cerebellar arteries.

293, 294. The answers are: 293-C, 294-A. *(Banna, pp 278–279, 311–313. Atlas, pp 540–542.)* Dural ectasia is most commonly associated with neurofibromatosis and connective tissue disorders. Bony erosion may occur in association with dural ectasia; for example, in patients with neurofibromatosis a common paraspinal mass is the lateral thoracic meningocele, which often erodes the adjacent ribs and vertebral body. Marfan syndrome is a congenital multisystem growth disturbance caused by a failure to produce normal collagen. Widening of the spinal canal and posterior scalloping of vertebral bodies results from the inherently defective dura.

The most common CNS neoplasm to arise in patients with type 1 neurofibromatosis is the optic nerve glioma, which occurs in 30–90% and is bilateral in 10–20%. Optic nerve gliomas are not associated with Marfan syndrome.

295, 296. The answers are: 295-C, 296-D. *(Barkovich, pp 108, 143.)* The Chiari I malformation consists of caudal extension of the cerebellar tonsils (tonsillar ectopia) below the foramen magnum. Tonsillar ectopia of 3 mm or less is rarely significant; however, the incidence of symptoms rises when the tonsils extend beyond 5 mm below the foramen magnum. About 20–25% of individuals with the Chiari I malformation have concurrent nonenhancing syringohydromyelia, which may involve the entire length of the spinal cord. Tectal "beaking" is associated with the Chiari II malformation. It refers to the pointed appearance of the mesencephalon, due to fusion of the colliculi and to compression by the cerebellum and temporal lobes; beaking is not a feature of the Chiari I malformation.

Cervical cord hemangioblastomas account for only 3% of intramedullary tumors, and 30% of these will arise in the setting of von Hippel–Lindau syndrome. Purely intramedullary lesions are associated with cyst/syrinx formation in two-thirds of cases. The cysts may be very extensive in comparison to the size of the tumor nodule. Indeed, the presence of a holocord cyst, with only small areas of enhancement, should raise the possibility of hemangioblastoma. Moreover, it may be difficult to differentiate idiopathic syringomyelia (e.g., due to Chiari I malformation) from syringomyelia secondary to hemangioblastoma without the use of gadolinium.

297, 298. The answers are: 297-C, 298-D. *(Schnitzlein, Murtagh, 2d ed., 1990, pp 104–120.)* MR has revolutionized the evaluation of lesions affecting the medial temporal lobe and hippocampal formation. Multiplanar imaging (particularly coronal views) and superb sensitivity and contrast resolution permit detection of diseases such as herpes encephalitis, hippocampal sclerosis, small gliomas, and choroidal fissure cysts.

The hippocampal formation consists of the dentate gyrus, hippocampus, subiculum, and parahippocampal gyrus. The choroid fissure lies above the dentate gyrus and the anterior and posterior choroidal arteries course through it. The hippocampus lies medial to the temporal horn of the lateral ventricle. The hippocampal sulcus is a potential space between the dentate gyrus and subiculum. Focal atrophy of the hippocampal formation (e.g., mesial temporal sclerosis) results in dilatation of the temporal horn and choroid fissure, whereas mass lesions compress these CSF-containing structures. Comparison of both medial temporal lobes should be performed routinely on all MR scans, particularly in patients with seizures.

The dentate *nucleus* is part of the cerebellum.

299, 300. The answers are: 299-C, 300-B. *(Atlas, pp 292–296, 640–644.)* Germinomas of the central nervous system generally develop in the midline, most frequently in the pineal region, followed by the suprasellar area and fourth ventricle. Rarely, they may arise in the basal ganglia or thalamus. Suprasellar germinomas occur either as a metastatic deposit from a pineal region tumor or as a primary suprasellar neoplasm. Unlike pineal germinomas, which show a 10:1 male predominance, germinomas of the suprasellar region affect males and females equally. There is a marked tendency for them to spread through cerebrospinal fluid pathways.

Craniopharyngiomas arise from remnants of the craniopharyngeal duct (Rathke's cleft). They account for approximately 50% of suprasellar tumors in children and occur almost exclusively in the region of the sella turcica and suprasellar cistern. Although the incidence of craniopharyngiomas peaks in childhood, a second, smaller peak occurs in the sixth decade of life. Craniopharyngiomas may extend into the anterior, middle, or posterior cranial fossa in 25% of cases.

Nuclear Medicine

DIRECTIONS: Each question below contains five suggested responses. Select the **one best** response to each question.

301. A 17-year-old male patient with neurologic abnormalities had the scan shown in the figure. The MOST likely diagnosis is

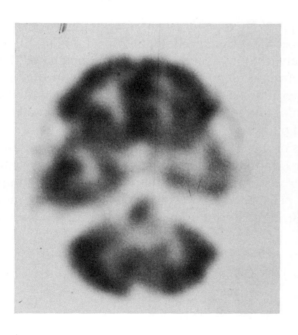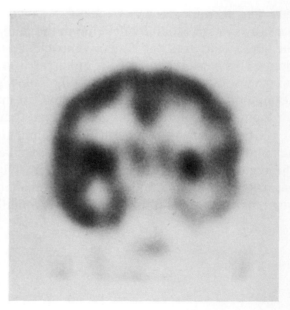

(A) Alzheimer disease
(B) infarct
(C) temporal lobe epilepsy
(D) AIDS dementia
(E) Pick disease

302. A young male patient presented with fever and abdominal pain. His scan shown in the figure is a

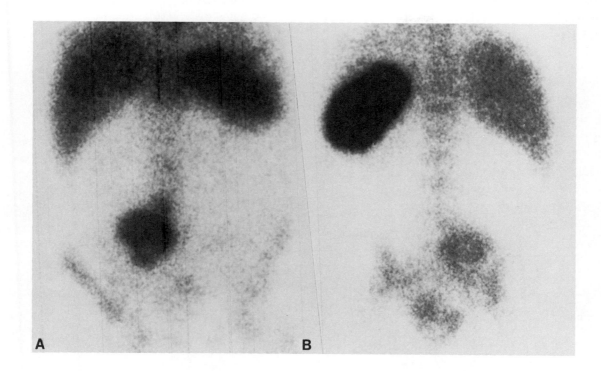

(A) positive Meckel scan
(B) gallium scan with normal bowel uptake
(C) indium scan which reveals an intraabdominal abscess
(D) gallium scan which reveals an intraabdominal abscess
(E) indium scan with swallowed phlegm mimicking an abscess

---

303. The maximum recommended energy for a low-energy collimator is ___ keV, and that for a medium-energy collimator is ___ keV.

(A) 81; 247
(B) 140; 296
(C) 150; 400
(D) 81; 388
(E) 180; 400

304. Pulmonary perfusion scanning with a standard dose (5 mCi) of macroaggregated albumin (MAA) will block what percentage of pulmonary arterioles?

(A) .01%
(B) 0.1%
(C) 1%
(D) 5%
(E) 10%

305. True statements regarding the responsibilities of the radiation safety officer (RSO) include ALL the following EXCEPT

(A) responsible for the investigation of incidents and accidents involving radionuclides
(B) establishes the policies for the delivery and disposal of radioactive products
(C) must be an "authorized user" of radionuclide
(D) must be a member of the Radiation Safety Committee of the facility where employed
(E) collects data on the appropriate calibration of instruments used to measure radiation

306. A whole-body bone scan was performed on this elderly man. The differential diagnosis includes ALL of the following EXCEPT

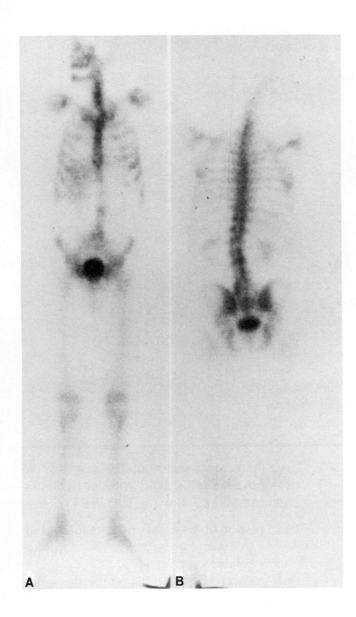

(A) colloid formation
(B) excess aluminum in the eluent or plasma
(C) metastatic disease
(D) free pertechnetate
(E) previous liver scan

307. Based on the figure, the MOST likely diagnosis is

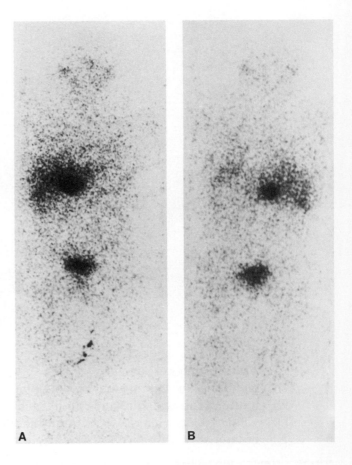

(A) pheochromocytoma
(B) neuroblastoma
(C) hepatoma
(D) hepatitis
(E) metastatic bladder carcinoma

308. In the case of a spill of radionuclide, the personnel in the room are required to do ALL the following EXCEPT

(A) put on gloves before handling potentially contaminated objects
(B) call the Radiation Safety Officer
(C) contain the spill by placing paper towels on it
(D) delineate the area of spill
(E) immediately remove themselves from the area and shower thoroughly

309. The pertechnetate and thallium scans shown in the figures are of a patient suspected of thyroid disease. The findings are consistent with ALL the following EXCEPT

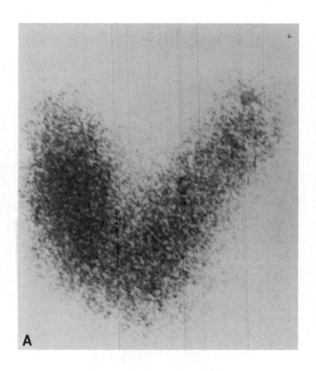 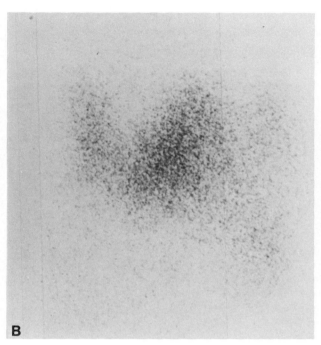

(A) parathyroid adenoma
(B) follicular carcinoma of the thyroid
(C) medullary carcinoma of the thyroid
(D) malignant lymphoma
(E) thyroid cyst

---

310. Choose the dose of ^{131}I that is appropriate for the therapy of Plummer disease.

(A) 3 to 5 millicurie (mCi)
(B) 8 to 15 mCi
(C) 20 to 30 mCi
(D) 75 to 100 mCi
(E) 150 to 200 mCi

311. Hyperthyroidism, thyromegaly, and auto-antibodies are characteristic of

(A) viral thyroiditis
(B) suppurative thyroiditis
(C) de Quervain disease
(D) Plummer disease
(E) Hashimoto thyroiditis

312. The physiologic mechanism underlying the captopril renogram in the diagnosis of renal artery stenosis

(A) causes afferent renal artery vasoconstriction and decreases glomerular filtration pressure
(B) blocks the release of renin by the juxtaglomerular cells
(C) blocks the formation of angiotensin II, impairing efferent renal arteriolar vasoconstriction
(D) blocks the conversion of angiotensinogen to angiotensin I, resulting in a decreased glomerular filtration pressure
(E) none of the above

313. The resolution phantom in the figure is presented to you as part of your routine quality control. It is

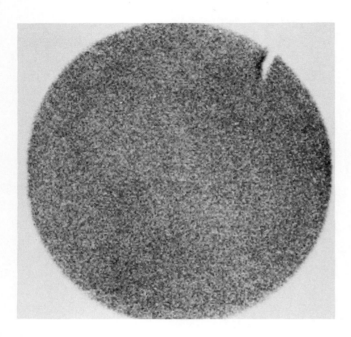

(A) acceptable
(B) abnormal because of a malfunctioning photomultiplier tube
(C) abnormal due to low resolution
(D) abnormal due to a cracked crystal
(E) abnormal due to a technical error in the acquisition

314. Which two diseases have similar findings by scrotal scintigraphy?

(A) Acute torsion and epididymitis
(B) Hydrocele and chronic torsion
(C) Abscess and late torsion
(D) Acute torsion and tumor
(E) Chronic torsion and epididymitis

315. After injection of a ^{99m}Tc diphosphonate compound, the contrast of an image peaks at

(A) 1 hour
(B) 2 hours
(C) 3 hours
(D) 4 hours
(E) 6 hours

316. The testicular scan in the figure may represent ALL the following EXCEPT

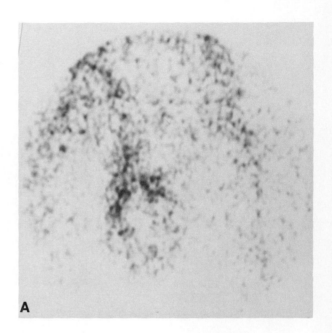

A

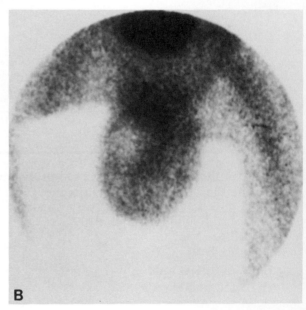

B

(A) acute torsion
(B) chronic (late) torsion
(C) tumor
(D) abscess
(E) incarcerated inguinal hernia

317. Twenty-four-hour anteroposterior and lateral images from a radionuclide cisternogram are presented in the left and right upper figures, respectively. The figures at bottom were taken at 48 hours. The MOST likely diagnosis is

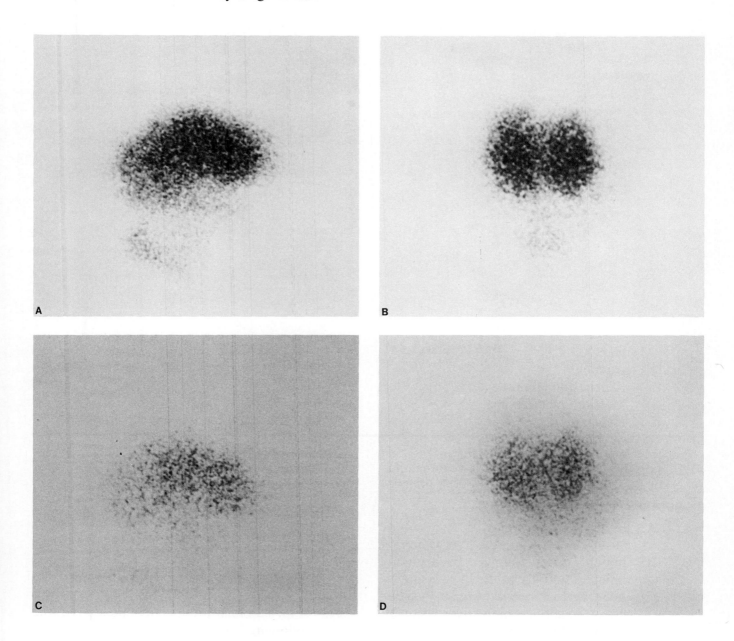

(A) normal examination
(B) severe atrophy
(C) normal pressure hydrocephalus
(D) transient ventricular penetration
(E) cerebrospinal fluid leak

318. Judging from the gallium and sulfur colloid scans in the figures, what would you say is the LEAST likely diagnosis?

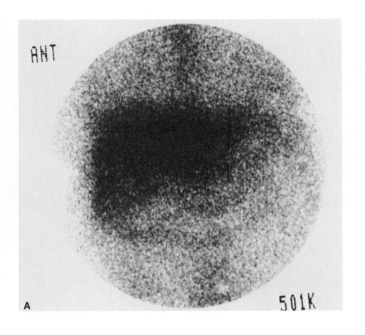 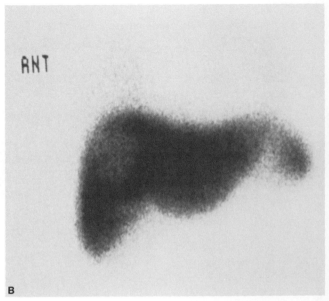

(A) Hepatoma
(B) Adenoma
(C) Regenerating nodule
(D) Metastatic carcinoma
(E) Hemangioma

---

319. For the diagnosis of hepatic hemangioma by ^{99m}Tc RBC scanning, one must demonstrate

(A) hyperperfusion followed by accumulation of activity in the liver lesion
(B) hypoperfusion followed by accumulation of activity in the liver lesion
(C) hyperperfusion followed by a decrease in activity in the liver lesion as compared to normal liver tissue
(D) hypoperfusion followed by a decrease in activity in the liver lesion relative to normal liver
(E) hypoperfusion, and then activity in the lesion equal to that of normal parenchyma

320. Metaiodobenzylguanadine (MIGB) is an analog of

(A) thyroxine
(B) norepinephrine
(C) aldosterone
(D) renin
(E) human chorionic gonadotropin

321. A misadministration is defined as ALL the following EXCEPT

(A) administration of the wrong radiopharmaceutical
(B) administration of a radiopharmaceutical to the wrong patient
(C) administration of a *diagnostic* dose greater or lesser than 10% of the prescribed dose
(D) administration of a *therapeutic* dose greater or lesser than 10% of the prescribed dose

322. Gastric emptying time depends on

   (A) radionuclide used
   (B) meal size
   (C) solid versus liquid food composition
   (D) B and C
   (E) A, B, and C

323. The "superscan" has been reported to occur in ALL the following cases EXCEPT

   (A) hyperparathyroidism
   (B) renal osteodystrophy
   (C) myelofibrosis
   (D) sickle cell disease
   (E) metastatic prostate carcinoma

324. Gated equilibrium blood pool imaging may be effectively performed using

   (A) ^{99m}Tc-labeled red blood cells
   (B) ^{99m}Tc-labeled diethylaminetriamine pentacetic acid (DTPA)
   (C) ^{99m}Tc-labeled human serum albumin
   (D) A and C
   (E) A, B, and C

325. A fixed inferior defect on cardiac thallium imaging may occur due to

   (A) diaphragmatic attenuation
   (B) a right coronary artery infarct
   (C) a left anterior descending artery infarct
   (D) A and B
   (E) A, B, and C

326. A 20-year-old jogger with bilateral leg pain had the bone scan shown in the figure. The MOST likely diagnosis is

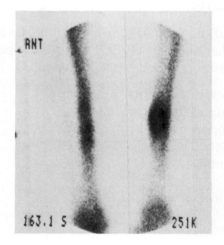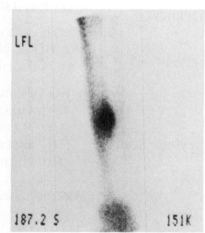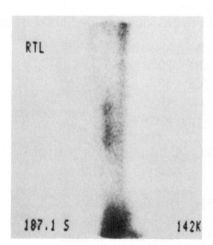

   (A) shin splints
   (B) stress fractures
   (C) both
   (D) neither

DIRECTIONS: Each group of questions below consists of lettered headings followed by a set of numbered items. For each numbered item select the **one** lettered heading with which it is **most** closely associated. Each lettered heading may be used **once, more than once,** or **not at all.**

Questions 327–329

Match each of the following investigative methods to the quality control item it is designed to evaluate.

(A) Dose calibrator, using a lead pig
(B) Rosolic acid paper
(C) Chromatography with acetone
(D) Hemocytometer
(E) Limulus amoebocyte lysate test

327. Molybdenum breakthrough

328. Aluminum breakthrough

329. Macroaggregated albumin particle size

Questions 330–332

For each type of thyroid nodule listed below, select the associated likelihood of malignancy.

(A) less than 10%
(B) 20%
(C) 30%
(D) 40%
(E) greater than 70%

330. Cold nodule in patient with previous head and neck radiation

331. Hot nodule

332. Discordant nodule

Questions 333–335

Match the following lung scan descriptions with the probability that pulmonary embolism has occurred.

(A) Low
(B) Intermediate
(C) High

333. Solitary lobar ventilation/perfusion (V/Q) matched defect, with a matching infiltrate on chest x-ray

334. Solitary segmental V/Q mismatch, with a substantially larger infiltrate on chest x-ray

335. Two segmental V/Q mismatches, with a normal chest x-ray

Questions 336–338

Match each of the following disease entities with the MOST characteristic SPECT brain scan pattern of distribution of decreased activity.

(A) Scattered small foci
(B) Unilateral frontoparietal
(C) Bitemporoparietal
(D) Bicerebellar
(E) Bifrontal

336. Alzheimer disease

337. Pick disease

338. AIDS encephalopathy

Questions 339–341

Match each of the following liver-spleen scan patterns with the entity with which it is MOST likely to be associated.

(A) Estrogen therapy
(B) SVC syndrome
(C) Budd-Chiari syndrome
(D) Hepatoma
(E) Portal hypertension

339. Increased uptake in the quadrate lobe

340. Increased uptake in the caudate lobe

341. Increased uptake in the lungs

Questions 342–345

Match each of the following drugs with the duration of its effect on the radioactive iodine uptake test.

(A) Several hours
(B) 1 week
(C) 4 to 8 weeks
(D) 6 months to 1 year
(E) Several years

342. Iohexol

343. Thyroxine (T_4)

344. Propylthiouracil

345. Pantopaque

DIRECTIONS: Each group of questions below consists of four lettered headings followed by a set of numbered items. For each numbered item select

A	if the item is associated with	(A) **only**
B	if the item is associated with	(B) **only**
C	if the item is associated with	**both** (A) and (B)
D	if the item is associated with	**neither** (A) nor (B)

Each lettered heading may be used **once, more than once,** or **not at all.**

Questions 346–348

(A) The count rate increases proportionately over a given distance
(B) The count rate decreases proportionately over a given distance
(C) Both
(D) Neither

346. Parallel hole collimator

347. Diverging collimator

348. Converging collimator

DIRECTIONS: Each question below contains five suggested answers. For **each** of the **five** alternatives listed, you are to respond either YES or NO. In a given item, **all, some,** or **none of the alternatives may be correct.**

349. Which of the following choices are TRUE regarding qualifications of physicians who administer radionuclides?

    (A) Certification by the American Board of Nuclear Medicine (ABNM) or the American Board of Radiology (ABR) is sufficient to become an authorized user
    (B) Only an authorized user may administer radionuclides
    (C) Any physician who has been reviewed by an authorized user and given training in Radiation Safety procedures may be permitted to handle radionuclides
    (D) 200 hours of training and 500 hours of experience are necessary for physicians who do not have ABNM or ABR board certification
    (E) The radiation safety officer may, at his or her discretion, appoint any physician as an authorized user

350. Decreased perfusion and function as demonstrated by a nuclear renogram may be seen in renal transplant patients in which of the following situations?

    (A) Hyperacute rejection
    (B) Cyclosporin toxicity
    (C) Ureteral obstruction
    (D) Acute tubular necrosis
    (E) Renal artery occlusion

351. Which of the following clinical features are compatible with benign thyroid disease?

    (A) Elderly male
    (B) History of head and neck irradiation
    (C) Nodule which feels hard at palpation
    (D) Solitary nodule
    (E) Elderly female

352. Which of the following statements regarding ^{99m}Tc MAG$_3$ is/are true?

    (A) ^{131}I orthoiodohippuran (OIH) provides superior images, as compared to studies using ^{99m}Tc MAG$_3$
    (B) MAG$_3$ and DTPA are both cleared by glomerular filtration
    (C) ^{99m}Tc MAG$_3$ provides superior images in patients with renal failure, as compared to other renal-imaging agents
    (D) ^{99m}Tc MAG$_3$ and ^{131}I OIH are used to measure effective renal plasma flow
    (E) The bladder is the critical organ for ^{131}I OIH, ^{99m}Tc MAG$_3$, and ^{99m}DTPA

353. Regarding ^{133}Xe ventilation studies, which of the following is/are TRUE?

    (A) The washout phase of a xenon ventilation study will return to baseline in 3 minutes
    (B) Thirty percent of all ventilation defects are seen on the single-breath portion of the lung scan only
    (C) The washout images are the most sensitive for detecting ventilatory abnormalities
    (D) Sensitivity for ventilation abnormalities is greater at 1 minute than at 3 minutes during the washout phase
    (E) Anterior segments are not well-evaluated in ^{133}Xenon ventilation studies

354. The "rim," or pericholecystic hepatic activity (PCHA), sign in hepatobiliary scanning may be positive in cases of

    (A) acute cholecystitis
    (B) chronic cholecystitis
    (C) ascending cholangitis
    (D) gangrene of the gallbladder
    (E) gallbladder perforation

355. Which of the following statements concerning dual isotope parathyroid scintigraphy is/are TRUE?

    (A) Comparison of ^{99m}Tc pertechnetate and ^{201}TI images is useful for identifying a parathyroid adenoma

    (B) The order of administration of isotopes is a critical factor for a successful examination

    (C) A false positive scan may occur with thyroid neoplasm

    (D) Both ^{201}TI and ^{99m}Tc pertechnetate accumulate in normal thyroid tissue

    (E) The study is particularly helpful for parathyroidectomy failures

356. Regarding antibody imaging, which of the following statements is/are TRUE?

    (A) ^{99m}Tc, ^{131}I, and ^{111}In are all capable of being used to label antibodies

    (B) Administering unlabeled antibodies mixed with labeled antibodies does not adversely affect imaging

    (C) SPECT imaging with radiolabeled antibodies rarely adds any additional information beyond planar imaging

    (D) ^{111}In-labeled antibodies tend to localize in the liver and spleen

    (E) Tumor detection using antibodies is approximately 80% at best

357. Regarding ^{111}In-labeled leukocytes, which of the following is/are TRUE?

    (A) They demonstrate an accuracy of greater than 90% for abdominal abscess

    (B) Surgical wound activity may persist for 6 months or longer

    (C) They are superior to gallium for the diagnosis of inflammatory bowel disease

    (D) A concomitant liver scan is often helpful in cases of abdominal abscess

    (E) Diffuse lung activity usually indicates a diffuse inflammatory or infectious process

358. Regarding right ventricular (RV) and pulmonary activity on a thallium cardiac scan,

    (A) RV activity which appears only during the stress portion is abnormal

    (B) substantial RV activity which appears only during a resting study is abnormal

    (C) RV redistribution is a significant finding

    (D) the RV is best visualized on the anterior view

    (E) immediately following a stress examination, the normal ratio of lung to cardiac activity is 30%

359. Which of the following statements about myocardial imaging agents is/are TRUE?

    (A) Thallium enters the myocardial cell utilizing an ATPase-dependent mechanism

    (B) Thallium has a 15% first-pass extraction by the myocardium

    (C) Fifteen percent of the injected thallium localizes in the heart

    (D) Once thallium enters the myocardial cells, it is modified intracellularly and becomes fixed

    (E) A 25% stenosis in a coronary artery is sufficient to produce a perfusion defect during a stress examination

360. Which of the following statements about gated blood pool imaging is/are TRUE?

    (A) An "endless loop" display is used

    (B) The diagnosis of a dyskinetic inferior wall segment is best made by the anterior view

    (C) The right ventricle is best evaluated in the left lateral view

    (D) Septal dyskinesis may occur following cardiopulmonary bypass surgery

    (E) The left atrium is best visualized in the left anterior oblique (LAO) view

361. Regarding hepatobiliary scanning,

    (A) the patient should be NPO for 6 hours

    (B) prolonged fasting (>24 hours) can affect the results

    (C) exogenous administration of cholecystokinin prior to the scan may be helpful

    (D) sincalide (Kinevac) may be used during an examination in order to exclude the diagnosis of acute cholecystitis

    (E) intravenous administration of morphine accelerates gallbladder filling

362. Regarding pertechnetate scanning for diagnosis of a Meckel diverticulum,

    (A) a false negative scan may occur in patients taking cimetidine (Tagamet)

    (B) intravenous glucagon administration is often helpful

    (C) pentagastrin (Pentavlon) has been reported to cause false negative scans

    (D) a Meckel diverticulum will concentrate ^{99m}Tc pertechnetate whether or not gastric mucosa is present

    (E) an intussusception may cause a false positive scan

363. Regarding benign bone lesions,

    (A) a "double density" sign on a bone scan is typical for osteoid osteoma

    (B) bone islands rarely demonstrate increased uptake

    (C) in a patient with Paget disease, decreasing bone uptake on serial scans indicates a response to therapy

    (D) the "double stripe" sign is found in patients with hypertrophic pulmonary osteoarthropathy

    (E) decreased flow on the first phase of a three-phase bone scan is typical for reflex sympathetic dystrophy

364. Which of the following statements about the detection of skeletal metastases with ^{99m}Tc-labeled methylene diphosphonate is/are true?

    (A) Multiple myeloma lesions are detected with greater sensitivity by plain radiography than by bone scanning

    (B) Thyroid carcinoma metastases to the skeleton are more likely to be detected using ^{131}I

    (C) Neuroblastoma metastases are more likely to be detected by radiographs than bone scan

    (D) Metastatic neuroblastoma is more likely to be detected by an MIBG scan as compared to a bone scan

    (E) Renal cell carcinoma metastases are detected by bone scan with a sensitivity approaching 90%

365. Regarding bone scanning,

    (A) in a patient with a known primary tumor, a solitary bone lesion has a 25% probability of being a metastasis

    (B) a single lesion in a rib has a 90% probability of being benign

    (C) a string of lesions in adjacent ribs is unlikely to represent tumor

    (D) sternal metastases are a typical pattern of spread for breast carcinoma

    (E) increased activity in a metastasis in a patient being treated for renal cell carcinoma indicates progression of disease

366. Which of the following statements regarding DTPA aerosol ventilation scans is/are TRUE?

    (A) The aerosol is deposited using a single-breath technique

    (B) Aerosolized particles of less than 0.5 μm are desirable

    (C) The aerosol ventilation study must be performed prior to the perfusion study

    (D) The count rates of the ^{99m}Tc DTPA aerosol and ^{99m}Tc MAA perfusion studies must have a ratio of at least 2:1

    (E) Aerosol studies are generally unsuccessful in ventilator patients

Nuclear Medicine

Answers

---

301. The answer is C. *(Devous, Sem Nucl Med, 20(4), pp 325–341, 1990.)* The axial and coronal views from the SPECT technetium-labeled (^{99m}Tc) HMPAO brain scan in the figure reveal decreased activity in the left temporal lobe, which corresponds to an EEG that localized abnormal activity to the same area in this patient with partial complex seizures. In the interictal state, there is decreased activity in the region of the seizure focus. During the ictus, increased activity is seen at the seizure focus and often also at remote sites.

The other diagnoses are unlikely. Alzheimer disease typically demonstrates bitemporal and biparietal defects. Pick disease is localized to the frontal lobes. Both occur primarily in the elderly. AIDS dementia tends to exhibit multiple small areas of decreased activity.

302. The answer is C. *(Mettler, ed. 3, pp 262–266.)* The figure shown is an indium-labeled leukocyte scan. There is a characteristic distribution of radiotracer activity in the spleen, liver, and bone marrow, and an absence of bowel activity. The figure at left is an anterior view, and the figure at right is a posterior view. The activity in the right lower quadrant represents a diverticular abscess.

Indium scans are the best means of looking for an intraabdominal abscess because of the lack of bowel activity, which might otherwise obscure foci of abnormal uptake. Intraabdominal pathology that can be diagnosed with ^{111}In-labeled leukocytes include inflammatory bowel disease, vasculitis, and abscess. Choice (E), swallowed phlegm, can be a cause of abnormal bowel activity; however, it is unusual for it to remain so intensely active by the time it has reached the right lower quadrant.

303. The answer is C. *(Mettler, ed. 3, p 16.)* The purpose of a collimator is to prevent scatter photons from reaching the scintillation crystal. It does this by attenuating those photons whose angle of approach is not perpendicular to the crystal. The collimator consists of a layer of lead which is perforated by multiple holes. The walls between the holes are called *septa;* their thickness varies with the energy of the scatter radiation they are required to intercept.

A low-energy collimator is designed to be used with radionuclides whose emissions are up to 150 kiloelectronvolts (keV); it is used for ^{99m}Tc and ^{201}Tl. A medium-energy collimator is designed for radionuclides with emissions of up to 400 keV; it is used for ^{131}Iodine and ^{111}In.

304. The answer is B. *(Taylor, p 257.)* In an adult, there are approximately 280 million pulmonary arterioles. Between 200,000 and 500,000 particles are injected for a lung scan, therefore approximately 1 in 1,000 or 0.1% are embolized. The biological $T_{1/2}$ of these particles is between 2 and 9 hours, depending on a number of factors.

In the infant or child, the number of arterioles is not as great and the number of particles is therefore reduced to 100,000. In patients with pulmonary hypertension, who have thickening of the arterial walls and pruning of the vascular tree, the number of particles must also be reduced.

305. **The answer is C.** *(Mettler, ed. 3, pp 269–270.)* The radiation safety officer (RSO) does not have to be an authorized user, but he or she is responsible for deciding who is an authorized user. The duties of the RSO include documentation of incidents and accidents involving radionuclides, radioactive waste disposal, and data collection during the calibration of instruments.

The RSO also reviews the cleanup of radionuclide spills, supervises the maintenance of departmental surveys and wipe-test routines, and investigates misadministrations. He or she is always a member of the facility's Radiation Safety Committee, which also includes an authorized user, an administrator, and a representative of nursing services.

306. **The answer is C.** *(Mettler, ed. 3, p 226)* The whole-body bone scan in the figure shows nonuniform increased liver activity. (The left and right figures are anterior and posterior views, respectively.) The uneven distribution of the hepatic uptake makes a malignancy in the liver the most likely choice. A liver spleen scan in this patient demonstrated a large photopenic defect in the right lobe of the liver, which proved to be a (mucinous) colon cancer metastasis. Breast carcinoma metastases may also pick up bone tracer, and widespread cholangiocarcinoma is another cause of this scintigraphic appearance.

Were this a case of free pertechnetate, activity would be expected in the bowel and thyroid. Colloid formation, which most commonly results from excess aluminum in the eluate, results in particles that are large enough to be picked up by the reticuloendothelial cells in the liver. Activity is usually uniform. Another common artifact that causes increased liver activity is a recent sulfur-colloid, hepatobiliary, or gallium scan.

307. **The answer is A.** *(Freeman, ed. 3, pp 2028–2067.)* The ^{131}I metaiodobenzylguanidine (MIBG) scan shown in the figure reveals intense activity in the region of the right adrenal gland (the figures at left and right are anterior and posterior views, respectively). MIBG scanning is used primarily for the imaging of pheochromocytoma, and uptake of the radionuclide occurs with both primary tumor and metastases. The sensitivity for detection of pheochromocytoma has been reported to be between 79 and 89%.

However, MIBG is not specific for pheochromocytoma. It is an analog of norepinephrine and is taken up by other neurosecretory tumors, such as neuroblastoma, carcinoid, paraganglioma, and medullary carcinoma of the thyroid.

308. **The answer is E.** *(Mettler, ed. 3, p 325.)* Following a radionuclide spill, the radiation safety officer (RSO) should be notified. All personnel involved in the immediate area should wait for the arrival of the RSO. It is the responsibility of the RSO to see that personnel and their clothing are not contaminated. Paper booties of the type worn in the operating room will help prevent contamination of shoes. Before helping to contain a spill, personnel should be gloved. The area of the spill should be clearly marked, and although personnel should wait outside the immediate area of the spill, it is vitally important that they not track radioactivity around the hospital.

309. The answer is E.   *(Freeman, ed. 3, p 2074.)*   Parathyroid scintigraphy is usually a combination of pertechnetate and thallium imaging. A pertechnetate (thyroid) scan is subtracted from a thallium (both thyroid and parathyroid) scan to reveal parathyroid activity alone, although the pathology is evident in most cases without subtraction. In the thyroid scan shown in the figure at left, there is a large mass effect on the lateral aspect of the left lobe of the thyroid. On the thallium scan in the figure at right, there is diffuse uptake adjacent to the left lobe of the thyroid corresponding to a palpable mass. This was found to be a medullary carcinoma of the thyroid. The differential diagnosis for false positives in parathyroid scintigraphy include thyroid carcinoma, goiter, and malignant lymphoma. A thyroid cyst would not be expected to take up thallium or pertechnetate.

Parathyroid adenomas may appear in various shapes: circular, oval, tubular, or irregular. They may be located in the thyroid, adjacent to the thyroid, or in a remote location (e.g., the mediastinum). Multiple areas of abnormal uptake on a thallium scan would suggest the diagnosis of parathyroid hyperplasia, a not-infrequent cause of hyperparathyroidism.

310. The answer is C.   *(Taylor, p 164.)*   Between 20 and 30 mCi is the appropriate therapeutic dose of radioactive iodine (RAI) for Plummer disease. Plummer disease, or toxic nodular goiter, consists of single or multiple autonomous nodules which may cause thyrotoxicosis. Since the nodules are autonomous, TSH is suppressed. This has a protective effect on normal thyroid tissue, which then does not avidly take up the radioactive iodine. Because the dose targets abnormal tissue, one may give a larger dose than is given for the treatment of Grave disease (8–15 mCi), with a lower risk of inducing subsequent hypothyroidism.

311. The answer is E.   *(Taylor, p 165.)*   Hashimoto thyroiditis is characterized by autoantibodies to thyroid tissue and thyromegaly. It may be accompanied by hyperthyroidism, hypothyroidism, or normal thyroid function. A thyroid scan may reveal uniform increased uptake, a multinodular goiter, or diffusely poor uptake. Sometimes, it may be difficult to distinguish from Grave disease.

De Quervain, or subacute, thyroiditis usually follows a viral illness. It presents with hyperthyroidism, thyromegaly, and can be painful. Suppurative thyroiditis results from bacterial infection and is rare. Plummer disease, or toxic multinodular goiter, occurs as a result of the development of one or more autonomously functioning nodules.

312. The answer is C.   *(Taylor, p 138. Mettler, ed. 3, p 242.)*   Captopril is an angiotensin I converting enzyme (ACE) inhibitor. If renal artery stenosis exceeds 60%, the drop in afferent arteriolar blood pressure will stimulate renin production by the juxtaglomerular cells and the subsequent production of angiotensin I. The conversion of angiotensin I to angiotensin II is blocked by the ACE inhibitors. Angiotensin II increases efferent renal arteriolar vasomotor tone. Patients with renal artery stenosis rely on efferent arteriolar constriction to maintain their glomerular filtration pressure. The use of an ACE inhibitor causes a deterioration in renal function.

If the renal artery stenosis is unilateral, the use of captopril will induce a discrepancy between the renogram curves of the two kidneys. When bilateral, both curves will be abnormal. Use of time-to-peak measurements and the $t_{1/2}$ clearance of radiotracer will help distinguish this situation.

313. The answer is D.   *(Sorenson, p 302.)*   In the figure, a crack in the crystal is evident in the 1 o'clock position. Scintillation crystals are typically made up of thallium-activated sodium iodine (NaI), and standard thicknesses are between one-quarter and one-half inch. The crystals are "grown" and are hence very expensive. They are also very fragile and may crack due to a direct blow or a rapid change in temperature.

Thinner crystals are preferred for technetium and thallium imaging because of better intrinsic resolution. Thicker crystals have a better detection efficiency and are useful for higher-energy radionuclides.

314. The answer is C. *(Mettler, ed. 3, p 249.)* Scrotal imaging is usually performed with 10 to 20 mCi of ^{99m}Tc pertechnetate. Dynamic (2-second) images will reveal increased perfusion in cases of infection or tumor. Normal flow or a "nubbin" sign may be seen in acute testicular torsion (the nubbin is the occluded artery). Static (5-minute) images reveal decreased activity in the testicle in cases of torsion, reactive hydrocele, abscess, and, occasionally, a necrotic tumor. Increased activity in the scrotal wall may also accompany cases of infection and tumor, giving the so-called halo sign.

315. The answer is E. *(Taylor, p 381.)* Contrast has been defined by Alazraki as the target-to-background ratio, after correction for compartment volume; it increases over 6 hours following injection of a bone tracer. Images, however, are usually obtained at 2 to 4 hours as a matter of practicality.

316. The answer is A. *(Mettler, p 249.)* The pertechnetate testicular scan in the figure reveals increased activity due to hyperemia in the flow phase (A) and a round, photopenic area in the right hemiscrotum on the delayed image (B). This is a case of late torsion, though an abscess or incarcerated inguinal hernia may have a similar scintigraphic pattern. A tumor may look similar, if central necrosis has occurred.

Acute torsion should have normal or decreased activity during the flow phase, and a photon-deficient area on the delayed scans. Epididymoorchitis typically demonstrates early hyperemia as well as increased activity on the delayed images.

317. The answer is C. *(Freeman, ed. 3, pp 679–703. Taylor, pp 310–314.)* In the ^{111}In nuclear cisternogram shown in the figure, there is persistent activity in the ventricles and no increase in activity over the convexity at either 24 or 48 hours. This is typical of normal pressure hydrocephalus (NPH), a type of obstructive, communicating hydrocephalus.

Normally, activity should ascend over the convexity by 24 hours. A delay in ascent is not specific for NPH, and may also be seen with severe atrophy.

Transient ventricular penetration may occur between 4 and 6 hours, but should not persist beyond that. CSF leaks may be diagnosed by nuclear cisternography, in which case pledgets are placed in the nares to collect tracer which has leaked through. These are then counted in a well counter. Occasionally, a leak may be large enough to detect visually.

318. The answer is E. *(Freeman, ed. 3, p 357. Mettler, ed. 3, p 257.)* The gallium scan in the figure at left reveals uniform activity throughout the liver. The anterior image from the sulfur colloid scan (see figure at right), however, shows a large photopenic area in the right lobe, which proved to be a hepatoma. Usually, hepatoma will have increased activity relative to the liver on a gallium scan, though it may be isointense, as in this case.

Adenomas, metastases, and regenerating nodules will take up gallium, but appear as defects on sulfur colloid imaging. A hemangioma will present as a defect on both types of scan.

319. The answer is B. *(Taylor, p 351.)* Cavernous hemangiomas typically demonstrate hypoperfusion on the angiographic phase, followed by a relative increase in activity in the liver lesion as compared to the normal liver tissue. It has been suggested that a 2-hour delayed scan may improve specificity. Hepatoma and metastases tend to be hypervascular and to have decreased activity on a delayed scan. Delayed increased activity alone, without hypoperfusion, is less specific than the combination of the two. SPECT imaging is useful in the diagnosis, because of the improved tissue contrast as compared to planar imaging.

320. The answer is B. *(Freeman, ed. 3, pp 2028–2067.)* Wieland et al. synthesized metaiodobenzylguanidine (MIBG) in 1979. It is taken up by adrenergic tissue through both sodium-dependent and sodium-independent mechanisms, in a manner similar to norepinephrine. It then localizes in intracellular storage granules.

321. The answer is C. *(Mettler, ed. 3, p 275.)* Administration of a diagnostic dose greater or less than 50% of the prescribed dose is considered a misadministration. Standard doses for adults and children should be posted in the department. The person administering the dose is the one responsible for its content. Either the syringe or syringe shield should be labeled as to radionuclide content. Doses should be measured by a dose calibrator immediately prior to injection, even if they are unit doses prepared by a remote laboratory. Records of a misadministration are required to be kept for 10 years.

322. The answer is D. *(Taylor, pp 351–353.)* Gastric emptying time depends on several factors. A radiopharmaceutical administered as a liquid will empty more rapidly than as a part of solid food. A solid, gastric emptying study, however, may find an abnormality which has been missed by a liquid study. Caloric content and meal size also affect the emptying time, but the radionuclide used has no affect.

In a biphasic gastric emptying study, one radionuclide is tagged to a solid and a different one is tagged to a liquid, which allows simultaneous evaluation.

323. The answer is D. *(Taylor, p 384.)* A "superscan" is the demonstration of intense tracer uptake in the skeleton, with no significant activity in the soft tissues. The most common cause of the superscan is metastatic disease from breast or prostate carcinoma. Among other causes are metabolic bone diseases, such as osteomalacia, hyperparathyroidism, and renal osteodystrophy.

Sickle cell disease causes increased activity in the skull on a bone scan because of marrow expansion, and in the long bones because of infarction. There is also increased activity in the kidneys and spleen.

324. The answer is D. *(Freeman, ed. 3, p 364. Mettler, ed. 3, p 318.)* Human serum albumin was the first agent used in the performance of gated equilibrium blood pool studies of the heart. Currently, tagged red blood cells (RBCs) are the most commonly used agent. In general, two methods are used to tag RBCs: (1) in vivo and (2) in vivo/in vitro, or in "viv-tro." In the first method, 2 mg of stannous pyrophosphate are injected intravenously. After 10 to 20 minutes, 20 mCi of ^{99m}Tc pertechnetate are injected. This results in 60–70% labeling. In the modified technique, stannous pyrophosphate is again injected intravenously. Rather than inject the pertechnetate, however, 3 cc of blood is withdrawn into a heparinized syringe which contains the pertechnetate. It is incubated for 10 to 15 minutes and then reinjected. This results in an 88% tag.

DTPA is excreted by the kidneys too rapidly to be of use as an imaging agent in these studies.

325. The answer is D. *(Iskandrian, p 90.)* Diaphragmatic attenuation typically causes a fixed inferior defect on thallium scans of the heart, which is indistinguishable from an inferior infarct. Some work has been done to show that diaphragmatic attenuation may be eliminated by the use of a prone view, which displaces the heart anteriorly.

An inferior wall infarct is typically caused by occlusion of the posterior descending artery (PDA) or right coronary artery disease (90%). In those patients in whom the PDA originates from the left circumflex artery, the inferior wall may be at risk for myocardial infarction in cases of circumflex disease. Left anterior descending occlusion characteristically causes an anterior wall or septal infarct.

326. The answer is C. *(Thrall, pp 127–129.)* In the static bone scan images of the legs in the figure, there is increased uptake in a long segment of the right tibial cortex. This is the characteristic appearance of shin splints. In the left mid-tibia, there is a fusiform focus of increased activity, which represents a stress fracture. A bone scan is more sensitive than a radiograph for the diagnosis of both shin splints and stress fractures, and often becomes positive earlier in the course of disease. A mixed injury is also not uncommon.

327–329. The answers are: 327-A, 328-B, 329-D. *(Mettler, ed. 3, pp 30–36.)* ^{99}Mo breakthrough is limited to 0.15 μCi/mCi^{99m}Tc, by NRC and USP regulations. It is measured by putting a sample of the generator eluate in a lead shield (pig) and placing it in a well counter. The ^{99m}Tc photons are attenuated by the shield, but the higher-energy ^{99}Mo (740 and 780 keV) penetrate the shield and are easily counted. ^{99}Mo has half-life of 66.7 hours as opposed to 6.03 hours for ^{99m}Tc. Thus, a sample that has an acceptable level of breakthrough initially will progressively demonstrate greater ^{99}Mo activity, relative to ^{99m}Tc activity, over time and eventually become unacceptable for human use.

Aluminum breakthrough is caused by the leaching of aluminum from the generator's elution column. When excess aluminum accumulates, it results in the formation of large particles, or colloid, which are then taken up by the liver. If used in the preparation of sulfur colloid, the particles that form may be large enough to be deposited in the lungs. The presence of aluminum is limited by USP standards to 10 μg/ml of eluate. The concentration may be tested by rosolic acid paper. A small sample of eluate is placed on the test strip next to a drop of a standard solution. If the eluate turns the paper a darker shade of red than the standard, aluminum "breakthrough" has occurred.

Macroaggregated albumin (MAA) particle size may be evaluated by using a hemocytometer slide. MAA particles are expected to have a maximum size of 150 μm, and 90% of them should be between 10 and 90 μm. The purpose of these particles is to embolize the pulmonary capillary bed, which consists of vessels measuring from 7 to 10 μm in diameter. Larger particles will embolize the pulmonary arterioles, which is undesirable.

330–332. The answers are: 330-D, 331-A, 332-E. *(Mettler, ed. 3, pp 80, 83–84. Taylor, p 167.)* Forty percent of patients who have had radiation treatment of the head and neck and who develop a poorly functioning, or "cold," nodule will have a malignancy. A cold nodule in a patient without antecedent radiation has only a 20% chance of being malignant.

A hyperfunctioning, or "hot," nodule has a less than 1% probability of being a malignancy; they are usually hyperfunctioning adenomas. They are not suppressible by thyroid hormone. A T$_3$ thyroid suppression test may be performed by obtaining radioactive iodine uptake studies before and after a 7-day course of triiodothyronine (Cytomel, T$_3$).

A discordant nodule is defined as one that demonstrates uptake on a ^{99m}Tc pertechnetate study, but not on a 24-hour ^{123}I examination. This represents normal trapping of iodine but failure of organification, and indicates a 78% probability of malignancy. Some institutions use ^{123}I routinely for all their thyroid examinations, though it is expensive because it is produced in a cyclotron. Some authors feel that a more practical alternative is for a hot nodule found on a pertechnetate scan to be followed up by an ^{123}I scan.

333–335. The answers are: 333-B, 334-A, 335-C. *(Taylor, p 274.)* The two most widely used sets of criteria for classification of lung scan findings are Biello's, published in 1976, and the Prospective Investigation of Pulmonary Embolism Diagnosis (PIOPED). The major difference between the two is the placement of a single V/Q mismatch into the indeterminate category by Biello, and into the low-probability category by PIOPED.

A lobar matched defect, with a corresponding infiltrate on chest x-ray, is indeterminate for pulmonary embolism, whereas if the infiltrate is substantially larger, the likelihood that embolism has occurred is reduced to only 7%. There is a probability of approximately 90% that two segmental mismatches, with a normal chest x-ray, represent pulmonary embolism.

336–338. The answers are: 336-C, 337-E, 338-A. *(Bonte, Sem Nucl Med 20(4), pp 344–345, 1990. Kramer, Sem Nucl Med 20(4), pp 353–363, 1990.)* In patients with Alzheimer disease, brain scans typically reveal bitemperoparietal defects. Accompanying bifrontal decreased activity has also been described. Sensitivities of 80–90% have been reported using either hexamethylpropylene amine oxime (HMPAO) or iodoamphetamine (IMP).

Pick disease is a form of dementia which is clinically similar to Alzheimer disease. The hallmark is severe atrophy of the anterior portions of both frontal lobes. With SPECT imaging, bifrontal defects are seen, accompanied by volume loss. Progressive supranuclear palsy may also demonstrate similar findings.

AIDS encephalopathy is due to infection of the brain by the HIV virus, and does not indicate an opportunistic infection. Multiple, small cortical defects are seen using SPECT imaging with either IMP or HMPAO. This pattern is not distinguishable from multi-infarct dementia.

339–341. The answers are: 339-B, 340-C, 341-A. *(Taylor, p 326.)* Focally increased activity in the quadrate lobe is typical of superior vena caval (SVC) obstruction. If the dose is injected in an arm, it is shunted into the portal venous system by the azygos and periumbilical veins. The quadrate lobe, for reasons not well-understood (probably flow-related), preferentially localizes the radiotracer.

Increased activity in the caudate lobe is typical of the Budd-Chiari syndrome (inferior vena caval (IVC) or hepatic vein thrombosis). The caudate lobe drains directly into the IVC and serves as the major route of hepatic drainage in the setting of hepatic venous obstruction. The increased flow through the caudate results in asymmetrical deposition of radiotracer.

Diffuse pulmonary activity during a sulfur-colloid liver-spleen scan, occurs with patients receiving estrogen therapy. This may be caused by a release of totipotential cells from the bone marrow, which travel to the lungs and assume the role of phagocytes, which trap the radiopharmaceutical. The differential diagnosis of increased lung activity on a sulfur-colloid scan includes cirrhosis, aluminum breakthrough, collagen vascular disease, Hunter syndrome, histiocytosis X, and widespread pulmonary metastases.

342–345. The answers are: 342-C, 343-C, 344-B, 345-E. *(Taylor, p 159. Freeman, ed. 3, p 1301.)* A large number of drugs can affect the radioactive iodine (RAI) uptake examination. The patient must be questioned about the use of iodine, thyroid hormone, antihyperthyroid drugs, and steroids, and a history of radiographic iodine administration should be obtained. Specifically, propylthiouracil (PTU) must be withheld for 1 week to 10 days. Triiodothyronine (T_3) should be withheld for at least 2 weeks. Thyroxine (T_4) must be stopped 6 weeks prior to studying the patient. No water-soluble iodinated contrast agent should be administered 4 to 8 weeks prior to an RAI uptake. Pantopaque, an oily contrast material once used for myelograms, can decrease the value of RAI uptake for many years.

346–348. The answers are: 346-D, 347-B, 348-C. *(Mettler, ed. 3, pp 16–17.)* When a parallel hole collimator is used, the count rate remains approximately the same as the distance between the collimator and the object increases. The loss of counts, which decreases with the square of the distance, is balanced by the increase in the size of the field-of-view. Furthermore, the objects in the image remain the same size.

With a diverging collimator, the septa diverge away from the collimator face, which results in a minified image. This type of collimator is sometimes used for whole-body bone scans. As the distance from the collimator increases, the number of counts decreases in proportion to the mean-square law. Unlike a parallel hole collimator, this is not compensated for by the increase in field-of-view, since the object occupies less of the field.

When a converging collimator is used, the count rate will increase initially until the focal zone is reached. At that point the count rate begins to decrease. A converging collimator produces a magnified image. The resolution of an object decreases with increasing distance.

349. **The answers are: A-Y, B-N, C-Y, D-Y, E-N.** *(Mettler, ed. 3, pp 271–272.)* Permission to handle radionuclides is not routine. The radiation safety officer (RSO) must determine if a physician is qualified to administer radiopharmaceuticals. Choices (A) and (D) are criteria which are used in this regard. The physician so certified is then considered an "authorized" user. Not every physician who handles radionuclides need be an authorized user. An authorized user may give permission to another physician to use radionuclides, but the latter must receive radiation safety training and be under the supervision of an authorized user.

350. **The answers are: A-Y, B-Y, C-Y, D-N, E-Y.** *(Mettler, ed. 3, p 247. Taylor, p 140.)* Both acute tubular necrosis (ATN) and cyclosporin toxicity typically present with preservation of renal perfusion but poor excretion of radiotracer. However, cyclosporin toxicity, hyperacute and chronic rejection, and ureteral or renal artery occlusion may all have diminished perfusion and function. If severe, the kidney may appear as a photopenic defect in the background blood-pool activity.

351. **The answers are: A-N, B-N, C-N, D-N, E-Y.** *(Mettler, ed. 3, p 84.)* Clinical features favoring a benign diagnosis of a thyroid mass include an older female, multiple nodules, a nodule which is soft to palpation, sudden onset, and a response to thyroid hormone administration. Clinical features of a malignancy include elderly male or young patient, a family history of thyroid cancer, a history of radiation to the head or neck, and a nodule which is hard to palpation.

352. **The answers are: A-N, B-N, C-Y, D-Y, E-N.** *(Mettler, ed. 3, p 238. Freeman [Annual], pp 1–35.)* The count rates per mCi for ^{131}I OIH and ^{99m}Tc MAG$_3$ are similar. However, the dose of a technetium agent can be much greater than a dose of an ^{131}I or ^{123}I agent due to superior dosimetry. The 140 keV photon is preferable for imaging, as compared to the high-energy 364 keV ^{131}I photon. Whereas DTPA is cleared by glomerular filtration only, ^{99m}Tc MAG$_3$ and ^{131}I OIH are both cleared by tubular extraction. Therefore, both agents can be used to measure the effective renal plasma flow. ^{99m}Tc MAG$_3$ is the preferred agent for imaging patients in renal failure because of its high extraction rate and superior target-to-background ratio. Although the bladder is the critical organ for both ^{99m}Tc-DTPA (0.60 R/mCi) and ^{99m}Tc MAG$_3$ 0.48 R/mCi), the thyroid is the critical organ (10–30 R/mCi) when ^{131}I OIH is used.

353. **The answers are: A-Y, B-N, C-Y, D-Y, E-Y.** *(Taylor, pp 262–267.)* The xenon study consists of three phases. First, a single-breath image is obtained, followed by 4 minutes of rebreathing (ending with a 300,000-count image), and 6 minutes of washout images. The lung fields should return to baseline after 3 minutes of washout.

   Only 7% of ventilation abnormalities are seen on the first-breath study alone. Overall, 64% of all ventilatory abnormalities are seen on the first-breath images. On the washout images, there is a 94% sensitivity for ventilatory abnormalities at 1 minute, accompanied by only a 62% specificity. At 3 minutes, the sensitivity decreases to 83%, but the specificity improves to 85%.

   Usually, only posterior images of the lungs are obtained on xenon studies. For this reason, anterior defects are sometimes poorly appreciated.

354. **The answers are: A-Y, B-N, C-N, D-Y, E-Y.** *(Mettler, ed. 3, p 200.)* The pericholecystic hepatic activity (PCHA) sign is a rim of increased activity in the hepatic tissue that surrounds the gallbladder fossa. It occurs in only 20% of hepatobiliary scans that are positive for acute cholecystitis. In 40% of these cases, the gallbladder is gangrenous or has perforated. This sign is not associated with chronic cholecystitis or ascending cholangitis.

355. The answers are: A-Y, B-N, C-Y, D-Y, E-Y. *(Taylor, pp 171–173. Mettler, ed. 3, pp 93–94.)* Pertechnetate scanning will image the thyroid, but thallium will accumulate in both the thyroid and parathyroid glands. Therefore, subtracting the pertechnetate scans from thallium image will reveal parathyroid activity alone. Often, though, parathyroid tissue is identified without the need for subtraction.

Either radionuclide may be administered first. The advantage of performing the thallium scan first is that it has a lower-energy photon which permits imaging without any downscatter from technetium. The disadvantage of this method, however, is that 10 to 20 minutes must elapse after injection of pertechnetate before the thyroid can be imaged. During that time, the patient may move, which may cause a misregistration of the subtraction image and result in a false positive scan. Either technique will work with care. Thallium may accumulate in thyroid malignancies, goiters, and lymphoma, and give a false positive scan.

About 95% of the time, an abnormal parathyroid gland can be found at surgery. When it is not, a parathyroid scan may help locate its position in the neck or mediastinum.

356. The answers are: A-Y, B-Y, C-N, D-Y, E-Y. *(Taylor, pp 187–199.)* SPECT imaging increases both resolution and contrast. This is particularly useful in antibody imaging, because the lesions are often small, superimposed by structures that normally localize antibody, or in areas where there is a lot of blood pool activity. New improvements in SPECT technology, including multihead cameras, faster computers, and new filters, continue to improve image characteristics.

^{99m}Tc, ^{131}I, and ^{111}In have all been used to label antibodies. Unlabeled antibodies help saturate nonspecific binding sites and also help clear antimurine antibodies from the serum, which may otherwise recirculate antigen.

Metastases to the liver can only be detected with difficulty using ^{111}In antibodies because of the nonspecific uptake of the radionuclide by the liver.

Overall, detection of tumor lesions by antibody imaging rarely exceeds 80%, which may be due to a number of causes: circulating antigen may bind antibody far from the tumor site; nonspecific binding of antibodies may occur; the tumor may be poorly vascularized, preventing delivery of antibodies to the tumor site; or the metastases may not express the same antigen as the primary tumor (antigenic heterogenicity).

357. The answers are: A-Y, B-N, C-Y, D-Y, E-N. *(Taylor, pp 210–217.)* The sensitivity for intraabdominal abscess exceeds 90%, which is comparable to CT and ultrasound. The specificity is high as well. Causes of false positive scans include intravenous and nasogastric tubing, colostomy or ileostomy, and inflammatory processes (e.g., Crohn disease and ulcerative colitis).

Gallium is poor for evaluating inflammatory bowel disease, because it produces activity in the gut normally. Tubular activity on an ^{111}In-labeled leukocyte scan, however, is a sensitive indicator of inflammatory bowel disease, though it is not specific for the underlying etiology.

Normal activity in the liver on ^{111}In scan may mask underlying liver or perihepatic pathology. A comparison liver spleen scan may be helpful in this situation.

Faint wound activity persists for approximately 10 days following surgery. After that, it is considered abnormal. Activity adjacent to a wound is also abnormal.

Diffuse lung activity corresponds to disease in only 10% of cases. One in six normal patients have increased pulmonary localization of ^{111}In-labeled WBCs, for reasons which are not clear. Gallium is very sensitive for infectious and inflammatory lung disease, and is the preferred radionuclide in this situation.

358. The answers are: A-N, B-Y, C-Y, D-N, E-Y. *(Mettler, ed. 3, pp 111.)* Activity in the right ventricle (RV) is best visualized on a 30° to 45° LAO view. It is often seen normally during the stress portion of the exam. Its absence, or a defect that later redistributes, should be regarded as suspicious for ischemia. During the redistribution study phase, RV activity is usually too minimal to be visualized in normal individuals. When there is RV activity on a rest-only study, it suggests RV hypertrophy or an increased RV workload, such as pulmonary hypertension.

The right and left chamber sizes are roughly equal by scintigraphy. The ratio of lung to heart activity is usually 30%. A value of 50% or greater is abnormal, and suggests left ventricular dysfunction on the basis of coronary artery disease.

359. The answers are: A-Y, B-N, C-N, D-N, E-N. *(Thrall, p 357. Mettler, p 104.)* Thallium is a potassium analog. It is taken up by the myocardium by a Na^+-K^+ ATPase-dependent pump. The exact mechanism, though, has not been elucidated. The uptake of thallium in the myocardium is directly proportional to coronary blood flow. The first-pass extraction of thallium is 85–90% and the plasma $t_{1/2}$ is 10 minutes.

Thallium moves readily from the intracellular to the extracellular compartment. Therefore, unlike isonitriles, it is not fixed in the cell, and planar imaging should be performed as soon as possible after injection. Thallium also washes out from the myocardial cell in relation to coronary blood flow. Thallium released from the organs of the body is taken up by the heart in a process described as "wash-in." The combination of wash-out and wash-in results in the redistribution image, taken 4 hours after the stress images.

Only 3 to 5% of thallium activity localizes in the heart. Other areas of distribution include the skeleton, liver, GI tract, kidneys, and muscles. Thallium is slowly cleared by urinary excretion. The target organ is the kidney, with a dose of 4 rad from a 3-mCi dose.

A stenosis of at least 50% is necessary to generate a perfusion defect on stress planar imaging.

360. The answers are: A-Y, B-N, C-N, D-Y, E-N. *(Freeman, ed. 3, pp 377–390, 393, 396.)* An endless loop is created to display the cardiac cycle during a gated blood pool study. A rate of 1 to 2 cardiac cycles per second is typically used.

The inferior wall is often partially obscured by the right ventricle (RV) on an anterior view; it is best evaluated on a left lateral view. The left atrium may be seen on a left anterior oblique (LAO) view, especially if it is enlarged, but it is best evaluated by a left lateral view, just as with chest radiography.

The RV is best seen on a shallow LAO view. Visualization of the right ventricle on a left lateral view may indicate RV enlargement; however, this finding must be judged against the rotation of the heart. For instance, if the septum is best seen on a 60°–70° LAO view, then the presence of the right ventricle contour on a left lateral view is expected.

Septal dyskinesis may follow cardiopulmonary bypass. Other causes include bundle branch block, RV pacing, RV volume overload, and septal infarction.

361. The answers are: A-Y, B-Y, C-Y, D-Y, E-Y. *(Taylor, pp 334–335. Mettler, ed. 3, p 200.)* A meal within 6 hours of a hepatobiliary scan results in the release of endogenous cholecystokinin (CCK). This can result in prolonged gallbladder contraction and may give a false positive scan.

Prolonged fasting (>1 day) causes bile stasis and decreased output of bile. This may cause delayed or absent filling of the gallbladder, again giving a false positive scan. A 24-hour follow-up scan may be helpful in this situation.

Sincalide, a synthetic compound, is the active octapeptide of CCK. It has a different physiologic effect on the gallbladder than does endogenous CCK, in that it causes only 5 minutes of contraction and then rapidly resolves. It is sometimes administered before a hepatobiliary scan, when gallbladder emptying is needed, such as with a patient who has been chronically fasting, which allows for more rapid filling. It may also be helpful in rare cases of acute cholecystitis in which there is delayed filling of the gallbladder, mimicking *chronic* cholecystitis; it is given 1 hour into the examination, and failure of the gallbladder to contract suggests an acute process.

A dose of 0.04 mg of morphine per kilogram causes contraction of the sphincter of Oddi, which accelerates gallbladder filling. This maneuver may be used after 1 hour, if the common bile duct and bowel are visualized, but the gallbladder is not.

362. The answers are: A-N, B-Y, C-N, D-N, E-Y. *(Mettler, ed. 3, p 196. Taylor, p 346.)* Pretreatment with cimetidine (Tagamet) for 48 hours before scanning blocks release, but not uptake, of ^{99m}Tc pertechnetate from any gastric mucosa present in a Meckel diverticulum. This useful pharmacologic intervention helps to increase the target-to-background ratio. Glucagon, administered just before the exam, will decrease bowel motility and result in pooling of pertechnetate, thereby improving chances of visualization. Pentagastrin (Pentavlon) increases the uptake of ^{99m}Tc pertechnetate in gastric mucosa by 30%, which serves to increase the target-to-background ratio.

Absence of gastric mucosa is a cause of a false negative examination (approximately 25% of Meckel diverticula contain ectopic mucosa). The secretory cells of the mucosa are thought to also concentrate the pertechnetate.

False positive scans may result from other sources of ectopic gastric mucosa, such as a duplication cyst, or may be due to areas of hyperemia (e.g., intussusception or appendicitis) or increased blood pool activity (e.g., hemangiomas). Pooling of urine, in a urinoma or in an obstructed system, may also cause a false positive.

363. The answers are: A-Y, B-N, C-Y, D-Y, E-N. *(Taylor, pp 395–397.)* The "double density" sign on a bone scan of osteoid osteoma refers to a center of intense activity (the nidus) and a less intense rim of activity due to reactive sclerosis. These lesions are hypervascular on a radionuclide angiogram.

Bone islands demonstrate increased activity approximately 30% of the time. Increased uptake correlates best with larger size. Growing bone islands also demonstrate increased uptake.

Paget disease typically presents with intensely increased activity at multiple sites during its active phase. In its quiescent phase, activity may normalize. In a positive response to therapy, the quantitative uptake of bone tracer will decrease.

Hypertrophic pulmonary osteoarthropathy (HPOA) will demonstrate increased cortical activity in the region of the diaphyses of long bones. The cortices are seen on tangent as two stripes of increased activity. Note that the lower extremities tend to be more involved than the upper extremities. Findings of HPOA may resolve when the primary lesion, usually a lung carcinoma, is resected.

On a three-phase bone scan, reflex sympathetic dystrophy typically demonstrates increased flow and blood pool activity. On the delayed images, increased activity is seen throughout the distal portion of the extremity.

364. The answers are: A-Y, B-Y, C-N, D-Y, E-N. *(Taylor, pp 385–386.)* Multiple myeloma lesions are detected 46% of the time by bone scanning and 82% of the time by x-ray. Similarly, 92% of patients with multiple myeloma will have a positive skeletal survey, as compared to only 78% on a bone scan.

Thyroid metastases to bone are best detected by whole-body ^{131}I images. Only 60% of the bone lesions seen on iodine scans are detected by diphosphonate bone scans.

Neuroblastoma metastases are better detected by a bone scan than by plain film, with a sensitivity of over 90%. Plain-film radiography has a sensitivity of only 67%. Although ^{131}I MIBG is more likely to detect skeletal neuroblastoma metastases than a bone scan, it unfortunately is also more likely to completely miss *all* the lesions in a given patient. Therefore, a bone scan is also usually obtained in a patient with neuroblastoma.

Bone scanning is relatively insensitive for bone metastases in metastatic renal cell carcinoma, with a true positive rate of 50% or less. However, the metastases are usually clinically apparent.

365. The answers are: A-N, B-Y, C-Y, D-Y, E-N. *(Taylor, pp 386–392.)* In a patient with a known malignancy, a single bone lesion on bone scan has a 54% chance of being a metastasis. Pain at the site of a bone lesion increases the likelihood of tumor being present. Half the solitary metastases discovered by bone scan will not be evident on plain film.

Solitary-rib lesions have a 90% chance of being benign. Elongated, horizontal areas of uptake are more likely to represent malignancy and pinpoint foci are more likely to be fractures. A single-rib lesion at the costochondral junction is most likely the result of cartilage injury.

Two lesions adjacent to each other in separate ribs are most likely fractures. Two lesions in the same rib are most likely metastases, unless a corroborative trauma history can be elicited.

Sternal lesions are typical of breast carcinoma. This is because of the propensity for tumor to spread along the internal mammary nodal chain. Typically, they are asymmetrical to the side of the primary lesion.

Increased uptake in metastatic lesions may occur in any patient being successfully treated for malignancy. It represents repair of bone damage and has been called the "flare" phenomenon.

366. The answers are: A-N, B-Y, C-N, D-N, E-N. *(Taylor, pp 261–262.)* ^{99m}Tc-labeled DTPA particles less than 0.5 μm in diameter are desirable for ventilation studies because they behave more like a gas. Larger particles will deposit in the trachea or bronchi. The aerosol is administered through a commercially available nebulizer, and the air is bubbled through at a preset rate. Patients are instructed to take deep breaths with end-inspiratory pauses. When a predetermined count rate is reached, the aerosol is turned off and the patient is imaged.

The order in which the ventilation and perfusion studies are done is not essential. However, the count-rate ratio between the second and first study must be 4:1 or greater. The ventilation study usually is done first. A patient on a respirator may be successfully ventilated with DTPA aerosol, although tracheal deposition will always occur.

Pediatric Radiology

DIRECTIONS: Each question below contains five suggested responses. Select the **one best** response to each question.

367. The MOST likely diagnosis in the figure is

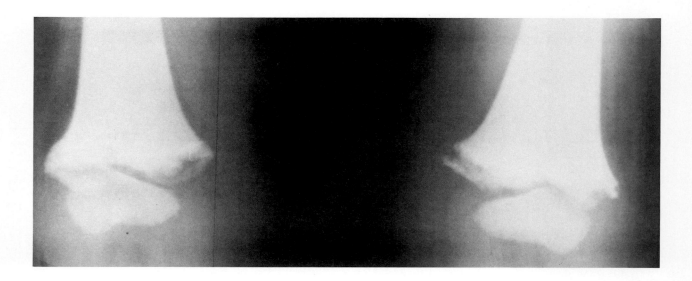

    (A)   syphilis
    (B)   scurvy
    (C)   child abuse
    (D)   rickets
    (E)   neonatal osteomyelitis

368. A newborn with respiratory distress had the chest x-ray shown in the figure. The MOST likely diagnosis is

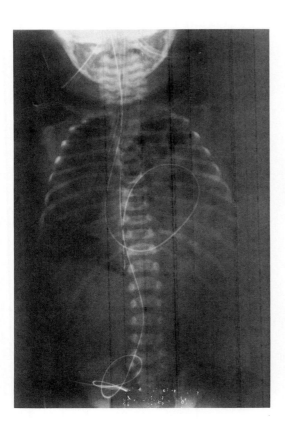

(A) congenital cystic adenomatoid malformation
(B) lobar emyphsema
(C) staphylococcal pneumonia
(D) congenital diaphragmatic hernia
(E) pulmonary interstitial emphysema

369. Cephalohematoma can be distinguished from a subgaleal hygroma by which ONE of the following?

(A) Presence of a depressed skull fracture
(B) Containment within suture lines
(C) Greater density on plain film
(D) Widening of sutures
(E) None of the above

370. A 4-year-old presented with 1 week of bilious vomiting (see figure). The MOST likely diagnosis is

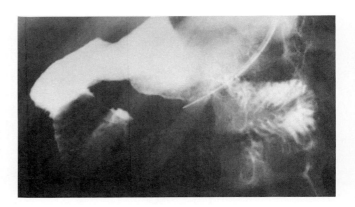

(A) intestinal malrotation
(B) intussusception
(C) duodenal hematoma
(D) Peutz-Jaeger syndrome
(E) Crohn disease

371. The MOST likely diagnosis of this teenage boy with long-standing lung disease (see figure) is

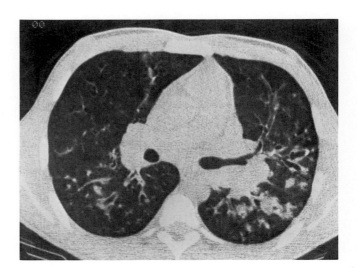

(A) recurrent pulmonary emboli
(B) cystic fibrosis
(C) aspergillosis
(D) metastatic Wilms tumor
(E) Wegener granulomatosis

372. The infant whose study is shown in the figure had failure to thrive. The MOST likely diagnosis is

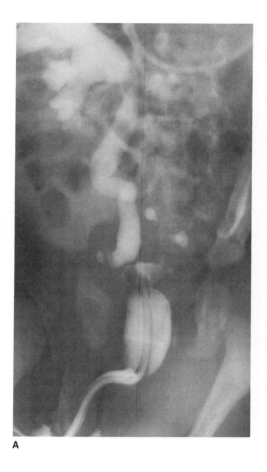
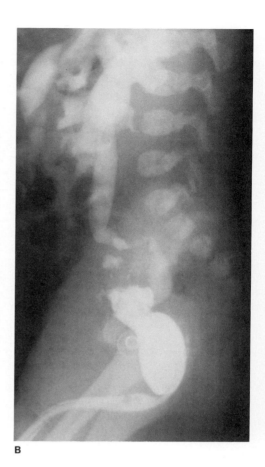

A   B

(A) prune-belly syndrome
(B) posterior urethral valves
(C) neurogenic bladder
(D) uteral reflux
(E) dilated utricle

---

373. Active rickets can be identified radiographically by which ONE of the following?

(A) Dense zones of provisional calcification
(B) Wimberger "rim" sign
(C) Widening and irregularity of the growth plate
(D) Thick periosteal new bone formation
(E) Metaphyseal sclerosis

374. Complications of cystic fibrosis include all the following EXCEPT

(A) bronchiectasis
(B) cirrhosis of the liver
(C) meconium ileus
(D) avascular necrosis
(E) sinus disease

375. A 7-year-old was found to have an abdominal mass. His CT scan is shown in the figure. The MOST likely diagnosis is

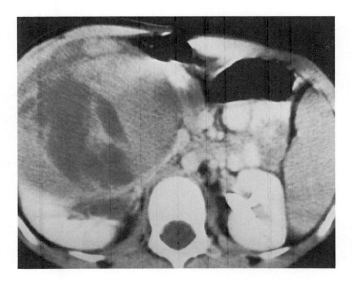

(A) Wilms tumor
(B) hepatoblastoma
(C) neuroblastoma
(D) ureteropelvic junction obstruction
(E) multicystic dysplastic kidney

376. The Weigert-Meyer rule states that in a duplicated renal collecting system,

(A) the upper pole ureter inserts medially and inferiorly to the lower pole ureter
(B) the upper pole ureter inserts laterally and inferiorly to the lower pole ureter
(C) the upper pole ureter inserts medially and superiorly to the lower pole ureter
(D) the upper pole ureter inserts laterally and superiorly to the lower pole ureter
(E) none of the above

377. The MOST likely diagnosis in this 6-year-old boy with 1 week of abdominal pain and fever (see figure) is

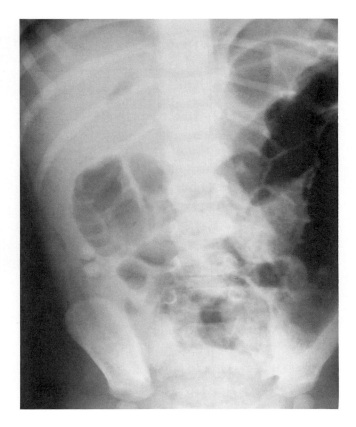

(A) intussusception
(B) gallstones
(C) appendicitis
(D) hemolytic uremic syndrome
(E) ulcerative colitis

378. An impression on the anterior aspect of the esophagus and posterior aspect of the trachea occurs in which ONE of the following entities?

(A) Aberrant left subclavian artery
(B) Aberrant right subclavian artery
(C) Pulmonary "sling"
(D) Double aortic arch
(E) None of the above

379. Judging from the figure, what would you say is the MOST likely diagnosis for this girl with cough and bad breath?

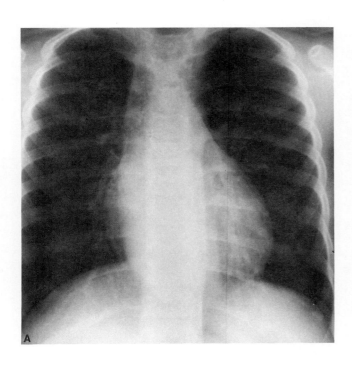

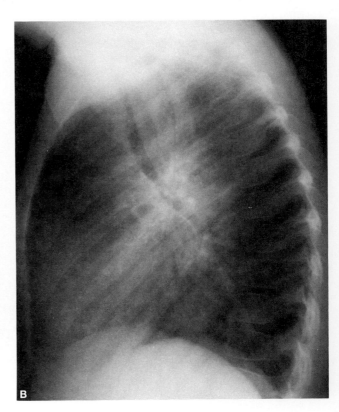

(A) Neuroblastoma
(B) Esophageal atresia
(C) Achalasia
(D) Aspirated foreign body
(E) Lymphoma

---

380. Anomalies of the radius are associated with ALL the following EXCEPT

(A) Fanconi anemia
(B) imperforate anus
(C) duodenal atresia
(D) thrombocytopenia
(E) none of the above

381. Secondary ossification centers that may be developed in a full-term infant include ALL the following locations EXCEPT

(A) proximal femur
(B) distal femur
(C) proximal tibia
(D) proximal humerus
(E) calcaneus

DIRECTIONS: Each group of questions below consists of lettered headings followed by a set of numbered items. For each numbered item select the **one** lettered heading with which it is **most** closely associated. Each lettered heading may be used **once, more than once,** or **not at all.**

Questions 382–384

Match each of the following complications to the disease with which it is most commonly associated.

- (A)   Mucocutaneous lymph node syndrome
- (B)   Histiocytosis X
- (C)   Hodgkin disease
- (D)   AIDS
- (E)   Varicella infection

382.   Coronary artery aneurysm

383.   Lymphocytic interstitial pneumonitis

384.   "Honeycomb lung"

Questions 385–387

For each of the following conditions, select the appropriate mode of inheritance.

- (A)   Autosomal recessive
- (B)   Autosomal dominant
- (C)   Sporadic
- (D)   X-linked recessive
- (E)   X-linked dominant

385.   Infantile polycystic kidney disease

386.   Hunter syndrome

387.   Ollier syndrome

Questions 388–390

Match each of the following conditions with the description which is MOST appropriate.

- (A)   Primarily metaphyseal in origin
- (B)   Round cell tumor
- (C)   Primarily epiphyseal in origin
- (D)   Associated with hemihypertrophy
- (E)   Associated with colonic polyps

388.   Osteochondroma

389.   Osteogenic sarcoma

390.   Osteomyelitis

Questions 391–393

Match the following disease entities with the ultrasound appearance most closely associated.

- (A)   Large, echogenic kidneys
- (B)   Noncommunicating cystic structures in a single kidney
- (C)   Communicating cystic structures
- (D)   Small echogenic kidneys
- (E)   Large hypoechoic kidneys

391.   Infantile polycystic kidney disease

392.   Multicystic dysplastic kidney

393.   Hydronephrosis

Questions 394–396

Match each of the following diseases with the tumor type with which it is MOST commonly associated.

- (A)   Wilms tumor
- (B)   Hemangioma
- (C)   Cardiac rhabdomyoma
- (D)   Prostatic rhabdomyosarcoma
- (E)   Medulloblastoma

394.   Tuberous sclerosis

395.   Beckwith-Weidemann syndrome

396.   Maffucci syndrome

Questions 397–399

Match each of the following tumor types with the MOST appropriate associate feature.

- (A)   Precocious puberty
- (B)   Opsoclonus/myoclonus
- (C)   Aniridia
- (D)   Hypertrophic pulmonary osteoarthropathy (HPOA)
- (E)   Hemiparesis

397.   Neuroblastoma

398.   Hepatoblastoma

399.   Wilms tumor

Questions 400–402

Match each of the following entities with the MOST commonly associated organism.

- (A)   *Hemophilus influenza*
- (B)   Staphylococcus
- (C)   Parainfluenza
- (D)   Streptococcus
- (E)   Actinomycosis

400.   Epiglottitis

401.   Croup

402.   Pneumatocele

DIRECTIONS: Each group of questions below consists of four lettered headings followed by a set of numbered items. For each numbered item select

A	if the item is associated with	(A) **only**
B	if the item is associated with	(B) **only**
C	if the item is associated with	**both** (A) and (B)
D	if the item is associated with	**neither** (A) nor (B)

Each lettered heading may be used **once, more than once,** or **not at all.**

Questions 403–405

(A) Trabeculated bladder
(B) Dilated posterior urethra
(C) Both
(D) Neither

403. Posterior urethral valves

404. Prune-belly (Eagle-Barrett) syndrome

405. Simple ureterocele

DIRECTIONS: Each question below contains five suggested answers. For **each** of the **five** alternatives listed, you are to respond either YES or NO. In a given item, **all, some,** or **none of the alternatives may be correct.**

406. True statements about slipped capital femoral epiphysis (SCFE) include which of the following?

(A) It is due to chronic stress on the growth plate
(B) There is a 5% incidence of bilaterality
(C) Males are more frequently affected
(D) It may be complicated by chondrolysis
(E) It typically occurs between 4 and 8 years of age

407. Which of the following statements regarding congenital hip dysplasia is/are TRUE?

(A) It occurs more commonly in males
(B) It more often follows vertex, rather than breech, presentation
(C) Most cases are bilateral
(D) The left hip is more often affected
(E) The diagnosis can be made by ultrasound

408. Regarding congenital cystic adenomatoid malformation (CCAM), which of the following statements are TRUE?

(A) It may appear as a solid or cystic chest mass
(B) The upper lobes are a favored location
(C) It is associated with polyhydramnios in utero
(D) Situs inversus is usually present
(E) It has malignant potential

409. True statements regarding ileal atresia include which of the following?

(A) It is a failure of normal intestinal recanalization
(B) Meconium peritonitis may result
(C) Microcolon is often associated
(D) It is more common than jejunal atresia
(E) It is associated with Down syndrome

410. Esophageal atresia is associated with which of the following?

(A) Duodenal atresia
(B) Imperforate anus
(C) Gastroschisis
(D) Down syndrome
(E) Cleft palate

411. Widened intracranial sutures are associated with which of the following?

(A) Achondroplasia
(B) Hyperthyroidism
(C) Stage IV neuroblastoma
(D) Deprivational dwarfism
(E) Neurofibromatosis

412. Meconium aspiration syndrome

(A) is characterized by hypoinflation and fine, granular pulmonary densities
(B) occurs only in preterm infants
(C) can result in pneumothorax or pneumomediastinum
(D) is commonly associated with pleural effusions
(E) may result in persistent fetal circulation

413. Syphilitic bone disease characteristically produces which of the following radiographic manifestations?

(A) Wimberger ring
(B) Periostitis
(C) Lytic lesions
(D) Lucent metaphyseal bands
(E) Widening and irregularity of the growth plate

414. Which of the following statements concerning lückenschädel (lacunar skull) are TRUE?

(A) It is associated with myelomeningocele
(B) It disappears by 6 months of age
(C) Hydrocephalus, from any etiology, is the common underlying cause
(D) It is present at birth
(E) Sclerosis of the temporal bone is typical

415. Delayed development of the epiphyses occurs with which of the following?

(A) Rickets
(B) Hypothyroidism
(C) Neurofibromatosis
(D) Hypervitaminosis A
(E) Hyperthyroidism

416. True statements about short-segment Hirschsprung disease include which of the following?

(A) It occurs more commonly in males
(B) Preterm infants are more commonly affected
(C) It is due to an absence of ganglion cells in the myenteric (Auerbach) plexus
(D) Biopsy is necessary for diagnosis
(E) The transition zone may be seen on barium enema

417. Posterior tibial bowing

(A) may result in pseudoarthrosis
(B) is typical of neurofibromatosis
(C) may be produced by abnormal fetal positioning
(D) is associated with Blount disease
(E) is typical of newborns with syphilis

418. Regarding intussusception, which of the following are TRUE?

(A) It occurs in infants between the ages of 1 week and 1 month
(B) Almost all are ileocolic or ileoileocolic
(C) The hydrostatic pressure of an enema often results in complete reduction
(D) In older children, a lead point is usually found
(E) There is a male predominance

419. True statements regarding Caffey disease include which of the following?

(A) The mandible is spared
(B) It is typically self-limited
(C) It occurs prior to 6 months of age
(D) Radiographic signs include cortical hyperostosis
(E) It is usually asymptomatic

420. Biliary atresia is characterized by which of the following?

(A) It is distinguishable clinically from neonatal hepatitis
(B) Choledochal cysts are occasionally associated
(C) The ultrasound diagnosis is supported by absence of the gallbladder
(D) It is associated with the asplenia syndrome
(E) The diagnosis is made by cholangiogram

421. Atlantoaxial instability may occur in which of the following conditions?

(A) Down syndrome
(B) Morquio disease
(C) Following trauma
(D) Klippel Feil syndrome
(E) Juvenile arthritis

422. Regarding Swyer-James syndrome, which of the following are TRUE?

(A) It is usually caused by adenovirus
(B) It is a form of bronchiolitis obliterans
(C) The volume of the affected lobe is increased
(D) The ipsilateral hilum is small
(E) It is usually unilateral

423. A retropharyngeal abscess

    (A) is typically caused by parainfluenza virus
    (B) occurs primarily in children over 3 years of age
    (C) may be simulated if a lateral radiograph is taken with the neck in flexion
    (D) can be differentiated from retropharyngeal cellulitis by plain film
    (E) may extend into the thorax

424. Skeletal findings in neurofibromatosis include which of the following?

    (A) Superior rib notching
    (B) Acute-angle kyphosis at the lumbosacral junction
    (C) Posterior bowing of the tibia
    (D) Lytic bone lesions
    (E) Sphenoid bone abnormalities

425. A 2-day-old infant fails to pass meconium. Which of the following diagnoses is/are likely?

    (A) Duodenal atresia
    (B) Ileal atresia
    (C) Hirschsprung disease
    (D) Intestinal malrotation
    (E) Meconium ileus

426. Regarding neuroblastoma,

    (A) it is commonly diagnosed in teenagers
    (B) it may present with bone pain
    (C) the age at presentation is an important prognostic indicator
    (D) primary tumors may arise in the mediastinum
    (E) it may occur congenitally

427. Cerebral calcifications may occur with which of the following?

    (A) Syphilis
    (B) Cytomegalovirus
    (C) Sturge-Weber disease
    (D) Toxoplasmosis
    (E) Craniopharyngioma

428. Complications of respiratory distress syndrome include

    (A) pulmonary interstitial emphysema
    (B) broncopulmonary dysplasia
    (C) Swyer-James syndrome
    (D) pneumomediastinum
    (E) congenital cystic adenomatoid malformation

429. Regarding pulmonary sequestration, which of the following are TRUE?

    (A) The right side is more commonly affected than the left
    (B) Upper lobe involvement predominates
    (C) Intralobar sequestrations contain a visceral pleural investment
    (D) The arterial supply is usually from the ipsilateral pulmonary artery
    (E) In the extralobar type, the venous drainage is through the pulmonary veins

430. Complications of foreign body aspirations include

    (A) recurrent pneumonia
    (B) pneumomediastinum
    (C) bronchiectasis
    (D) atelectasis
    (E) emphysema

431. Associations with myelomeningocele include

    (A) clubfeet
    (B) maternal diabetes
    (C) Chiari II malformation
    (D) dislocation of the hips
    (E) lipomas of the spinal cord

432. Pyloric stenosis

    (A) usually presents in the first week of life
    (B) can produce bilious vomiting
    (C) is more common in girls
    (D) ultrasound diagnosis requires a pyloric wall thickness of greater than 1 mm
    (E) the upper GI series diagnosis rests on delayed gastric emptying

433. Necrotizing enterocolitis

(A) most commonly presents due to bowel perforation
(B) is characterized by pneumatosis intestinalis
(C) may feature diffuse bowel-loop distention
(D) generally occurs in full-term infants
(E) is a common complication of failure to pass meconium

434. Down syndrome is associated with

(A) eleven ribs
(B) AV canal
(C) duodenal atresia
(D) small left colon syndrome
(E) ileal atresia

435. Which of the following are manifestations of histiocytosis X?

(A) Vertebra plana
(B) Interstitial lung disease
(C) Lytic skull lesions
(D) Sclerotic vertebral pedicles
(E) Soft-tissue tumors

436. Manifestations of hemophilia include

(A) symmetrical joint involvement
(B) fragmented patella
(C) epiphyseal overgrowth
(D) early growth plate closure
(E) leg length deformity

437. Radiographic findings in patients with sickle cell disease include

(A) dactylitis
(B) avascular necrosis of the hips
(C) increased splenic density by CT
(D) radioopaque gallstones
(E) "rugger-jersey" spine

438. TRUE statements regarding adrenal masses include which of the following?

(A) In the newborn, they require immediate surgery
(B) They should be followed by ultrasound in the older child
(C) They are always benign if discovered prenatally
(D) The most common tumor is a pheochromocytoma
(E) They are benign if endocrinologically active

439. Regarding cranial ultrasound (USG),

(A) it can only be done in the premature infant
(B) germinal matrix hemorrhage is generally hypoechoic
(C) Dandy-Walker cysts may be diagnosed by USG
(D) germinal matrix hemorrhage is often indistinguishable from a bulky choroid plexus
(E) intracranial bleeding invariably results in ventriculomegaly

440. Regarding Hurler syndrome,

(A) affected children are generally dwarfed
(B) intelligence is normal
(C) hepatosplenomegaly is typical
(D) vertebral body heights are uniformly decreased
(E) the first metacarpal is hypoplastic

441. Which of the following should be considered in the differential diagnosis of bilious vomiting?

(A) Intestinal volvulus
(B) Intussusception
(C) Gardner syndrome
(D) Pyloric stenosis
(E) Kawasaki disease

442. Urinary incontinence occurs in

(A) girls with neurogenic bladders
(B) boys with ectopic ureters
(C) girls with ectopic ureters
(D) boys with duplicated collecting systems
(E) girls with duplicated collecting systems

443. Which of the following occur in patients with Gaucher disease?

(A) Renal tumors
(B) Undertubulation of bones
(C) Avascular necrosis of the hips
(D) Thrombocytopenia
(E) Cyclical vomiting

444. Which of the following are characteristic of renal osteodystrophy?

(A) "Rugger-jersey" spine
(B) Slipped capital femoral epiphysis
(C) Rickets
(D) Subperiosteal resorption
(E) Dactylitis

Pediatric Radiology

Answers

367. The answer is C. *(Silverman, ed. 8, pp 780.)* The figure reveals bilateral femoral metaphyseal fractures of the "corner" or "bucket handle" type. The bones are normally mineralized. These injuries result from strong pulling and twisting forces and are very suspicious for child abuse, since normally active children never fracture their limbs in this way. Violent shaking of a child also may produce these characteristic fractures as well as fractures of the posterior ribs. When these types of injury are encountered, especially with multiple fractures in varying stages of healing and repair, the radiologist should suspect child abuse and the proper authorities should be notified.

368. The answer is D. *(Silverman, ed. 8, pp 1785–1787.)* The figure shows a complex, cystic mass in the left chest, representing multiple loops of air-filled bowel. The nasogastric tube fails to reach the abdomen. This is a case of congenital diaphragmatic hernia; most occur on the left and cause a shift of the mediastinum to the right. The patients' abdomens are scaphoid, because the bowel is in the chest. This is best appreciated on a cross-table lateral view.

The continuity of the gas-filled mass with air-filled loops within the abdomen establishes the diagnosis.

369. The answer is B. *(Silverman, ed. 8, p 55.)* Cephalohematomas usually occur as a result of trauma to the fetal head during birth. Because they are subperiosteal hemorrhages, they do not cross the suture lines, where the periosteum is tightly bound. Radiographically, their density is that of soft tissue. Fine, linear skull fractures may be found in association.

Subgaleal hygromas may result from skull fracture, wherein a tear in the dura and arachnoid allows cerebrospinal fluid (CSF) to escape into the subgaleal space. Unlike the cephalohematoma, the fluid accumulation is superficial to the periosteum and therefore may extend across the suture lines.

370. The answer is C. *(Silverman, ed. 8, pp 1575–1576.)* An upper GI study (done through a naso-gastric tube) shows a mass effect in the second and third portions of the duodenum. The mucosal folds are stretched around it, suggesting that it is intramural. An intramural mass in this region in a child most likely represents a hematoma.

Following blunt abdominal trauma, the most common gastrointestinal injury involves the du-odenum.

The duodenum is fixed in the retroperitoneum along its second portion, allowing it to be compressed against the vertebral column during blunt trauma. The radiographic findings may be those of partial or complete obstruction. The duodenal hematoma causes an intramural mass with stretched, but otherwise intact, mucosal folds. If a history of blunt trauma, such as a motor-vehicle accident or bicycle handlebar injury, is *not* clearly established, child abuse should be considered.

371. The answer is B. *(Silverman, ed. 8, pp 1157–1162.)* The CT scan in the figure shows diffuse bronchiectasis, a common feature of cystic fibrosis. Cystic fibrosis is an autosomal recessive disease that affects the cellular Na^+-K^+-ATPase pump. The exocrine glands of the body produce abnormally thick secretions, leading to bronchiectasis and recurrent infections in the lung, as well as the gastrointestinal complications of pancreatic insufficiency, malabsorption, and meconium ileus. The diagnosis is made by sweat test or DNA analysis.

None of the other illnesses listed commonly result in bronchiectasis. Patients with pulmonary emboli either have normal films or pleural-based infiltrates. Aspergillosis may give focal infiltrates, interstitial prominence, cavitary lesions, or mucus-filled bronchi. Metastatic tumors usually result in nodular densities. Wegener granulomatosis results in nodules or patchy densities.

372. The answer is B. *(Silverman, ed. 8, pp 1674–1675.)* Anteroposterior and lateral views from a voiding cystourethrogram show a small trabeculated bladder, a hypertrophied bladder neck, and a dilated posterior urethra. Reflux into a moderately tortuous right ureter and mildly dilated right pelvocalyceal system is present, as is a urinoma around the right kidney.

Posterior urethral valves are the most common cause of urethral obstruction in the male infant. They are remnants of the Wolffian duct, and form obstructing folds at the level of the verumontanum. The prostatic urethra is distended during voiding and the bladder wall becomes hypertrophied and trabeculated. Bilateral renal dysplasia results from reflux and back pressure, and unfortunately the damage is usually irreparable by the time an ultrasound can detect the problem.

373. The answer is C. *(Silverman, [Essentials], p 895.)* Rickets is due to a deficiency of calcium, which results in a failure of growing bones and cartilage to calcify. It may result from a variety of causes, including dietary lack of calcium or vitamin D, renal failure, and hepatobiliary disease. Radiographic findings include osteopenia, rarefaction and irregular fraying of the provisional zone of calcification, apparent widening of the growth plates, and "cupping" of the metaphyses. Periosteal new bone formation occurs during the healing phase.

Increased density in the zones of provisional calcification and the Wimberger "rim" sign (the faint dense line which represents the cortex of a rarified epiphysis) are radiographic manifestations of scurvy.

374. The answer is D. *(Silverman, [Essentials], p 258.)* Cystic fibrosis is an autosomal recessive disease which predominantly affects white children, causing abnormally thick exocrine gland secretions. The respiratory tract, gastrointestinal tract, and reproductive organs are most severely affected. Respiratory complications include bronchitis, bronchiectasis, and pulmonary abscess formation, which, when combined, often lead to cor pulmonale. Gastrointestinal involvement may result in meconium ileus, rectal prolapse, pancreatic insufficiency and malabsorption, as well as biliary cirrhosis, portal hypertension, and variceal hemorrhage. Avascular necrosis is not associated with cystic fibrosis.

375. The answer is A. *(Silverman, ed. 8, p 1639.)* The abdominal CT in the figure reveals a large partially cystic mass on the right, which is intrarenal, as suggested by a "claw" of renal parenchyma posteriorly that extends around to the right. The most likely diagnosis is Wilms tumor, which is felt to arise from rests of nephrogenic blastema. Wilms tumor generally occurs between the ages of 3 months and 7 years, with a peak incidence of 3½ years. It is bilateral approximately

5% of the time, in which case it is more likely to be associated with chromosomal abnormalities and other anomalies, such as aniridia.

Hepatoblastoma and neuroblastoma are extrarenal in origin. A rim of kidney would not be seen extending around the tumor. A large, irregularly shaped cystic mass would be expected in a case of UPJ obstruction, which represents the dilated pelvocalyceal system.

Multicystic dysplastic kidneys generally show no normally functioning parenchyma. In the newborn, multiple cysts are seen in the renal fossa. In the older child, often a small calcified nubbin is the only remnant of the affected kidney.

376. The answer is A. *(Silverman, ed. 8, p 1661, 1664.)* In complete ureteral duplication, the Weigert-Meyer rule states that the ureter draining the upper pole moiety of the kidney inserts below and medial to the ureter of the lower pole moiety.

Reflux is more common in completely duplicated ureters than in nonduplicated systems, and reflux more often occurs into the lower pole ureter. The upper pole ureter may or may not be associated with a ureterocele, which is a dilatation and protrusion of the submucosal segment of the ureter into the bladder lumen. The ureterocele orifice is frequently stenotic and therefore often obstructs the upper pole system.

377. The answer is C. *(Silverman, ed. 8, pp 1554–1557.)* The x-ray in the figure demonstrates two fecaliths in the right lower quadrant. In the setting of acute abdominal pain, the presence of a fecalith is diagnostic of appendicitis. In addition, there is a mass effect on the ascending colon, pushing it away from the lateral abdominal wall, as well as gas, which is not clearly in a viscus, lateral to the ascending colon. These are caused by gas-forming organisms in a periappendiceal abscess.

Intussusceptions, classically on plain films, result in a gasless right lower quadrant, but are not associated with calcific densities. These "stones" are in the wrong position for gallstones. Hemolytic-uremic syndrome causes bleeding in the bowel wall. This results in "thumbprinting" on both plain-film examination and barium enema. Ulcerative colitis may result in a featureless bowel, which may sometimes be appreciated on plain films. It should not be associated with calcific densities.

378. The answer is C. *(Silverman, [Essentials], pp 469.)* In the anomaly often referred to as the pulmonary "sling," the left pulmonary artery arises from the right pulmonary artery and crosses between the trachea and esophagus. If a lateral esophagogram is performed, the impression on the anterior aspect of the esophagus will be visible. The indentation of the posterior aspect of the trachea should be evident.

An aberrant subclavian artery causes an oblique defect on the *posterior* aspect of the esophagus. The double aortic arch displaces the trachea posteriorly and narrows it, while it also impresses on the posterior aspect of the esophagus.

379. The answer is C. *(Silverman, ed. 8, p 1422.)* The plain films in the figure reveal an extra density in the mediastinum with an air-fluid level superiorly. A double density overlies the right heart. The most likely diagnosis is esophageal achalasia, which is an obstruction at the level of the esophageal-gastric junction. Fluid and debris accumulate in the esophagus, creating the extra density in the mediastinum. The barium swallow shown in the figure reveals the dilated esophagus which ends in the characteristic distal "beak."

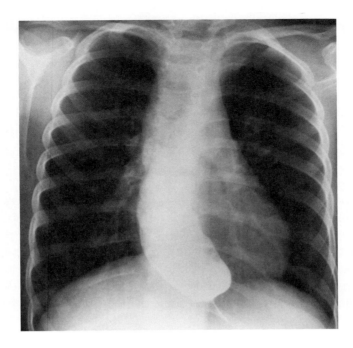

Neuroblastoma should not be considered in the differential. It arises from the sympathetic chain and therefore would be in the posterior mediastinum. Esophageal atresia presents in the newborn, and therefore would not be considered in this older child. Aspirated foreign bodies, by definition, are in the airway and cause lung disease such as focal emphysema or atelectasis. Lymphomas generally are located in the anterior mediastinum and are often associated with hilar adenopathy.

380. The answer is C. *(Silverman, ed. 8, p 501.)* Radial ray abnormalities, which include the thumb, occur as part of the Holt-Oram and TAR (*t*hrombocytopenia *a*bsent *r*adius) syndromes, Fanconi anemia, Cornelia de Lange syndrome, and trisomies 13 and 18. They are also part of the VATER association and frequently occur in conjunction with imperforate anus. There is no association with duodenal atresia.

381. The answer is A. *(Silverman, [Essentials], p 757.)* The ossification centers of the distal femoral, proximal tibial, and proximal humeral epiphyses are present in almost all full-term infants. The talus and calcaneus are also usually ossified at birth. The femoral head, however, usually does not ossify before 6 months of age.

382–384. The answers are: 382-A, 383-D, 384-D. *(Silverman, ed. 8, pp 1072, 1279.)* Kawasaki disease, or mucocutaneous lymph node syndrome, is an acute illness characterized by fever, desquamative rash of the palms and soles, conjunctivitis, and fissures around the mouth. The cervical lymph nodes are usually enlarged. Occasionally patients develop coronary artery aneurysms as a delayed complication, which may cause coronary thrombosis or cardiac ischemia.

Lymphocytic interstitial pneumonitis is a complication of AIDS that is more common in children than adults. The chest x-ray generally reveals a reticular-nodular pattern, but may have a more patchy (even lobar) distribution. With the reticular-nodular pattern, the differential diagnosis includes tuberculosis; however, these patients are usually not acutely ill.

Histiocytosis X refers to a spectrum of clinical diseases, including Letterer-Siwe, Hand-Schüller-Christian disease, and eosinophilic granuloma, which are caused by an abnormal proliferation of histiocytes. All three varieties of disease may involve the lung. Alveolar-wall invasion by histiocytes may result in pulmonary fibrosis and the development of multiple cysts. This may lead to end-stage "honeycomb lung."

385–387. The answers are: 385-A, 386-D, 387-C. *(Silverman, ed. 8, pp 606, 689–693, 1630–1632.)* Infantile polycystic kidney disease is characterized by severe renal disease, with milder involvement of the liver. It is inherited as autosomal recessive and is generally a bilateral process with symmetrically enlarged, poorly functioning kidneys. Histopathologically, normal parenchyma is replaced by dilated and elongated collecting ducts and tubules. By ultrasound, the kidneys are echogenic, without clearly discernible cysts. Excretory urograms show delayed function, with streaky or irregular changes on the delayed nephrograms.

Hunter syndrome is a form of mucopolysaccharidosis that is inherited as an X-linked recessive. The other mucopolysaccharidoses are all autosomal recessive. Radiographically, the patients resemble those of Hurler disease, though the features are generally less severe: The patients are dwarfed; the hands characteristically have metacarpals which are pinched and pointed at their proximal ends and hypoplastic distally; the ribs are widened laterally, while they are thin nearer the spine; the clavicles are short and thick; the lower thoracic and upper lumbar vertebral bodies, when viewed laterally, have a hooklike projection inferiorly; and the iliac bones are hypoplastic.

Ollier syndrome is also known as multiple enchodromatosis. Cartilage rests are deposited throughout the developing skeleton, which then grow as the child matures. The ends of the involved bones become irregularly dilated, calcified, and deformed. The changes are often more dramatic on one side of the body than the other, causing a growth disturbance. Malignant potential is present but low. The more central the lesion, the greater the risk of malignant degeneration, which does not usually occur until adulthood.

388–390. The answers are: 388-A, 389-A, 390-A. *(Silverman, ed. 8, pp 819–822, 851–852, 866–867.)* An osteochondroma, or exostosis, is a common benign tumor of childhood, and usually arises in the metaphysis. It is covered with a cap of cartilage. It may continue to grow while the skeleton matures. Radiographically, it may be bulky and sessile or it may arise on a slender stalk. Although individual lesions may arise sporadically, there is also a generalized condition of multiple exostoses, which is inherited as an autosomal dominant syndrome.

Osteogenic sarcomas are malignant tumors, which also arise in the metaphysis of bone. They are most common in the second decade of life. The tumor is bone-forming, as well as destructive of bone, and there is often a large soft-tissue mass associated. The most common location is around the knee. Metastases most commonly spread to the lungs, but other bones may be involved as well.

Osteomyelitis is generally bacterial in origin; the most common organism is *Staphylococcus aureus*. Infection favors the metaphyses because of capillary loops which form hairpin turns, causing the organisms to become lodged. Early on, radiographs are normal, though the bones may be demineralized. The diagnosis at that time, however, can be made by three-phase bone scan. Bone destruction generally occurs after about 2 weeks, which may be visible on plain films. Periosteal reaction then develops, which represents the start of healing.

391–393. The answers are: 391-A, 392-B, 393-C. *(Silverman, ed. 8, pp 1629, 1633.)* Infantile polycystic kidney disease is an autosomal recessive condition in which infants present with symmetrically enlarged kidneys that are echogenic due to the myriad tissue interfaces presented by the dilated tubules and collecting ducts. Oliguria and secondary pulmonary hypoplasia may occur in utero, leading to respiratory distress shortly after birth.

Communicating cystic structures, representing the dilated renal collecting system, are the ultrasound hallmark of hydronephrosis. In contrast, the multicystic dysplastic kidney consists of noncommunicating cysts of varying sizes separated by varying amounts of dysplastic parenchyma. The ureter is often atretic in the region of the ureteropelvic junction.

394–396. The answers are: 394-C, 395-A, 396-B. *(Silverman, ed. 8, p 494, 607, 1077.)* The Beckwith-Weidemann syndrome consists of visceromegaly, macroglossia, and omphalocele. Nephroblastomatosis may be present at birth, and Wilms tumor may develop later in life. Patients are also at increased risk for hepatoblastoma, adrenal cell carcinomas, and adrenal cystic lesions.

Multiple enchondromas and soft-tissue cavernous hemangiomas comprise Maffucci syndrome. The malignant potential of the enchondromas in Maffucci syndrome is approximately 30%.

Cardiac rhabdomyomas often arise in the setting of tuberous sclerosis. They frequently involve the septum and produce a variety of rhythm disturbances. A neonate with a cardiac tumor should also have a head CT scan to look for intracranial tubers and an abdominal ultrasound to look for a renal and/or liver cyst. Angiomyolipomas, common in tuberous sclerosis, are usually not present at birth.

397–399. The answers are: 397-B, 398-A, 399-C. *(Silverman, ed. 8, pp 1377, 1638, 1733.)* Patients with neuroblastoma (NB) may present with an encephalopathy of uncertain etiology which produces acute cerebellar ataxia and a syndrome known as opsoclonus/myoclonus. The latter is characterized by acute cerebellar ataxia and "dancing eyes." Other syndromes may be produced by different hormones secreted by the tumor: paroxysmal tachycardia, flushing, and sweating may result from elevated catecholamine levels; in others, an intractable watery diarrhea occurs due to secretion of vasoactive intestinal polypeptide (VIP).

Hepatoblastomas occasionally produce gonadotropin, which can lead to precocious puberty in males.

Wilms tumor has an association with hemihypertrophy, aniridia (with or without the Beckwith-Wiedemann syndrome), and Drash syndrome (male pseudohermaphroditism and progressive nephritis).

400–402. The answers are: 400-A, 401-C, 402-B. *(Silverman, [Essentials], p 186, 303.)* Epiglottitis is most frequently due to *Hemophilus influenza*. It occurs in children between the ages of 3 and 6 years. A lateral radiograph is typically diagnostic, revealing thickening of the epiglottis and aryepiglottic folds. Twenty-five percent of children have subglottic edema, which is identical to that seen in croup.

Croup occurs in a younger age group, usually between 6 months and 3 years of age and usually follows a viral infection, most notably parainfluenza, but respiratory syncytial virus (RSV) and adenovirus are also common causes. The subglottic narrowing of the trachea which develops is best appreciated by the frontal radiograph.

Pneumatoceles, thin-walled air-filled cysts, develop from a variety of causes, including infection, trauma, and hydrocarbon aspiration. Staphylococcal pneumonia is the most common infectious cause. The majority of pneumatoceles are self-limited and resolve spontaneously.

403–405. The answers are: 403-C, 404-B, 405-D. *(Silverman, [Essentials], p 703.)* Posterior urethral valves (PUV) obstruct the flow of urine and cause the posterior urethra to dilate. Working against the obstruction, the bladder wall becomes thickened and trabeculated, and diverticula may form. In addition, obstruction may cause hydroureteronephrosis which, if severe, causes irreparable damage to the kidneys. The diagnosis is made by voiding cystourethrography (VCUG).

Prune-belly (Eagle-Barrett) syndrome is characterized by the triad of abdominal wall muscular deficiency, cryptorchidism, and urinary tract abnormalities (e.g., renal dysplasia, hydronephrosis, and hydroureter). The bladder is thick-walled, but smooth. A urachal remnant or utricle is often discovered. By VCUG, dilatation of the posterior urethra may simulate PUV, although no obstruction is present.

A simple ureterocele is thought to occur from obstruction of the distal ureteral orifice. It can occur in a nonduplicated collecting system. The bladder wall is not affected, since there is no bladder outlet obstruction. The urethra is also not involved.

406. The answers are: A-Y, B-N, C-Y, D-Y, E-N. *(Silverman, ed. 8, p 774.)* Slipped capital femoral epiphysis (SCFE) occurs in boys ages 12 to 15 years and girls ages 10 to 13 years. Boys are more commonly affected than girls by a ratio of 2.5 to 1. A fracture-separation (Salter I type injury) occurs at the epiphyseal plate in relation to chronic stress. The cause is unknown, but there is a 25% incidence of bilaterality. SCFE may occur simultaneously in both hips or may occur in one hip several months prior to occurring in the opposite hip.

Complications include avascular necrosis of the femoral head and chondrolysis of the affected hip. The latter appears as joint-space narrowing.

407. The answers are: A-N, B-N, C-N, D-Y, E-Y. *(Silverman, ed. 8, p 344.)* Congenital hip dysplasia is far more common in female infants, and usually follows a breech presentation at birth. The left side is more commonly affected. It is believed to be related to high levels of maternal hormones which produce ligamentous laxity in the infant.

The diagnosis is made clinically, by the use of the Ortolani or Barlow test, or by ultrasound or plain film. Correction is essential to normal development of the femoral head and acetabulum. This is often done simply by placing the child in a Pavlik harness to keep the hips abducted. Surgery is occasionally necessary.

408. The answers are: A-Y, B-Y, C-Y, D-N, E-N. *(Silverman, ed. 8, p 1143.)* Congenital cystic adenomatoid malformation (CCAM) of the lung is a type of hamartoma—disordered but otherwise normal pulmonary tissue—which arises from the terminal portion of the bronchial tree. It occurs with equal frequency in both lungs, but has an upper lobe predominance. It is not associated with situs inversus and is not premalignant.

Three histologic types are described. Type I is the most common and consists of multiple large cysts of varying sizes. Type II consists of multiple small cysts (1–2 cm) and is associated with other congenital abnormalities. Type III is the rarest form and consists of a mass of tiny cysts that may appear solid. Polyhydramnios and fetal anasarca may be associated. CCAM is usually surgically removed.

The differential diagnosis includes congenital lobar emphysema, congenital diaphragmatic hernia, and pulmonary sequestration.

409. The answers are: A-N, B-Y, C-Y, D-Y, E-N. *(Silverman, ed. 8, p 1838.)* Ileal atresia and the less common jejunal atresia are due to bowel ischemia which occurs in utero. Duodenal atresia is due to a failure of the bowel lumen to recanalize normally during development. Unlike duodenal atresia, ileal atresia is not associated with Down syndrome. Ileal atresia may result in perforation and meconium peritonitis, which is usually self-limited. The meconium may calcify in as little as 1 week.

Ileal atresia, by obstructing the passage of succus entericus, is one of the causes of microcolon. Meconium ileus is another cause.

410. The answers are: A-Y, B-Y, C-N, D-Y, E-N. *(Silverman, ed. 8, p 1408.)* Esophageal atresia may be part of the VATER constellation of anomalies (*v*ertebral and *v*ascular (i.e., cardiac), *a*nal, *tra*cheal, and *e*sophageal, and *r*enal or *r*adial abnormalities), which is also sometimes referred to as the VACTEREL syndrome (*v*ertebral *a*nal *c*ardiac *t*racheal *e*sophageal *r*enal and *l*imb, especially the radius), or it may occur as an isolated abnormality.

Duodenal atresia is also associated with esophageal atresia, and both are associated with Down syndrome.

Gastroschisis is an anomaly of midline closure and is not associated with esophageal atresia. Cleft palate also bears no association with the VATER anomalies.

411. The answers are: A-N, B-N, C-Y, D-Y, E-N. *(Silverman, ed. 8, p 494, 1737.)* Deprivational dwarfism and Stage IV neuroblastoma may cause widening of the cranial sutures. In deprivational dwarfism, widening of the sutures is evident in the recovery phase due to accelerated brain growth. In Stage IV neuroblastoma, the widened sutures reflect the presence of extradural metastases.

Any cause of increased intracranial pressure can also cause splitting of the sutures.

Hyperthyroidism causes accelerated maturation of the skeleton and premature synostosis of the cranial sutures. The achondroplastic skull has a small-sized foramen magnum, but is otherwise normal.

412. The answers are: A-N, B-N, C-Y, D-N, E-Y. *(Felman, p 82.)* Meconum aspiration syndrome occurs in full-term and postterm infants. Meconium is expressed by the infant into the amniotic fluid during stress, such as hypoxia or a difficult prolonged labor. Fetal respiratory efforts, as well as the first breaths after birth, cause aspiration of meconium into the airways. Depending on the severity of the aspiration, the chest x-ray can be normal or demonstrate coarse pulmonary densities and hyperinflation. Complications include pneumothorax and pneumomediastinum, but pleural effusions are uncommon. Persistent fetal circulation may result from the high pulmonary arterial pressure, which causes blood to shunt from right to left through the patent ductus arteriosis.

413. The answers are: A-N, B-Y, C-Y, D-Y, E-N. *(Silverman, ed. 8, p 835.)* Syphilitic disease of bone results in areas of destruction, lucent metaphyseal bands (which represent a trophic response to the infection), and periostitis. Wimberger "notch" sign, a focal destruction of the proximal medial tibial metaphysis, is characteristic. Wimberger "ring," however, is a sign of scurvy. Widening and irregularity of the growth plate are features of rickets, not syphilis.

414. The answers are: A-Y, B-Y, C-N, D-Y, E-N. *(Silverman, ed. 8, p 32.)* Lückenschädel, or lacunar skull, is associated with meningocele and myelomeningocele. It is present at birth and disappears by 6 months of age. Characteristically, it appears as "soap bubble" lucencies in the upper calvaria. It is a dysplasia of the bone and underlying dura, and is not the result of increased intracranial pressure.

415. The answers are: A-N, B-Y, C-N, D-N, E-N. *(Silverman, [Essentials], p 991.)* In hypothyroidism, skeletal growth and maturation are retarded, leading to delayed and often irregular ossification of the epiphyses. Other bony abnormalities include cortical thickening, which results in osteosclerosis and narrowing of the medullary arteries in tubular and flat bones. Enlargement of the sella turcica from pituitary hypertrophy offers a clue to the diagnosis.

Rickets causes widening of the epiphyseal plate and fraying and splaying of the metaphyses. Neurofibromatosis is a dysplasia of bone which does not affect maturation of the skeleton. Hypervitaminosis A causes periosteal reaction and premature fusion of growth plates. Hyperthyroidism causes early maturation of the skeleton.

416. The answers are: A-Y, B-N, C-Y, D-Y, E-Y. *(Stringer, p 379.)* In Hirschsprung disease, there is an absence of ganglion cells in the myenteric plexus of the distal bowel, resulting in impaired peristalsis and abnormal muscle tone in the affected segment. The condition is rarely seen in preterm infants and males are more often affected.

In 65% of patients, a transition zone between the normal-caliber aganglionic bowel and the dilated normal bowel is discovered in the rectosigmoid or sigmoid colon (short-segment Hirschsprung disease). The transition zone is found in the rectum in 8% of cases, in the descending colon in 14%, and in the more proximal colon in 10%. The diagnosis is suggested by barium enema, which must then confirmed by suction or full-thickness rectal biopsy.

417. The answers are: A-N, B-N, C-Y, D-N, E-N. *(Silverman, [Essentials], pp 806, 858.)* Posterior tibial bowing is due to fetal positioning and resolves spontaneously as the bones respond to weight bearing. Anterior tibial bowing occurs in neurofibromatosis, which is due to an intrinsic bone dysplasia, and may result in a pseudoarthrosis.

Blount disease is due to a growth disturbance of the proximal tibial metaphysis and epiphysis. Varus deformities of the tibias result, whereas anterior or posterior bowing is not a feature. Blount disease may require surgical correction to correct bowing deformities.

Babies with syphilis have periosteal reactions and metaphyseal changes, and may even fracture easily; however, they do not typically present with bowing.

418. The answers are: A-N, B-Y, C-Y, D-Y, E-Y. *(Silverman, ed. 8, p 1501.)* Most intussusceptions are ileocolic or ileoileocolic and are idiopathic, though hypertrophy of lymphoid tissue following viral infection is thought to play a role in many cases. The most common age is between 2 months and 3 years and there is a male predominance. Patients present with crampy abdominal pain, and, clinically, an abdominal mass may be palpable or the infant may pass bloody stools. Intussusceptions in very young infants or children over 3 years of age often have a lead point, such as a Meckel diverticulum. Reduction is performed by air or barium enema, though in some cases surgery may be required.

419. The answers are: A-N, B-Y, C-Y, D-Y, E-N. *(Silverman, ed. 8, p 841.)* Infantile cortical hyperostosis, or Caffey disease, is an idiopathic self-limited condition which equally affects males and females under the age of 6 months. The average age of onset is 7 weeks. Clinically, infants present with irritability, soft-tissue swelling, and cortical thickening of the underlying bones. The condition may have a recurring course. The mandible, clavicle, and ulna are the most common bones to be involved, but any tubular bone, except the phalanges, may be affected.

420. The answers are: A-N, B-Y, C-Y, D-N, E-Y. *(Stringer, p 476–477. Torrisi, AJR 155(6): 1273–1276, 1990.)* Biliary atresia is difficult to distinguish from neonatal hepatitis, since both present in the first weeks of life with jaundice and hepatomegaly.

The diagnosis is suggested by hepatobiliary scintigraphy or biopsy but is made definitively only by cholangiography. Up to 10% of infants with biliary atresia have associated anomalies, including *poly*splenia, preduodenal portal vein, and azygous continuation of the inferior vena cava. On sonography, the gallbladder may be absent or small (less than 1.5 cm in length), but is occasionally normal or even enlarged. A recent article describes the association between biliary atresia and the presence of a choledochal cyst.

421. The answers are: A-Y, B-Y, C-Y, D-N, E-N. *(Silverman, ed. 8, pp 288, 291, 321.)* Atlantoaxial instability occurs in Down syndrome because of inherent ligamentous laxity. It also is a feature of Morquio disease, because of absence or hypoplasia of the dens, which reduces skeletal support. Trauma can disrupt the transverse alar ligament or fracture the dens, both of which contribute to instability.

In Klippel Feil syndrome, there is fusion of the cervical vertebral bodies. Atlantoaxial instability is not a problem. Associated features include Sprengel deformity (scapular elevation, due to an omohyoid bone or fibrous connection), short neck, and low hairline.

Juvenile arthritis is characterized by destruction of the facet joints with subsequent fusion of the articular processes of the cervical spine, usually in the upper portion, but it may extend to involve the entire cervical spine.

422. The answers are: A-Y, B-Y, C-N, D-Y, E-Y. *(Silverman, ed. 8, p 1169.)* Swyer-James syndrome is felt to be a type of bronchiolitis obliterans which results from an infectious insult (typically adenovirus) to the lung early in childhood. Other causes include measles, tuberculosis, pertussis, and mycoplasma. The result is a reduction in the number of alveoli and capillaries, and hypoplasia of the pulmonary arteries to the affected segment. The volume of the affected lung is normal to decreased. Radiographically, there is hyperlucency of the affected lung due to decreased perfusion, and the ipsilateral hilum is often small.

423. The answers are: A-N, B-N, C-Y, D-N, E-Y. *(Silverman, [Essentials], p 185.)* The majority of retropharyngeal abscesses occur in children between 6 and 12 months of age and most are caused by oral bacteria. There is no way to differentiate retropharyngeal cellulitis from an abscess by plain film; CT is the best means for that purpose. Plain-film findings include thickening of the prevertebral soft tissues, anterior displacement of the esophagus and trachea, and straightening or reversal of the normal lordotic curve of the cervical spine. Rarely, a retropharyngeal abscess may track down into the thorax.

424. The answers are: A-N, B-N, C-N, D-Y, E-Y. *(Edeiken, ed. 3, p 1357.)* The skeletal findings of neurofibromatosis are myriad and include *inferior* rib notching, a sharp-angled kyphoscoliosis in the lower *thoracic* spine, anterior tibial bowing, and multiple cystic or lytic areas within bone. Additional features include macrocranium, absence or hypoplasia of the greater wing of the sphenoid bone, characteristic defects in the posterior parietal calvaria, enlargement of optic and neural foramina, posterior scalloping of the vertebral bodies, ribbon ribs, and pseudoarthroses (especially in the tibias).

425. The answers are: A-N, B-Y, C-Y, D-N, E-Y. *(Silverman, ed. 8, pp 1828–1858.)* Infants who fail to pass meconium usually have a distal obstruction. The differential diagnosis includes imperforate anus, Hirschsprung disease, meconium ileus, small left colon, and ileal atresia. The diagnosis is made by enema.

When the anus is imperforate, the superficial anatomy is obvious, and a catheter cannot be placed. In patients with Hirschsprung disease, the rectum is of normal caliber. A "transition zone" occurs, usually in the rectosigmoid, at which point the "normal"-caliber bowel (the diseased segment) joins the dilated bowel (which functions normally). Small left colon features dilated ascending and transverse colons, and a narrow, meconium-plug-filled descending colon. Meconium ileus and ileal atresia are both associated with the enema finding of "microcolon."

Patients with duodenal atresia and intestinal malrotation present with vomiting, not failure to pass meconium.

426. The answers are: A-N, B-Y, C-Y, D-Y, E-Y. *(Silverman, ed. 8, p 1733.)* Neuroblastoma is a tumor of infancy and early childhood with a peak of 2 to 3 years of age. It may be congenital in origin and has been identified by prenatal ultrasound. The tumor arises from neural crest tissue and, therefore, may arise anywhere along the sympathetic chains as well as in the adrenal gland. Prognosis is multifactorial, depending on age and tumor site as well as stage. There are five stages: stage I is confined to the organ of origin; stage II is confined to the organ of origin and ipsilateral nodes; in stage III, the mass crosses the midline; in stage IV, there are distant bone metastases discovered on plain films or by bone scan; in stage IV S disease, tumor cells may be found in the bone marrow, skin and/or liver, as well as a primary site. In general, patients under 1 year of age have an improved chance of survival, as compared to older children.

427. The answers are: A-N, B-Y, C-Y, D-Y, E-Y. *(Silverman, ed. 8, pp 137, 183, 218.)* Pathologic calcifications of the brain occur for a variety of reasons. Cytomegalovirus (CMV) and toxoplasmosis are two common infections that cause intracranial calcifications to form, with those in CMV being primarily periventricular in location.

Sturge-Weber disease, also known as *encephalotrigeminal angiomatosis,* is a neurocutaneous disorder characterized by a vascular nevus ("port wine stain") on the face in the distribution of the trigeminal nerve, seizures, hemiatrophy of the ipsilateral brain hemisphere, and mental retardation. Curvilinear "tram-line" calcifications are characteristic and usually predominate in the posterior parietal and occipital regions.

Craniopharyngiomas are suprasellar tumors which contain calcifications 60–80% of the time.

Babies with syphilis may present with cardiac disease, pneumonia, hepatosplenomegaly, and bone changes. Cerebral involvement is not associated with calcification.

428. The answers are: A-Y, B-Y, C-N, D-Y, E-N. *(Silverman, ed. 8, pp 1143, 1169, 1771.)* Respiratory distress syndrome (RDS) is a disease of premature infants. Immature lungs lack surfactant which is made by type II pneumocytes and therefore cannot keep inflated because of the high surface tension. Stiff lungs require high pressures to ventilate and may develop "air block" complications such as pulmonary interstitial emphysema, pneumothorax, and pneumomediastinum. Late complications include bronchopulmonary dysplasia, which is thought to result from a combination of barotrauma and oxygen toxicity.

Swyer-James syndrome, or unilateral hyperlucent lung, is a bronchiolitis obliterans due to prior infection, and is not related to RDS. Congenital cystic adenomatoid malformation is disorganized lung tissue that is classified as a pulmonary hamartoma. It is also unrelated to RDS.

429. The answers are: A-N, B-N, C-N, D-N, E-N. *(Felman, pp 29–34.)* Pulmonary sequestrations occur as a result of bronchopulmonary (foregut) malformations. They have aberrant arterial supply, usually from the aorta, and abnormal or absent connection to the tracheobronchial tree. Sequestrations are categorized as intralobar or extralobar. The extralobar type has its own visceral pleural investment and generally drains into the azygos or hemiazygos system. Intralobar sequestrations have no distinct pleural covering and drain normally into the pulmonary venous system. Both types occur more commonly in the left lower lobe.

430. The answers are: A-Y, B-Y, C-Y, D-Y, E-Y. *(Felman, pp 273–274.)* Children, particularly infants and toddlers, commonly put foreign bodies into their mouths and often swallow or aspirate them. The majority of aspirated foreign bodies are not radioopaque, so that their recognition rests solely on appreciation of the plain-film findings of air-flow obstruction. Objects that partially obstruct a bronchus cause air trapping or emphysema. An expiratory film reveals no emptying of the lung on the affected side. Complete obstruction will result in atelectasis and volume loss. Atelectatic lung may develop pneumonia which, if chronic or relapsing, may lead to bronchiectasis. Air-block disease may cause air to dissect into the interstitium and produce a pneumomediastinum.

431. The answers are: A-Y, B-N, C-Y, D-Y, E-Y. *(Kirks, p 148.)* A myelomeningocele is a protrusion of spinal cord, nerve roots, and meninges, which results from a failure of the neural tube to close, usually at the caudal end. Associated abnormalities include rib deformities, Chiari malformation, clubfeet, vertical talus, hip dislocation, anorectal malformations, ureteral reflux and hydronephrosis, and sacral agenesis. The spinal cord often has a lipoma at the end.

432. The answers are: A-N, B-N, D-N, D-N, E-N. *(Kirks, pp 644–645.)* Hypertrophic pyloric stenosis is an abnormality of the circular musculature of the pylorus. Its etiology is uncertain, though it runs in families. It rarely occurs before 2 weeks of age, and it is seen most frequently between the ages of 4 to 6 weeks. Boys are affected four times as frequently as girls.

Though delayed gastric emptying is present on upper GI series, the visualization of a narrow enlongated canal is necessary to make the diagnosis. By ultrasound, the hypertrophied pyloric muscle is seen as an anechoic ring surrounding the bright echoes produced by the mucosa. The muscle thickness must be greater than 4 mm for the diagnosis to be made.

Pyloric stenosis prevents bile from refluxing into the stomach, hence bilious vomiting indicates another diagnosis. Care should be taken to rule out a malrotation or volvulus.

433. The answers are: A-N, B-Y, C-Y, D-N, E-N. *(Silverman, ed. 8, pp 1859–1862.)* Necrotizing enterocolitis is a disease that predominantly occurs in the premature infant several days after birth. The patients present with signs of physical deterioration, abdominal distention, blood-streaked stools, and bilious gastric aspirates. Radiographs commonly show distended loops of bowel and intramural gas (pneumatosis). Gas may gain access to the portal venous system and travel to the liver, where it assumes a peripheral location. Perforation occurs, but is not the most common presentation. The pathogenesis is uncertain, but is probably related to a combination of a weakened mucosal barrier (due to poor blood flow) and bacterial colonization of the GI tract.

434. The answers are: A-Y, B-Y, C-Y, D-N, E-N. *(Kirks, pp 230–233.)* Down syndrome, or trisomy 21, is the most frequent chromosomal abnormality. Radiographic features include hypoplasia of the nasal bones and paranasal sinuses, clinodactyly, eleven pairs of ribs, multiple manubrial ossification centers, flattened acetabular roofs, and flared iliac wings.

Endocardial cushion defects (specifically of the AV canal type) and ventricular septal defects (VSD) are the most common congenital heart disease. Infants with Down syndrome have an increased frequency of duodenal atresia, duodenal stenosis, annular pancreas, Hirschsprung disease, anorectal malformations, and umbilical hernias.

435. The answers are: A-Y, B-Y, C-Y, D-N, E-N. *(Silverman, ed. 8, pp 899–900.)* Histiocytosis X refers to a group of related conditions which include eosinophilic granuloma, Letterer-Siwe disease, and Hand-Schüller-Christian disease. The common feature is an abnormal proliferation of histiocytes. Bone involvement usually produces lytic areas, and the skull is the most commonly affected bone. Vertebral body infiltration may result in collapse, the "vertebra plana," which may reconstitute if the disease regresses. Sclerotic pedicles are not an association.

Hepatosplenomegaly, interstitial lung disease, and skin rash occur due to infiltration of the tissues by histiocytes. Soft-tissue tumors are not described.

436. The answers are: A-N, B-N, C-Y, D-Y, E-Y. *(Silverman, ed. 8, pp 896–899.)* Hemophilia refers to a group of inherited bleeding diatheses; factor VIII deficiency is the most common. Acute and recurrent bleeding into joints results in hyperemia, which leads to epiphyseal overgrowth and early growth plate closure. A leg length deformity can result, and chronic hemarthroses may deform the joints. The large joints are more commonly affected, because they are prone to trauma and stress, although the disease is often asymmetrical. The patellas are typically "squared" inferiorly, and do not have a fragmented appearance.

437. The answers are: A-Y, B-Y, C-Y, D-N, E-N. *(Silverman, ed. 8, pp 889–893.)* Sickle cell anemia most severely affects individuals who are homozygous for S hemoglobin. The red cells become sickle-shaped under conditions of reduced oxygen tension. The abnormal shape of the red cells causes microvascular occlusion, typically at the capillary level, which leads to further tissue hypoxia and exacerbates the problem. Bone and bone marrow are particularly affected. Bone infarction results in focal destruction and sclerosis of cortical bone, with a reparative periosteal reaction.

In very young children (6 months to 2 years), infarction most often affects the small bones of the hands and feet. Dactylitis is the syndrome of pain and soft-tissue swelling that results. Infarction of the femoral head (avascular necrosis) may mimic Legg-Calvé-Perthe disease. The H-shaped vertebrae that are so characteristic represent central collapse due to infarction.

Patients with sickle cell disease also have a diminished resistance to infection because the spleen is generally infarcted by the second or third decade. It becomes dense due to the deposition of iron and calcium. Sometimes the changes of osteomyelitis are radiographically indistinguishable from those of osteonecrosis from infarction. Cholelithiasis occurs commonly, due to hemolysis and a rapid turnover of bilirubin, but the stones are of the "pigment" type and are usually not radioopaque.

438. The answers are: A-N, B-N, C-N, D-N, E-N. *(Silverman, ed. 8, pp 1733–1743.)* When an adrenal mass is identified in a fetus or a newborn, the differential diagnosis is between neuroblastoma and adrenal hemorrhage. Both may occur prenatally. Imaging is useful for identifying a mass, but no modality is able to distinguish uncomplicated hemorrhage from neuroblastoma, since the latter may bleed and not be identifiable in the hematoma.

A baby with an adrenal mass should be followed for several months to allow for resolution of hemorrhage. If the mass completely resolves, no further treatment is needed. If the mass does not resolve, surgery is recommended.

In the older child, since adrenal hemorrhage is less common, any adrenal mass should be removed upon discovery. The most common tumor of the adrenal gland in childhood is a neuroblastoma. Adrenal cortical carcinoma is very rare; it often brings the patient to attention because of its hormonal activity.

439. The answers are: A-N, B-N, C-Y, D-N, E-N. *(Leo & Rao, pp 178–179. Sarti, pp 1200–1239.)* Ultrasound (USG) is a useful modality in the evaluation of babies with open anterior fontanelles, which usually do not fuse until 1 year of age. Premature infants have an increased risk of intracranial hemorrhage. Hemorrhage usually arises in the germinal matrix and acutely is echogenic. It can be differentiated from the echogenic choroid plexus by its location; choroid plexus runs in the floor of the posterior aspect of the lateral ventricles and roof of the third ventricle, whereas the germinal matrix is located anteriorly, between the head of the caudate and anterior horn of the lateral ventricle. Hemorrhage may extend into the ventricular system, but does not invariably cause hydrocephalus.

The Dandy-Walker syndrome consists of midline hypoplasia of the cerebellum in association with a posterior fossa cyst. Even though scanning is routinely performed through the anterior fontanelle, the midline cerebellum is well seen. A cyst in the posterior fossa can also be appreciated with careful scanning.

440. The answers are: A-Y, B-N, C-Y, D-N, E-N. *(Silverman, ed. 8, pp 689–693.)* Hurler disease is an autosomal recessive mucopolysaccharidosis. Patients are normal at birth, but develop progressive disease and generally die by the second decade. Coarse features and dwarfism are characteristic. Kyphosis near the thoracolumbar junction results from hypoplasia of the lower thoracic and/or upper lumbar vertebral bodies. The hands are broad and the fingers are short and stubby. The second, third, and fourth metacarpals appear "pinched" at their proximal ends. Infiltration of organs with mucopolysaccharide material may lead to organomegaly, typically most severe in the liver and spleen. There is usually mental retardation and developmental delay.

441. The answers are: A-Y, B-Y, C-N, D-N, E-N. *(Silverman, ed. 8, pp 1072–1073, 1444–1449, 1501–1507, 1562, 1830–1831.)*   Bilious vomiting in the child can be seen in numerous conditions ranging from severe, prolonged gastroenteritis to surgical emergencies, such as volvulus and intussusception. Midgut volvulus should be the leading diagnosis in a baby who presents with acute onset of bilious vomiting in the first week of life. It is due to a malrotation of the gut and improper fixation within the peritoneum.

Intussusception is the invagination of one portion of the intestine into the contiguous distal segment. Though bilious vomiting due to small-bowel obstruction is not the usual presentation of intussusception, it is common enough in the 6-month to 2-year group that it belongs in the differential diagnosis.

Gardner syndrome is a hereditary colonic polyposis that also features osteomas and soft-tissue tumors. It should not cause bilious vomiting. Pyloric stenosis causes gastric outlet obstruction, and therefore the vomiting that results is nonbilious. Kawasaki disease presents with constitutional symptoms, a skin rash, and lymphadenopathy. Vomiting is not a feature.

442. The answers are: A-Y, B-N, C-Y, D-N, E-Y. *(Silverman, ed. 8, pp 1662–1664, 1687.)*   Urinary incontinence occurs with neurogenic bladders, of either the flaccid or spastic type.

Ectopic ureters are usually seen in the context of duplication; only 10% of ectopic ureters occur in nonduplicated systems. In girls, the ectopic orifice is most commonly in the vestibule or urethra. It only occasionally enters the vagina, and even more rarely the uterus. Therefore, the common presentation is continuous leakage of urine. In males, the ectopic ureter may end in the posterior urethra, seminal vesicle, or vas deferens, but because it always enters above the external sphincter, incontinence does not occur.

443. The answers are: A-N, B-Y, C-Y, D-Y, E-N. *(Silverman, ed. 8, p 699.)*   Gaucher disease is a storage disease that results in the accumulation of glucocerebroside in reticuloendothelial cells. Marked splenomegaly is characteristic, which results in platelet trapping and a tendency to bleed. Infiltration of bones by Gaucher cells results in undertubulation, producing the "Ehrlenmeyer flask" deformity, which is often best appreciated in the distal femurs. Osteonecrosis may also occur. Renal tumors are not a feature of this disease, nor is cyclical vomiting.

444. The answers are: A-Y, B-Y, C-Y, D-Y, E-N. *(Kirks, pp 313–314.)*   Renal osteodystrophy and secondary hyperparathyroidism produce a variety of bony changes, which include rickets, osteomalacia, osteosclerosis, and soft-tissue calcification. Rickets is a manifestation of deficient mineralization of growing bone in children, and children with rickets have an increased incidence of slipped capital femoral epiphysis at any age. The "rugger-jersey" spine refers to the bands of density which appear in the spine when osteosclerosis involves the endplates. Hyperparathyroidism typically causes subperiosteal bone resorption, especially of the radial aspects of the second and third metacarpals.

Ultrasonography

DIRECTIONS: Each question below contains five suggested responses. Select the **one best** response to each question.

445. Of the following, which is the LEAST likely disease to have caused the condition of the kidney shown in the figure?

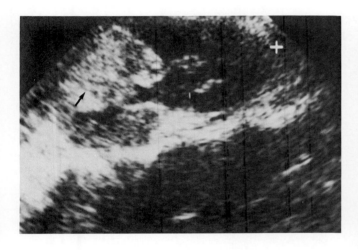

    (A)   Angiomyolipoma
    (B)   Renal lymphoma
    (C)   Focal pyelonephritis
    (D)   Hypernephroma
    (E)   Renal tuberculosis

446. A 1-year-old infant presents with vomiting for 24 hours and a distended abdomen on physical exam. An ultrasound (see figure) is obtained. The MOST likely diagnosis is

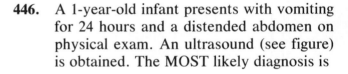

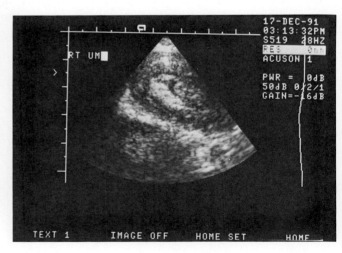

    (A)   Ladd bands
    (B)   fecalith
    (C)   omphalomesenteric duct remnant
    (D)   Wilms tumor
    (E)   idiopathic

447. The LEAST likely explanation for the appearance of the uterus pictured in the figure is

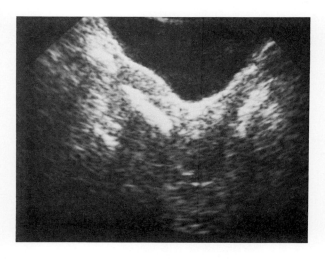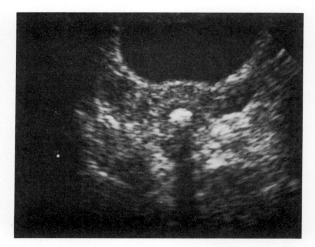

(A)   recent instrumentation
(B)   Asherman syndrome
(C)   an IUD
(D)   the secretory phase of the menstrual cycle
(E)   a fistula to bowel

448. A 5-year-old girl with a recent history of several urinary tract infections had a renal and pelvic ultrasound study (see figure). Given that the other kidney was normal, which of the following is the MOST likely explanation?

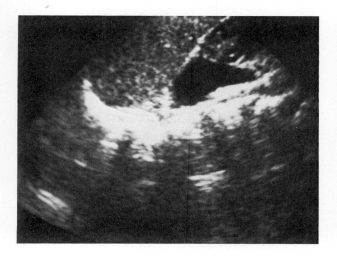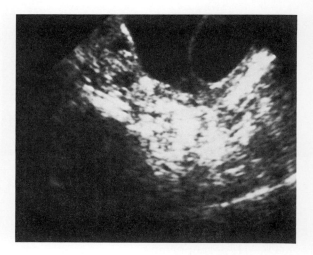

(A)   Partial duplication and a simple ureterocele
(B)   Complete duplication and an ectopic ureterocele
(C)   Ureteropelvic junction obstruction
(D)   Multicystic dysplastic kidney
(E)   Posterior urethral valves

449. An elderly man is brought to the emergency room with right upper quadrant pain. An ultrasound (see figure) is performed. The MOST likely diagnosis is

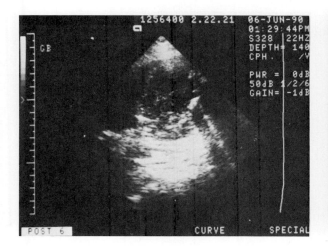 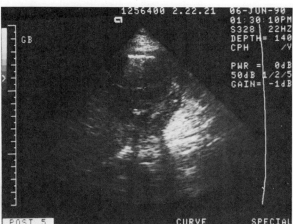

(A) gallbladder carcinoma
(B) chronic cholecystitis
(C) passage of a gallstone through the ampulla
(D) emphysematous cholecystitis
(E) perforated duodenal ulcer

---

450. A 45-year-old man presents with acute flank pain. His serum and urinary calcium are normal. A renal ultrasound is performed (see figure). Which is the MOST likely diagnosis?

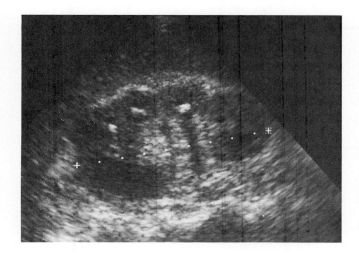

(A) Medullary sponge kidney
(B) Xanthogranulomatous pyelonephritis
(C) Ethylene glycol poisoning
(D) Type I renal tubular acidosis
(E) Multiple myeloma

451. Generalized decreased renal echogenicity is LEAST likely to be caused by

(A) retroperitoneal fibrosis
(B) renal lymphoma
(C) acute pyelonephritis
(D) global infarction
(E) renal vein thrombosis

452. Ultrasound diagnosis of deep vein thrombosis in an extremity relies most heavily on which ONE of the following features?

(A) Noncompressibility
(B) Lack of augmentation
(C) Loss of respiratory phasicity
(D) Visualization of clot within the vein
(E) Visualization of venous collaterals

453. The MOST common risk factor for placenta percreta is

(A) placenta previa
(B) prior cesarean section
(C) multiple gestations
(D) previous IUD
(E) prior molar pregnancy

454. The obstetric ultrasound in the figure was obtained during the 34th week of gestation. The MOST likely diagnosis is

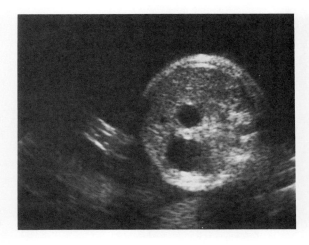 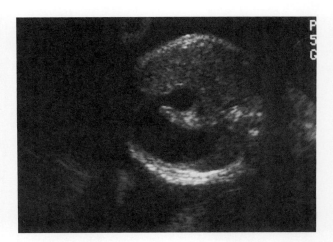

(A) meconium ileus
(B) duodenal stenosis
(C) ileal atresia
(D) duodenal atresia
(E) annular pancreas

455. Based on your diagnosis in Question 454, ancillary sonographic findings might include ALL the following EXCEPT

(A) polyhydramnios
(B) endocardial cushion defects
(C) meconium ileus
(D) IUGR
(E) biliary atresia

---

456. The MOST common neural tube defect associated with an elevated alpha fetoprotein (αFP) is

(A) anencephaly
(B) myelomeningocele
(C) encephalocele
(D) Dandy-Walker malformation
(E) gastroschisis

457. Fetal ascites and peritoneal calcifications are MOST commonly associated with

(A) intestinal volvulus
(B) cystic fibrosis
(C) TORCH infections
(D) neuroblastoma
(E) duodenal atresia

458. Which type of twinning is depicted in the figure?

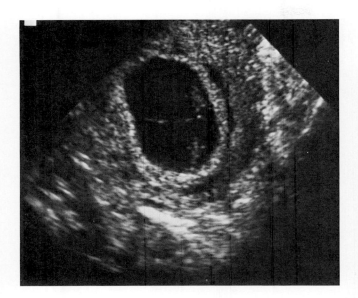

(A) Monozygotic dichorionic diamniotic
(B) Monozygotic dichorionic monoamniotic
(C) Monozygotic monochorionic diamniotic
(D) Dizygotic dichorionic diamniotic
(E) Monozygotic monochorionic monoamniotic

459. Of the following, the MOST common type of twinning is

(A) monozygotic dichorionic diamniotic
(B) monozygotic monochorionic diamniotic
(C) monozygotic dichorionic monoamniotic
(D) monozygotic monochorionic monoamniotic
(E) dizygotic dichorionic monoamniotic

460. A patient presents with diarrhea, intermittent intestinal obstruction, and severe peripheral edema. The ultrasound of his right upper quadrant is shown in the figure. The MOST likely diagnosis is

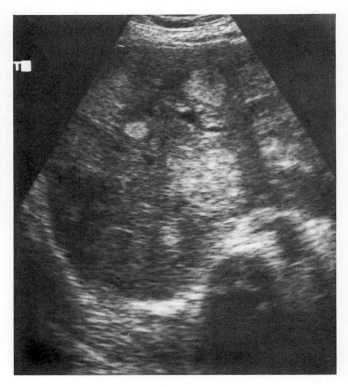

(A) metastatic colon carcinoma
(B) lymphoma
(C) metastatic carcinoid
(D) multiple hemangiomas
(E) multifocal hepatoma

461. A duplex Doppler ultrasound is performed on a kidney transplanted less than 24 hours before. Judging from the figure, a velocity spectrum obtained from an arcuate vessel, which ONE of the following processes would you say is MOST likely?

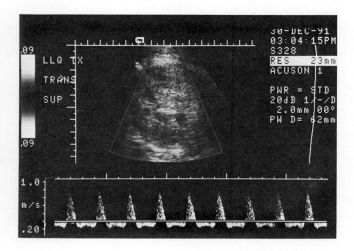

(A) Stenosis of the arterial anastomosis
(B) Acute tubular necrosis
(C) Arteriovenous fistula
(D) Cyclosporine toxicity
(E) Renal vein thrombosis

462. Based on the spectrum given in the figure accompanying Question 460, the resistive index is approximately

(A) 0%
(B) 50%
(C) 75%
(D) 100%
(E) 125%

DIRECTIONS: Each group of questions below consists of lettered headings followed by a set of numbered items. For each numbered item select the **one** lettered heading with which it is **most** closely associated. Each lettered heading may be used **once, more than once,** or **not at all.**

Questions 463–466

For each of the following renal diseases, choose the MOST common association.

(A) Hepatic cysts
(B) Ureteral atresia
(C) Renal cell carcinoma
(D) Duplication anomalies
(E) Hepatic fibrosis

463. Multicystic dysplastic kidney disease

464. Juvenile polycystic kidney disease

465. Autosomal dominant polycystic kidney disease

466. Dialysis-acquired renal cysts

Questions 467–469

An echogenic uterine mass is discovered by ultrasound. For each of the following additional features, what is the MOST likely diagnosis?

(A) Dermoid cyst
(B) Leiomyoma
(C) Molar pregnancy
(D) Incomplete abortion
(E) Ovarian hyperstimulation syndrome

467. Cystic adnexal mass(es)

468. Curvilinear calcification(s)

469. Open cervical os

Questions 470–472

For each of the following syndromes, select the feature with which it is commonly associated.

(A) Ectopia cordis
(B) Neonatal hypoglycemia
(C) Patent urachus
(D) Azygos continuation of the inferior vena cava
(E) Polydactyly

470. Beckwith-Wiedemann

471. Polysplenia

472. Eagle-Barrett ("prune belly")

DIRECTIONS: Each group of questions below consists of four lettered headings followed by a set of numbered items. For each numbered item select

A	if the item is associated with	(A)**only**
B	if the item is associated with	(B) **only**
C	if the item is associated with	**both** (A) and (B)
D	if the item is associated with	**neither** (A) nor (B)

Each lettered heading may be used **once, more than once,** or **not at all.**

Questions 473–477

(A) Pancreatic microcystic cystadenoma
(B) Pancreatic macrocystic cystadenoma
(C) Both
(D) Neither

473. Female predominance

474. Malignant potential

475. Associated with von Hippel-Lindau syndrome

476. Central stellate scar

477. May appear echogenic

Questions 478–482

(A) Hydranencephaly
(B) Alobar holoprosencephaly
(C) Both
(D) Neither

478. Monoventricle

479. Fused thalami

480. Cyclopia

481. Preservation of the hippocampal ridge

482. May resemble massive hydrocephalus

Questions 483–486

(A) Omphalocele
(B) Gastroschisis
(C) Both
(D) Neither

483. Reliably diagnosable at 10 to 12 weeks' gestation

484. Covered by a membrane

485. Elevated alpha fetoprotein

486. Chromosomal abnormalities

DIRECTIONS: Each question below contains five suggested answers. For **each** of the **five** alternatives listed, you are to respond either YES or NO. In a given item, **all, some,** or **none of the alternatives may be correct.**

487. Which of the following is/are part of Meckel-Gruber syndrome?

(A) Macroglossia
(B) Renal cysts
(C) Polydactyly
(D) Endocardial cushion defect
(E) Microcephaly

488. In a fetus with congenital cystic adenomatoid malformation of the lung, which of the following might be seen by ultrasound?

(A) Ascites
(B) Pulmonary mass with numerous cysts of varying size
(C) Pulmonary mass with numerous small (<2 cm) cysts
(D) An echogenic, solid-appearing pulmonary mass
(E) Bowel in a normal location in the abdomen

489. Which of the following statements regarding the spleen are TRUE?

(A) Hemangiosarcomas are the most common primary splenic neoplasm
(B) Splenomegaly in Hodgkin disease indicates tumor involvement
(C) Epidermoid splenic cysts are associated with cysts in other organs
(D) Pseudocysts are distinguished from true splenic cysts on the basis of size and wall thickness
(E) Splenic infarcts characteristically evolve from hypoechoic to hyperechoic

490. Which of the following features help to differentiate the fibrolamellar type of hepatocellular carcinoma from typical hepatoma?

(A) Absence of underlying liver disease
(B) Older patient
(C) Higher serum alpha-fetoprotein level
(D) Central fibrous scar or calcification
(E) Satellite nodules

491. Increased renal echogenicity in a fetus may represent

(A) a normal variant
(B) multicystic dysplastic kidney
(C) autosomal recessive polycystic kidney disease
(D) early sickle cell nephropathy
(E) autosomal dominant polycystic kidney disease

492. Regarding fetal cranial ultrasound, which of the following are TRUE statements?

(A) The width of the lateral ventricular atrium increases at a constant rate throughout gestation
(B) Hydrocephalus is the most sensitive indicator of a CNS abnormality
(C) The cerebral hemisphere nearer to the transducer is usually better visualized
(D) The "lemon sign" is a sensitive indicator of myelomeningocele
(E) The most common cause of hydrocephalus is aqueductal stenosis

493. Which of the following statements concerning vein of Galen aneurysms is/are true?

(A) They are the most common type of cranial vascular malformation
(B) Hydrocephalus is the most common presenting sign in the neonate
(C) Ultrasound diagnosis can be made during the second trimester
(D) Heart failure can develop because of a high-output state
(E) Doppler examination is diagnostic

494. Which of the following statements are TRUE regarding the Doppler frequency shift?

   (A) It is inversely proportional to the incident frequency
   (B) It is directly related to the cosine of the insonating angle
   (C) It approaches 0 at 180°
   (D) It varies with the size of the gate
   (E) It is inversely proportional to the speed of sound in air

495. Aliasing may be eliminated by

   (A) adjusting the spectral scale
   (B) adjusting the time gain compensation curve
   (C) using a higher-frequency transducer
   (D) widening the sample gate
   (E) increasing the angle of insonation toward 90°

496. A low resistive index may result from which of the following?

   (A) Relative increase in diastolic flow
   (B) Absolute increase in systolic flow
   (C) Arteriovenous shunting
   (D) A Doppler gate that is too wide
   (E) Poor angle correction

497. Regarding disease of the scrotum, which of the following statements are TRUE?

   (A) Scrotal hydroceles are located within the tunica albuginea
   (B) Testicular rupture is usually detectable by the visualization of a fracture plane
   (C) The nondescended testis is usually intraabdominal, just above the inguinal ring
   (D) Seminomas usually appear as an echogenic mass within the testis
   (E) Doppler examination may be helpful in evaluation of inflammatory disease of the scrotum

498. Regarding breast ultrasound, which of the following statements are TRUE?

   (A) Mammographically suspicious calcifications may be confirmed by sonography
   (B) Ultrasound is definitive in characterizing certain solid lesions as benign fibroadenomas
   (C) Cysts with debris may be difficult to distinguish from solid lesions
   (D) Solid lesions are readily distinguished from normal breast tissue
   (E) Sonography is useful in characterizing a palpable mass as solid

499. Which of the following are TRUE statements regarding encephaloceles?

   (A) They are commonly associated with the Arnold Chiari II malformation
   (B) An off-midline location suggests amniotic band syndrome
   (C) An encephalocele must be present to diagnose Meckel syndrome
   (D) Encephaloceles are most commonly frontal
   (E) They are readily distinguishable from other neck masses

500. Which of the following statements are TRUE regarding complete agenesis of the corpus callosum?

   (A) It is excluded by visualization of a cavum septum pellucidum
   (B) The "banana" sign is a sensitive sonographic indicator
   (C) It is characterized by midline cerebellar (vermian) hypoplasia
   (D) Medial displacement of the lateral ventricular walls by Probst's bundles is a feature
   (E) It may be associated with nonobstructive colpocephaly

501. Which statements concerning the biliary tree are TRUE?

(A) The most common noniatrogenic cause of pneumobilia is choledocho-duodenal fistula

(B) A common hepatic duct caliber of greater than 1 cm indicates ongoing obstruction

(C) The common hepatic duct normally decreases in size after a fatty meal

(D) The sonographic "too many tubes," or "shotgun sign," sign is a specific indicator for intrahepatic ductal dilatation

(E) The diagnoses of cholelithiasis and choledocholithiasis are easily made by ultrasound

502. Which statements regarding pancreatic sonography are TRUE?

(A) Diffuse calcifications within the pancreatic duct are highly specific for chronic pancreatitis

(B) A dilated pancreatic duct is a relatively specific sign of pancreatic carcinoma

(C) Functional islet cell tumors are reliably localized with ultrasound

(D) A unilocular mucinous cystadenoma is not distinguishable from a unilocular pseudocyst

(E) Splenic vein thrombosis may result from inflammatory or neoplastic pancreatic disease

503. Dense shadowing emanates from the gallbladder fossa, but no gallbladder lumen is visualized. Which of the following is/are possible?

(A) Agenesis of the gallbladder

(B) Chronic cholecystitis

(C) Emphysematous cholecystitis

(D) Porcelain gallbladder

(E) Diffuse cholesterolosis

504. Which of the following statements is/are TRUE regarding sonography of the AIDS patient?

(A) Bulky hypoechoic adenopathy is characteristic of CMV infection

(B) Cholangitis, with thickening of the bile duct walls, may result from *Cryptosporidium* infection

(C) Cystic changes within enlarged lymph nodes suggests disseminated *Pneumocystis carinii* infection

(D) Renal ultrasound characteristically demonstrates large hypoechoic kidneys secondary to glomerular and tubular changes

(E) Hepatosplenomegaly is relatively specific for HIV infection in children with AIDS

Ultrasonography

Answers

445. The answer is B. *(Taveras & Ferrucci, vol 4, chap 117.)* The sonogram in the figure demonstrates an echogenic renal mass (arrow). The most likely diagnosis is an angiomyolipoma, which is a benign hamartoma of the kidney that frequently occurs in patients with tuberous sclerosis. Since it has vascular, muscular, and lipomatous elements, it generates many acoustic interfaces, resulting in an echogenic appearance. CT is required to prove the presence of fat within the lesion, otherwise renal cell carcinoma cannot be excluded.

Although pyelonephritis usually appears as a hypoechoic mass, it may on occasion be echogenic. Renal tuberculosis results in parenchymal granulomas which frequently appear as echogenic masses.

Renal lymphoma, on the other hand, appears as solitary or multiple hypoechoic renal masses or may present as hypoechoic retroperitoneal masses enveloping and sometimes invading the kidney. It is rarely echogenic, since the homogeneous nature of the tumor results in few acoustic interfaces.

446. The answer is E. *(Kirks, pp 662–667.)* The sonogram of the child's abdomen in the figure demonstrates a hyperechoic circular mass with an echogenic center, giving the lesion a "target," or "bull's-eye," appearance. This is most compatible with a diagnosis of intussusception, in which proximal bowel (intussusceptum) invaginates into distal bowel (intussuscipiens). The echogenic area within the mass shown represents the mesenteric fat of the intussusceptum within the intussuscipiens, and should not be confused with renal sinus fat.

In children under 2 years of age, there is usually no definable lead point (fewer than 10% of cases), and the intussusception is attributed to hypertrophy of the lymphoid tissue comprising Peyer patches which have been stimulated by viral exposure. Therefore, the correct answer is idiopathic. Pathologic lead points include omphalomesenteric duct remnant (Meckel diverticulum), polyp, duplication cyst, lymphoma, and appendiceal stump.

A fecalith, to aid in the diagnosis of acute appendicitis, is not evident on the images. Wilms tumors are renal masses, which usually arise in older children, typically 2- to 5-year-olds.

447. The answer is D. *(Callen, ed. 2, pp 393–411.)* The pelvic ultrasound shown in the left and right figures demonstrates a highly echogenic endometrium and distal shadowing. This is typical of an IUD, though retained products of conception (fetal parts or calcified placental tissue) may sometimes create this appearance. Alternatively, air in the uterine cavity, from instrumentation or a fistula to bowel, might result in shadowing, but it is usually less intense and its gray appearance has been referred to as "dirty" shadowing.

The entity which does not account for this degree of echogenicity, or for the shadowing, would be the endometrium in the secretory phase of the menstrual cycle. This is the time when the thickness of the endometrium increases in preparation for menses. Although more echogenic, it does not produce nearly as bright echoes as those associated with air or calcification, and shadowing does not occur.

448. **The answer is B.** *(Taveras & Ferrucci, vol 4, chap 108.)* The figure at left demonstrates differential hydronephrosis in the two poles of a kidney. The upper pole is markedly hydronephrotic, and the cortex is almost completely atrophic. The images of the bladder (see figure at right) reveal a cystic structure near the trigone. This constellation of findings is characteristic of a complete duplication of the collecting system on that side, and a ureterocele which is obstructing the upper pole ureter.

In a complete duplication, the ureter of the pole moiety usually inserts ectopically low in the bladder, bladder neck, or posterior urethra, but sometimes into the seminal vesicle or ejaculatory duct in boys or into the vagina in girls. The ureter of the lower pole moiety inserts more cephalad (Weigert-Meyer rule) and assumes a horizontal path through the bladder wall. Typically, there is hydronephrosis in both poles, but it is greater in the upper moiety because of obstruction, and less in the lower pole, which tends to reflux. The ectopic ureteral orifice is often stenotic and causes the intramural portion of the ureter to dilate into a ureterocele, which appears sonographically as a cystic bladder mass.

449. **The answer is D.** *(Taveras & Ferrucci, vol 4, chap 67.)* The ultrasound in the figure at left demonstrates a markedly thick-walled and distended gallbladder. The discrete foci of shadowing represent gallstones. There is also an echogenic line along the anterior aspect of the gallbladder (see figure at right), indicating air within the lumen. The correct diagnosis is therefore emphysematous cholecystitis, a form of acute cholecystitis that occurs in elderly or diabetic patients, which has a much higher morbidity and mortality.

In chronic cholecystitis, the gallbladder wall is usually not as thick as it is in the acute form, and the lumen is usually small. Since no focal mass is visualized, gallbladder carcinoma is not likely. Perforated duodenal ulcer and ampullary passage of a gallstone may allow air into the gallbladder and biliary tree, but neither is likely to account for the diseased condition of the gallbladder.

450. **The answer is A.** *(Taveras & Ferrucci, vol 4, chap 110.)* The figure demonstrates highly echogenic renal pyramids, one of which is so dense as to cause shadowing. This is typical of medullary nephrocalcinosis, for which there are numerous etiologies. Of the choices given, only medullary sponge kidney occurs in the setting of normal serum and urinary calcium levels. The stasis of urine in congenitally dilated tubules causes the calcium to precipitate.

Multiple myeloma, hyperparathyroidism, vitamin D toxicosis, and sarcoidosis may all cause medullary nephrocalcinosis, but do so as a result of hypercalcemic hypercalcuria. Renal tubular acidosis (distal—type I) results in impaired hydrogen ion secretion and a loss of calcium in the urine. Hyperoxaluria develops in patients because of increased ingestion or absorption of oxalate, ethylene glycol toxicity, or pyridoxine deficiency; and also following methoxyfluorane anesthesia. It predisposes to cortical, not medullary, nephrocalcinosis. Xanthogranulomatous pyelonephritis is a chronic inflammatory condition resulting from long-standing obstruction (usually by a staghorn calculus) and is unrelated to nephrocalcinosis.

451. The answer is A. *(Mittelstaedt, pp 416–417. Pollack, vol I, chap 12.)* The entity which is least likely to produce generalized decreased renal echogenicity is retroperitoneal fibrosis. The ureters and vessels are enveloped, but not displaced, by hypoechoic fibrous tissue, resulting in an obstructive uropathy. Although it is most often idiopathic, it may arise secondary to drug toxicity (methysergide) or desmoplastic tumor reaction. The kidneys most often appear normal, even in the presence of high-grade obstruction, but may be hydronephrotic.

A generalized decrease in cortical echogenicity and a loss of corticomedullary distinction, in a patient with acute symptoms, should lead to the following differential diagnosis: renal vein thrombosis, renal arterial occlusion, and acute pyelonephritis. The latter two entities can both produce echogenic foci within the renal parenchyma as well. In the absence of acute symptoms, infiltrative tumors such as lymphoma should also be considered.

452. The answer is A. *(Appleman, Radiology 163:743–746, 1987.)* The most important diagnostic sign of deep venous thrombosis (DVT) is lack of compressibility of the vein. The sensitivity of this finding is over 90%. Although visualization of the thrombus is the ultimate proof of DVT, ultrasound is not a very sensitive means of detecting it, since recent thrombus is often isoechoic with blood.

Lack of augmentation, loss of respiratory phasicity, and visualization of collaterals are secondary signs of deep venous thrombosis.

453. The answer is B. *(Callen, ed. 2, pp 297–322.)* Placenta percreta results from a deficiency of decidualization, which allows the chorionic villi to penetrate through the myometrium and uterine serosa. Lesser forms include placenta accreta, in which the villi begin to grow into the myometrium, and placenta increta, where they extend through it. The most common predisposing factor is the uterine scar resulting from a prior cesarean section.

The major clinical problem results from retained placental tissue following delivery, which causes persistent postpartum bleeding. The diagnosis of placenta percreta may be suggested when myometrium is not identified beneath the placenta, which is an observation more easily made if the placenta is located anteriorly. Sometimes placental tissue is visualized extending into the urinary bladder. The milder forms (increta and accreta) are usually not identifiable sonographically.

454. The answer is D. *(Callen, ed. 2, pp 207–239.)* This third-trimester ultrasound demonstrates two cystic structures in the midabdomen of this fetus unrelated to the kidneys; the so-called double-bubble sign. It reflects obstruction of the midduodenum and dilatation of the stomach and duodenal bulb. The most common cause is duodenal atresia, a failure of recanalization of the duodenum, which normally occurs at 10 weeks' gestation. Duodenal stenosis, duplication cysts, and annular pancreas are less common entities which may cause duodenal obstruction. Ileal atresia results in a distal small-bowel obstruction, which produces many dilated loops of bowel.

455. The answer is C. *(Callen, ed. 2, pp 207–239.)* Duodenal atresia is frequently associated with polyhydramnios (45%) because the obstruction impairs fetal swallowing. It is highly associated with symmetrical growth retardation (50%) and is found in 30% of patients with trisomy 21 (Down syndrome). Ancillary sonographic findings in Down syndrome might also include endocardial cushion cardiac defects and biliary atresia. Meconium ileus is a consequence of cystic fibrosis and is not related to duodenal atresia.

456. The answer is A. *(Callen, ed. 2, pp 83–135.)* Neural tube defects are among the most common congenital anomalies in the U.S., estimated at 16 per 10,000 births. The most common anomaly affecting the nervous system is anencephaly, which is also the most severe defect. The absent cranial vault is sonograpically obvious above normally formed orbits, which gives the facies a striking appearance. Anencephaly results from a failure of the cephalad end of the neural tube to close completely, which occurs between the second and third weeks of fetal development. The cranial surface is covered by a thick angiomatous stroma instead of normal skin, which allows alpha fetoprotein (αFP), a glycoprotein synthesized by normal fetal liver tissue, to leak into the amniotic fluid. It then appears in the maternal serum in higher concentrations. The αFP is also elevated in other conditions in which the fetal nervous system is uncovered, such as myelomeningocele (the second-most-common open neural tube defect) and encephalocele (the least common). Gastroschisis and omphalocele are also associated with an elevated αFP, however, these are defects of the body wall, not the neural tube.

457. **The answer is A.** *(Callen, ed. 2, pp 207–239.)* The combination of fetal ascites and peritoneal calcifications occurs in meconium peritonitis, which is a sterile chemical peritonitis that follows small-bowel perforation in utero. The calcifications may take 10 days or so to form. Predisposing factors include obstructive bowel lesions such as volvulus, atresia, and malrotation, and less commonly follows meconium ileus in the setting of cystic fibrosis. Atresia of *distal* small intestine is necessary for meconium spillage to occur. The TORCH infections result in visceral and cerebral calcification, not meconium peritonitis. If there is an associated mass, then fetal neuroblastoma or teratoma should be included in the differential diagnosis.

458. **The answer is C.** *(Sanders, ed. 3, pp 321–332.)* The sonogram in the figure depicts an early twin gestation in a single gestational sac which has been divided by a membrane. The single gestational sac therefore has only one chorion, and the pregnancy is therefore monochorionic. Since the thin dividing membrane is made up of two abutting layers of amnion, this is a diamniotic pregnancy. A monochorionic pregnancy must be monozygotic (one sperm fertilizing one ovum).

For dichorionic pregnancies, however, a monozygotic gestation is indistinguishable sonographically from a dizygotic one when both fetuses have the same sex. Dizygotic gestations (two ova fertilized by two sperm) will always be *dichorionic* and *diamniotic*.

459. **The answer is B.** *(Sanders, ed. 3, pp 321–332.)* The incidence of twin gestations is 1 in 90 live births. Two-thirds of these are dizygotic (two sperm fertilizing two ova) and one-third are monozygotic (one sperm and one ovum). All dizygotic twins, however, must be dichorionic and diamniotic (i.e., two gestational sacs, each with its own amnion), and so choice (E) (dizygotic dichorionic monoamniotic) is not physiologically possible.

In two-thirds of monozygotic twins, cleavage occurs in the blastocyst stage, 4 to 8 days following fertilization, which results in one chorion and two amnions. In the other one-third of monozygotic twin gestations, the zygote cleaves earlier, within 4 days of fertilization, resulting in a dichorionic/diamniotic gestation, which appears sonographically identical to a dizygotic pregnancy. Monochorionic monoamniotic pregnancies result from a later cleavage of the zygote, 8 to 13 days following fertilization (3% of monozygotic twins).

460. **The answer is C.** *(Taveras & Ferrucci, vol 4, chap 61. Wilson, ed. 12, pp 1388–1389.)* The differential diagnosis of multiple echogenic liver masses, as shown in the figure, includes metastases from gastrointestinal malignancy, especially colon, and vascular/endocrine tumors, most notably carcinoid. Multicentric hepatoma and multiple benign hemangiomas are also considerations.

The symptoms lead one to the correct diagnosis: metastatic carcinoid. The syndrome results when metastases to the liver release serotonin, which causes diarrhea, flushing, valvular heart disease, and paroxysmal hypotension. The primary tumor in this case also acts as a lead point, producing intermittent intussusception. The severe peripheral edema is the result of right heart failure due to the associated valvular disease caused by endocardial fibroelastosis.

The patient's symptoms could be caused by lymphoma, which can cause diarrhea and obstruction secondary to small-bowel involvement; however, the lesions are most often hypoechoic.

461. The answer is E. *(Reuther, Radiology 170:557–558, 1989.)* The arterial Doppler spectrum shown in the figure demonstrates normal systolic flow. However, blood flow is directed *out* of the transplant during diastole, as the velocity curve is below the baseline. This reversal of flow indicates a dramatic elevation of vascular resistance, which occurs primarily in the setting of renal vein thrombosis or severe rejection (not given as a choice).

An inflow stenosis would result in increased systolic velocities across the anastomosis and dampened flow in the arcuate arteries and peripherally. Acute tubular necrosis and cyclosporine toxicity may increase resistance, but rarely if ever to such a degree. Also, cyclosporine toxicity requires time to develop and would not be expected in a newly transplanted kidney. An arteriovenous fistula, such as may occur following biopsy, would result in elevation of both systolic and diastolic flow, with a reduced vascular resistance.

462. The answer is E. *(Nelson, AJR 151:439–447, 1988.)* The equation to calculate a resistive index (RI) is given by

$$RI = \frac{PSV - EDV}{PSV}$$

where PSV = peak systolic velocity and EDV = end diastolic velocity.

Therefore, if the EDV is negative (below the baseline), then its absolute value is effectively added to the PSV which produces a resistive index over 100%. Thus the correct answer is 125%. If the EDV is zero, then the RI = 100%. If the EDV approaches the PSV (in cases of extremely high flow states, i.e., an arteriovenous fistula), then the RI approaches 0%.

463–466. The answers are: 463-B, 464-E, 465-A, 466-C. *(Taveras & Ferrucci, vol 4, chap 120.)* Multicystic dysplastic kidney disease is a nonfamilial entity which is most often unilateral. Sonographically, it appears as a dysmorphic kidney with multiple cysts of varying sizes and no discernible renal pelvis or continuity with the distal ureter. The ipsilateral renal artery is hypoplastic.

Juvenile polycystic kidney disease is a later expression of the infantile (autosomal recessive) form of polycystic disease. Although the disorder is usually lethal early in childhood, some variants have lesser renal disease and present later in childhood with progressive hepatic fibrosis, leading to portal hypertension, splenomegaly, and variceal bleeding.

Autosomal dominant polycystic renal disease usually arises in adulthood, and is sonographically characterized by numerous large renal cysts bilaterally. At least 30% of patients have cysts in other locations, particularly the liver and spleen and, less commonly, the pancreas. Associated abnormalities include intracranial "berry" aneurysms. Presentation may be due to hypertension, hematuria, and/or progressive renal failure.

Small renal cysts progressively develop in patients on long-term dialysis. The kidneys are usually shrunken from the underlying end-stage renal disease. Although the mechanism is not well understood, there is an increased incidence of renal cell carcinoma in these patients, which has prompted some investigators to advocate screening them with routine sonography or CT scanning.

467–469. The answers are: 467-C, 468-B, 469-D. *(Callen, ed. 2, pp 393–422.)* Cystic adnexal masses and an echogenic uterine mass is most consistent with the diagnosis of gestational trophoblastic disease. There are three forms—hydatidiform mole, invasive mole, and choriocarcinoma. The first is the most common, with an incidence of approximately one in 1200 to 2000 pregnancies. Risk factors include prior molar pregnancy and increasing age. Sonographically, a hydatidiform mole appears as an echogenic soft-tissue mass within the uterine cavity. Myriad small vesicles develop later, as the mole matures. Associated findings include hemorrhage, which is isoechoic with the mass when acute but which later appears as anechoic regions surrounding the tumor. Approximately 20–50% of patients with molar pregnancy develop theca-lutein cysts in the ovaries, secondary to the high levels of βHCG secreted by the molar tissue. Although ovarian hyperstimulation syndrome (caused by exogenous hormonal therapy) is also characterized by large cystic ovaries, there is no associated uterine mass.

Leiomyomas are the most common benign neoplasm of the uterus and are frequently multiple. Curvilinear calcification, though not the most common form, is virtually pathognomonic of a leiomyoma. Locations include submucosal (least common, but most likely to produce symptoms), intramural (most common), and subserosal (most likely to appear as an adnexal mass). The appearance of a myoma depends on the relative amounts of stromal and muscular elements and on the occurrence of any secondary changes such as hyalinization, fatty degeneration, calcification, hemorrhage, or necrosis. Immature leiomyomas are classically hypoechoic with little through transmission, but may become echogenic as the content of fibrous tissue increases. Degeneration often leaves cystic spaces that have increased through transmission. Dystrophic calcification forms, which is coarse and usually focal.

If an echogenic uterine mass is detected in association with an open cervical os, this is most suspicious for an incomplete abortion. The echogenic material may represent merely hemorrhage within the endometrial cavity or may represent retained products of conception, including fetal parts or placental tissue.

A dermoid cyst is an ovarian, not a uterine, mass, and is echogenic because of its fatty elements.

470–472. The answers are: 470-B, 471-D, 472-C. *(Callen, ed. 2, pp 246. Pollack, vol I, chap 19.)* Beckwith-Wiedemann syndrome is a disorder characterized by fetal hemimacrosomia, macroglossia, and omphalocele. Islands of hypertrophic pancreatic tissue (within the pancreas) produce insulin, which results in hypoglycemia shortly after birth.

Polysplenia and asplenia are syndromes of visceral heterotaxy, with a tendency for organs which are normally asymmetrical to have mirror-image counterparts. Both have a male predominance. Polysplenia is characterized by bilateral left-sidedness, including two left lungs and multiple spleens. There is often absence of the intrahepatic inferior vena cava, in which case blood from the lower half of the body returns to the heart via "continuation" of the azygos vein.

Eagle-Barrett, or "prune belly," syndrome is a disorder of uncertain pathogenesis which almost exclusively affects males. It is usually a triad consisting of lax abdominal musculature, undescended testes, and various urinary tract abnormalities. The renal collecting systems are atonic, which produces a nonobstructive hydronephrosis the resultant dilatation of the ureters, bladder and posterior urethra, can be mistaken for a case of posterior urethral valves. Associated urologic abnormalities include patent urachus and urachal remnants.

Ectopia cordis is not associated with any of the options given, but is a feature of pentalogy of Cantrell. It is a complex midline body-wall anomaly characterized by omphalocele, diaphragmatic defect, and a sternal cleft with location of the heart outside of the thorax.

473–477. The answers are: 473-C, 474-B, 475-A, 476-A, 477-A. *(Friedman, Radiology 149:45–50, 1983.)* Cystic pancreatic tumors may be classified into two broad categories—microcystic adenoma (serous) and mucinous cystadenoma (macrocystic). Both are found more commonly in women, but only the microcystic adenomas are associated with the von Hippel-Lindau syndrome. The microcystic type is more likely to occur in the head of the pancreas whereas the mucinous type is more commonly found in the body and tail.

The microcystic adenoma has no malignant potential. It is characterized by numerous small cysts, usually under 2 cm, but may have several larger cysts. When the cysts are numerous and very small, the mass may appear echogenic, due to the high number of tissue interfaces. It is usually vascular, and may demonstrate a central stellate scar, with or without calcification.

The mucinous cystadenoma, on the other hand, does possess a malignant potential and may develop into a cystadenocarcinoma. The cysts which characterize this lesion are usually large, and the tumor is typically hypo- or avascular.

478–482. The answers are: 478-B, 479-B, 480-B, 481-A, 482-C. *(Callen, ed. 2, pp 83–135.)* Holoprosencephaly refers to a spectrum of congenital abnormalities of normal development of the prosencephalon (forebrain). The most severe form is the alobar type in which there has been a failure for normal cleavage to occur, creating a single mass of brain tissue with a monoventricle. The thalamus and basal ganglia are also fused. Midline structures such as the corpus callosum, falx, optic tracts, and olfactory bulbs fail to develop. The more caudal structures (midbrain, brainstem, and cerebellum) are normal, unless significant hydrocephalus arises. Less severe developmental distortion results in the semilobar and lobar forms, in which the appearance of the brain approaches normal. The septum pellucidum does not form in any type of holoprosencephaly and its identification helps to exclude the diagnosis. Any remaining cerebral tissue which surrounds the monoventricular cavity is displaced cephalad and anteriorly, and the hippocampal ridge is rostrally displaced. No cerebral tissue surrounds the dorsal sac. Severe facial dysmorphism may be present.

Hydranencephaly is the massive destruction or atrophy of the cerebral hemispheres and basal ganglia, resulting from occlusion of internal carotid circulation. The thalami are usually preserved, but are never fused as they are in holoprosencephaly, and the choroid plexus may also be spared. Some temporal cortex may remain intact, including the hippocampi and parahippocampal gyri, which usually retain their normal location.

483–486. The answers are: 483-D, 484-A, 485-C, 486-A. *(Callen, ed. 2, pp 240–253.)* Between 9 and 12 menstrual weeks, the fetal bowel physiologically herniates into the base of the umbilical cord, appearing there as an echogenic mass, and begins a complex series of rotations. Therefore, the diagnosis of an omphalocele or gastroschisis may be difficult prior to 12 weeks. After that time, however, a mass at the base of the cord is most certainly abnormal. The omphalocele is reliably diagnosed by its midline location and by whether or not it contains liver tissue and has a covering membrane. In contrast, a gastroschisis occurs to the right of midline, and rarely if ever contains liver tissue, and it has no overlying membrane.

There is an increased incidence of polyhydramnios and genetic abnormalities with omphaloceles, specifically cardiovascular defects (trisomy 18) and cranial anomalies (trisomy 13), which are both rare with gastroschisis. Alpha-fetoprotein levels are elevated in both, but are higher in the setting of a gastroschisis, since there is no peritoneal membrane covering the defect. Additionally, the free-floating bowel loops are irritated by the amniotic fluid and become thick-walled and matted.

487. The answers are: A-N, B-Y, C-Y, D-N, E-Y. *(Callen, ed. 2, pp 254–276.)* Meckel-Gruber syndrome is a fatal autosomal recessive disease which is characterized by bilateral multicystic dysplastic kidneys (95% of cases), occipital encephaloceles (80%), and polydactyly (75% of cases). The presence of at least two of the features is required for diagnosis. Additional associations include cleft lip and palate, microcephaly, and the development of oligohydramnios secondary to renal dysfunction.

488. The answers are: A-Y, B-Y, C-Y, D-Y, E-Y. *(Rosado-de-Christenson, Radiographics 11:865–886, 1991.)* Congenital cystic adenomatoid malformation (CCAM) is a hamartoma arising from fetal lung, and is classified into three types. Type I malformation, the most common, contains one or more dominant cysts surrounded by multiple smaller cysts (2–10 cm). Type II is a multicystic mass with numerous small cysts smaller than 2 cm and is associated with renal agenesis. Type III is the type originally described by Ch'in and Tang in 1949; it appears as a solid echogenic mass because the cysts are microscopic and present the ultrasound beam with myriad tissue interfaces. Polyhydramnios and fetal anasarca are commonly associated. Prognosis in cystic adenomatoid malformation depends upon the condition of the contralateral lung, which is often hypoplastic, and upon any associated abnormalities.

The differential diagnosis of a multicystic thoracic mass includes congenital diaphragmatic hernia. However, fetal stomach or bowel would not maintain their normal positions within the abdomen.

489. **The answers are: A-N, B-N, C-N, D-N, E-Y.** *(Ros, Radiology 162:73–77, 1987. Georg, Radiology 174:803–807, 1990. Dachman, AJR 147:537–542, 1986.)* Hemangiomas, although rare, are the most common primary splenic neoplasm. They may be predominantly echogenic, but also cystic and complex. Calcifications, similar to phleboliths, may be present. Histologically, they are characterized by a proliferation of endothelial-lined vascular channels filled with erythrocytes. Lymphangiomas may appear similar, but the cystic spaces are filled with lymphatic fluid.

The spleen is a common site of lymphoma of all types. In patients with non-Hodgkin lymphoma, splenomegaly is a good indicator of organ involvement (even without focal masses), but in Hodgkin lymphoma, the size of the spleen does not correlate with disease. When focal, the splenic lesions are usually hypoechoic.

Traumatic splenic cysts are not true cysts, since they do not have an epithelial lining. Pancreatic pseudocysts can insinuate themselves into the splenic hilum and may mimic splenic cysts. Neither is sonographically distinguishable from a true congenital cyst, which does have an epithelial lining. Congenital cysts usually occur sporadically and are not associated with cysts in other organs.

Acute splenic infarcts are invariably hypoechoic and may either be wedge-shaped or round, most often with irregular borders. They routinely decrease in size and increase in echogenicity with time.

490. **The answers are: A-Y, B-N, C-N, D-Y, E-N.** *(Friedman, Radiology 157:583–587, 1985.)* Fibrolamellar hepatocellular carcinoma is distinguished from the usual variety in that it is most often sporadic and tends to occur in younger patients who have no predisposing liver disease. The alphafetoprotein (αFP) level is usually normal. Sonographically, the lesions are usually echogenic and well-demarcated, with central hypoechoic or echogenic regions that may correspond to the histologic findings of a central fibrous scar or stellate calcifications, respectively. Fibrolamellar tumors have an overall better prognosis than those with the usual histology, but nevertheless can metastasize. Satellite nodules should be looked for, as well as portal vein invasion.

491. **The answers are: A-Y, B-Y, C-Y, D-N, E-N.** *(Estroff, Radiology 181:135–139, 1991.)* Increased renal echogenicity in a fetal kidney may be normal, but it may represent a multicystic dyplastic kidney or infantile (autosomal recessive) polycystic disease. Autosomal dominant polycystic renal disease is rarely manifest antenatally, but may produce one or more macroscopic cysts, which represent dilated nephrons. Sickle cell disease has no in utero manifestations, since circulating fetal hemoglobin is all type F, but in adults the disease may produce large, echogenic kidneys.

492. **The answers are: A-N, B-Y, C-N, D-Y, E-N.** *(Filly, Radiology 181:1–7, 1991.)* The width of the atrium of the lateral ventricle is a useful measurement in pregnancy because its value remains stable during the second and third trimesters. The normal size upper limit is approximately 10 mm. This measurement is obtained at the level of the glomus of the choroid plexus, which should fill or nearly fill the atrium. If the value obtained is greater than 1 cm, then hydrocephalus is present, which is the most sensitive indicator of CNS abnormality (88%). However, 15% of open spinal dysraphisms, most of the closed spinal dysraphisms, and some Dandy-Walker variants and anomalies of neuronal migration may all retain a normal ventricular size.

Performance of antenatal cranial ultrasound is somewhat hindered by the fact that the far hemisphere is better visualized, as compared to the near hemisphere, because reverberation artifact from the fetal skull obscures the near field. Symmetry is assumed to be present unless asymmetry can be documented.

Although the pathogenesis of the "lemon sign" is unknown, it has a high association with spina bifida, particularly in fetuses under 24 weeks of age. Hydrocephalus occurs in a wide variety of CNS anomalies; the most common underlying etiology is a Chiari II malformation with an associated myelomeningocele.

493. The answers are: A-Y, B-N, C-N, D-Y, E-Y. *(Comstock, J Ultrasound Med 10:361–365, 1991.)* The vein of Galen aneurysm is the most common cranial vascular malformation. A key perinatal clue to the presence of a vein of Galen malformation is high-output heart failure, but it may be so severe as to cause fetal hydrops. However, there is also a high incidence of associated cardiovascular anomalies, so that if congestive heart failure develops, it should not be presumed to be solely on the basis of a high-output state. The sonographic diagnosis is made by demonstration of a cystic mass (the nidus) in the region of the quadrigeminal plate cistern, which has a high Doppler signal, indicating rapid flow. To date, this has not been documented prior to the third trimester. Hydrocephalus may not be present in the neonate, but is the major presenting sign after the neonatal period. The lesion may also compromise cerebral perfusion since it acts as a siphon. Brain infarction and leukomalacia may result. Unfortunately, little can be done postnatally to prevent these sequelae, and mortality is high.

494. The answers are: A-N, B-Y, C-N, D-N, E-N. *(Taylor, Radiology 174:297–307, 1990.)* The Doppler equation is given by

$$\Delta v = \left(\frac{2vs}{v}\right)\cos v$$

where

Δv = Doppler frequency shift
v = incident frequency of Doppler pulses
s = speed of moving object
Θ = angle of sound beam insonation
v = speed of sound in tissue (1540 m/sec).

The frequency shift is therefore directly proportional to the incident frequency and cos Θ and inversely related to the speed of sound in tissue (not air). Since cos 90° is 0, and cos 0°, or 180°, is 1, the Doppler shift is maximized by insonating at angles closer to 0 or 180°. The frequency shift is independent of the size of the Doppler gate, which simply determines the sample volume of tissue being insonated.

495. The answers are: A-Y, B-N, C-N, D-N, E-Y. *(Taylor & Holland, Radiology 1990; 174:297–207.)* The pulse repetition frequency is the frequency at which a series of tones is emitted by a probe. When a pulse is transmitted, the system must receive the last echo from this pulse before it can transmit the next one. This is necessary to preserve unambiguous determination of source location. The maximum measurable frequency is half the pulse repetition frequency (PRF), since the signal must reach the object and return. Therefore, the maximum velocity measurable (V_{max}) by a system with a fixed pulse repetition frequency is

$$V_{max} = \left(\frac{PRF}{4}\right)\left(\frac{v}{v\cos\Theta}\right)$$

where v = the speed of sound in tissue
v = the incident frequency
Θ = angle of insonation

So, the maximum measurable velocity can be increased by increasing the PRF, decreasing the incident frequency of doppler pulses, or decreasing cos Θ (i.e., increasing the angle toward 90°).

Aliasing occurs when the velocities measured exceed the V_{max} and PRF of a system. When plotted on a graph, the peak velocities in the forward direction are misregistered below the baseline as slow velocities in a reverse direction. Changing to a lower-frequency transducer will reduce aliasing. Another alternative is to switch to continuous-wave pulsed Doppler, which has a PRF of infinity. But there are two ways to eliminate aliasing with a given transducer. The first is to increase the sampling rate, which is automatically done using most systems by adjusting the spectral scale. However, depending on the depth of the vessel and the fixed speed of sound in tissue, it may be impossible to increase the PRF sufficiently, especially for fast flow in deep vessels. The other method is to obtain a greater angle of insonation in order to reduce the Doppler shift and allow it to fit the scale.

496. The answers are: A-Y, B-N, C-Y, D-N, E-N. *(Nelson, AJR 151:439–447, 1988.)* The resistive index is a measure of resistance in a vascular bed, which has a direct impact on diastolic flow; as the resistance decreases, there is an increase in diastolic flow. The resistive index is relative, however, and does not reflect the absolute amount of systolic flow, nor is it specific. For instance, diastolic flow is also increased by shunting, such as in an arteriovenous malformation or neoplasm.

Widening the Doppler gate does not affect the value of the index, but does result in a wider range of velocities being sampled. Poor angle correction results in inaccurate absolute velocities. However, since both peak systolic velocity and end diastolic velocity are affected equally by changes in angle, the resistive index remains unchanged.

497. The answers are: A-N, B-N, C-N, D-N, E-Y. *(Taveras & Ferrucci, vol 4, chap 134.)* The tunica *albuginea* is the dense connective tissue which surrounds each testis. The tunica *vaginalis* is an extension of parietal peritoneum that covers the posterior portion of each testis. It contains a potential space which may accumulate fluid, forming a hydrocele.

Testicular rupture is characterized by disorganization of the echotexture of the testis. Fracture planes are rarely, if ever, visualized by ultrasound even when rupture is later found at operation. The integrity of the tunica albuginea is also not reliably evaluated by ultrasound.

Most (80%) of undescended testes are located within the inguinal canal. Only 20% are intraabdominal, but this difference is important to the operative approach for orchiopexy. Testicular agenesis, incidentally, is quite rare.

Seminomas are the most common neoplasm arising in the testis and most often appear as hypoechoic masses. The other germ cell tumors, including embryonal cell carcinoma and choriocarcinoma, more frequently appear as heterogeneous masses, with areas of cystic necrosis or calcification.

Although Doppler ultrasound has only recently been applied to diseases of the scrotum, it holds promise for distinguishing acute torsion of the testis from epididymoorchitis.

498. The answers are: A-N, B-N, C-Y, D-N, E-Y. *(Jackson, Radiology 177:305–311, 1990.)* Microcalcifications which appear malignant on mammography are rarely, if ever, visualized on ultrasound because of their small size. Breast calcifications coarse enough to be visualized sonographically are those associated with fibroadenomas or, occasionally, mammary duct ectasia. Unfortunately, it is not possible for ultrasound to distinguish between benign and malignant solid breast masses. There are features which favor a benign lesion, typically a fibroadenoma, which include good definition, homogeneous echotexture, and enhanced through transmission. Irregular margins and acoustic shadowing favor a diagnosis of malignancy.

Cysts with debris may be quite difficult to distinguish from solid lesions, just as the most common benign solid lesion, the fibroadenoma, may appear hyperechoic and have acoustic enhancement posteriorly. Solid lesions may be difficult to locate with ultrasound, since they are often isoechoic with breast tissue. Conversely, normal breast tissue may sometimes be lobular and dense, mimicking a breast mass.

One of the most useful applications of ultrasound in the breast is the characterization of palpable masses as cystic or solid, and it complements mammography well in this capacity.

499. The answers are: A-Y, B-Y, C-N, D-N, E-Y. *(Callen, ed. 2, pp 83–135.)* Encephaloceles result from a failure of closure of the neural tube, and occur at a rate of 4 per 10,000 births. They occur in the midline and are most common in the occipital region (75%), but may be frontal (13%) or parietal (12%). Basal skull encephaloceles are quite rare. Arnold Chiari malformation is a common association, as is Dandy-Walker malformation and agenesis of the corpus callosum. Encephaloceles are also common in Meckel syndrome (80% of cases).

Off-midline encephaloceles are invariably the result of the amniotic band syndrome, and may accompany limb amputations and body wall defects. A bony defect helps distinguish them from other fetal neck lesions.

500. The answers are: A-Y, B-N, C-N, D-N, E-Y. *(Callen, ed. 2, pp 83–135.)* The corpus callosum is the largest fiber tract in the nervous system; it develops from anterior to posterior between the eighth and seventeenth weeks. Since the septum pellucidum forms concomitantly, its visualization excludes a complete agenesis of the corpus callosum. When partial, dysgenesis affects the posterior aspect, which forms later. So far, only complete agenesis of the corpus callosum has been documented in utero. Since the fibers cannot cross into the contralateral hemisphere, they run in thick longitudinal bundles (of Probst) along the medial walls of the lateral ventricles, characteristically indenting them and displacing the ventricles laterally. The absence of the large callosal tract over the roof of the ventricles allows them to extend more cranially. The third ventricle similarly may expand and "herniate" upward between the hemispheres. Enlargement of the ventricular atria and occipital horns from underdeveloped white matter tracts is termed *colpocephaly,* which is a focal nonobstructive type of hydrocephalus. Abnormalities associated with agenesis of the corpus callosum include all forms of holoprosencephaly, Dandy-Walker malformation, hypoplastic falx cerebri, intracranial lipoma, heterotopic gray matter, and certain trisomies.

The "banana" sign is not a characteristic of agenesis of the corpus callosum. It is associated with the Arnold-Chiari malformation and myelomeningocele. Midline cerebellar (vermian) hypoplasia is a characteristic of the Dandy-Walker malformation, which results in a large fourth ventricle and appears as a large posterior fossa cystic structure or mass. Although the Dandy-Walker anomaly may coexist with agenesis of the corpus callosum, vermian hypoplasia, which is integral to Dandy-Walker, occurs independently.

501. The answers are: A-N, B-N, C-Y, D-N, E-N. *(Mittelstaedt, pp 81–162. Taveras & Ferrucci, vol 4, chap 68.)* The most common cause of air in the biliary tree is a surgically created biliary-enteric anastomosis. Of the noniatrogenic causes, the most frequent is chole*cysto*duodenal fistula, followed by cholecystocolic fistula. Both result from cholelithiasis and erosion of a gallstone into the adjacent bowel. Tumors of the gastrointestinal tract or biliary tree are a rare cause of pneumobilia.

A diameter of 6 mm is the upper limit of normal for the common hepatic duct. However, a larger diameter does not necessarily indicate current obstruction. Dilatation is frequently seen in the elderly because of reduced elasticity of the duct walls. Additionally, following high-grade obstruction, duct caliber may not return to preobstruction dimensions.

When a fatty meal is consumed, the gallbladder normally contracts and the sphincter of Oddi relaxes. The bile duct caliber either does not change or it decreases. In the presence of obstruction, the duct paradoxically increases in caliber.

The "too many tubes" sign refers to the demonstration of linear structures which parallel the portal vein. It was originally felt to indicate intrahepatic biliary ductal dilatation, but is now considered unreliable because, as ultrasound resolution has improved, nondilated ducts are also sometimes visualized. Also, in the setting of portal hypertension, the hepatic arteries carry increased flow and may be seen as parallel tubes.

Ultrasound is the method of choice for the diagnosis of cholelithiasis, but its role in choledocholithiasis is less certain. The diagnosis of a common duct stone is only made in 25% of cases.

Reasons for poor specificity include the deep location of the common duct, obscuration of the duct by air in adjacent duodenum, and lack of fluid surrounding the stone.

502. **The answers are: A-Y, B-N, C-N, D-Y, E-Y.** *(Mittelstaedt, pp 163–220.)* Approximately 20 to 40% of patients (often alcoholic) with chronic pancreatitis develop stone disease. The stones are usually within the pancreatic ducts rather than in the parenchyma.

Pancreatic ductal dilatation indicates an abnormality, but may be seen in carcinoma or chronic pancreatitis. If ductal calcifications are seen, the latter diagnosis is favored. Even when a mass is visible, differentiating these two entities may be impossible unless distant metastases are discovered.

Since functional islet cell tumors are frequently small (most under 2 cm), ultrasound is not reliable in localization unless the study is performed in the operating room. Twenty percent of islet cell tumors are nonfunctional, and become evident only because of mass effect. These lesions are more easily visualized by ultrasound.

A unilocular mucinous cystadenoma may be indistinguishable from a pseudocyst, and the clinical history is usually vital in making the diagnosis. Pseudocysts are usually located in the lesser sac or the left anterior pararenal space, but they may track into unusual locations.

Both inflammatory and neoplastic disease may result in splenic vein thrombosis. Collateral venous channels may develop around the stomach or in the porta hepatis. Inflammation around the splenic artery may also result in pseudoaneurysm formation.

503. **The answers are: A-Y, B-Y, C-Y, D-Y, E-N.** *(Mittelstaedt, pp 81–157.)* Shadowing from the gallbladder fossa, with no visible gallbladder lumen, is a commonly encountered clinical problem. The shadowing results from air or calcification.

In gallbladder agenesis, the fossa is occupied by bowel (frequently the colon), resulting in dense shadowing from air within the bowel lumen. Even when the gallbladder is present, bowel directly adjacent may contain air which scatters the sound beam and causes shadowing.

Chronic cholecystitis is usually a sequela of cholelithiasis, which is a common cause of dense shadowing. The lumen may not be visualized in this setting since the gallbladder is often small and contracted. Porcelain gallbladder is a subtype of chronic cholecystitis, in which the gallbladder wall is densely calcified and is considered premalignant. Emphysematous cholecystitis is a much rarer entity. It is a form of acute cholecystitis which is found in elderly or diabetic patients, and results from gangrenous infection of the biliary tree. By definition, air is found in the lumen and/or wall of the gallbladder.

In cholesterolosis (the "strawberry gallbladder") the gallbladder lumen is well-visualized, but small echogenic nonmobile foci protrude into the lumen. "Ring down" artifact may emanate from many of them.

504. **The answers are: A-N, B-Y, C-N, D-N, E-N.** *(Federle, Radiology 166:553–562, 1988. Haney, AJR 152:1033–1042, 1989. Radin, AJR 154:27–31, 1990.)* Mesenteric and retroperitoneal adenopathy is a common finding in patients with lymphoma, Kaposi sarcoma, or *Mycobacterium avium-intracellulare* (MAI) infection. The last entity may be distinguished from the others by identifying cystic areas within the adenopathy secondary to caseation or necrosis. Cytomegalovirus (CMV) infection does not characteristically produce adenopathy.

AIDS-related cholangitis consists of the typical triad of pain, fever, and jaundice. Sonography may show irregularly beaded ducts with thickened walls, including gallbladder-wall thickening, even in the absence of calculi. The more common organisms are *Cryptosporidium* and CMV.

Visceral and nodal calcifications have been identified in patients with disseminated *Pneumocystis carinii* infection. The calcifications may be punctate and so fine that they do not produce shadowing. The organs involved include the liver, spleen, kidneys, adrenal glands, and lymph nodes.

The cause of AIDS nephropathy has not been entirely elucidated, but pathologic changes include glomerulosclerosis as well as tubular dilatation, both of which result in increased renal echogenicity.

Hepatosplenomegaly is a common, but nonspecific abnormality in the pediatric AIDS patient. It may be caused by the HIV virus itself, but CMV, hepatitis B, and MAI are often found. All produce chronic liver infections and may progress to liver failure and portal hypertension.

Cardiovascular and Interventional Radiology

DIRECTIONS: Each question below contains five suggested responses. Select the **one best** response to each question.

505. Judging from the angiogram shown in the figure, what would you say is the MOST likely diagnosis for this 23-year-old male patient?

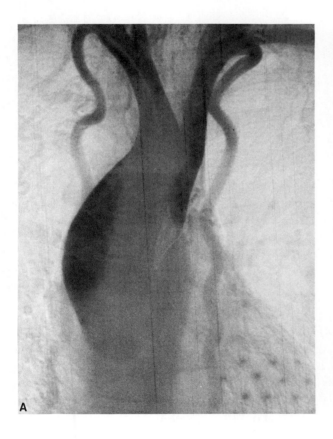 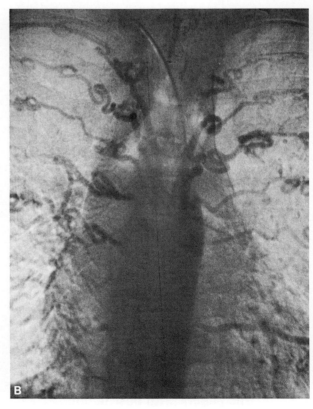

(A) Marfan syndrome
(B) Interrupted aortic arch
(C) Superior vena cava obstruction
(D) Pulmonic stenosis
(E) Postductal coarctation of the aorta

506. The 31-year-old woman, whose angiogram is shown in the figure was the unrestrained driver in a motor vehicle accident. The MOST likely diagnosis is

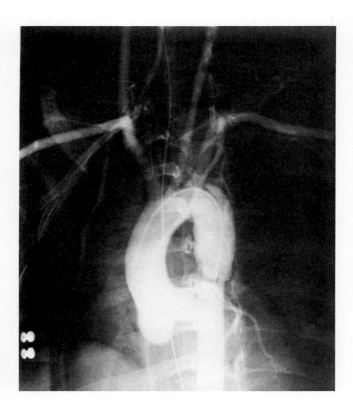

(A)   aortic dissection
(B)   congenital aortic web
(C)   pseudocoarctation of the aorta
(D)   previous open heart surgery
(E)   laceration of the aorta

507. Antibiotic prophylaxis both during and after treatment is routinely used in ALL the following clinical situations EXCEPT

(A)   hepatic abscess drainage
(B)   nephrostomy for afebrile patient with obstructing calculus
(C)   gastrostomy tube placement in patient with prosthetic mitral valve
(D)   hepatic cyst aspiration
(E)   transhepatic biliary drainage for afebrile patient with obstruction

508. The patient whose angiogram is shown in the figure has MOST likely had which type of operative shunt?

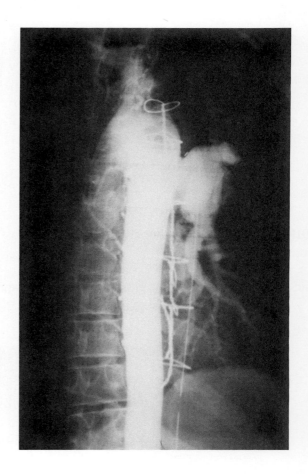

(A)   Glenn
(B)   Potts
(C)   Waterston
(D)   Blalock-Taussig
(E)   None of the above

509. A 2-day-old infant is brought to the emergency room with severe cyanosis. The LEAST likely diagnosis is

(A)   tetralogy of Fallot
(B)   total anomalous pulmonary venous return (TAPVR) below the diaphragm
(C)   complete transposition of the great vessels
(D)   Ebstein anomaly
(E)   hypoplastic left heart syndrome

510. A 21-year-old male had a sudden cardiac arrest while exercising. Angiograms of the right (A) and left (B) coronary arteries, shown in the figure, were obtained. The MOST likely diagnosis is

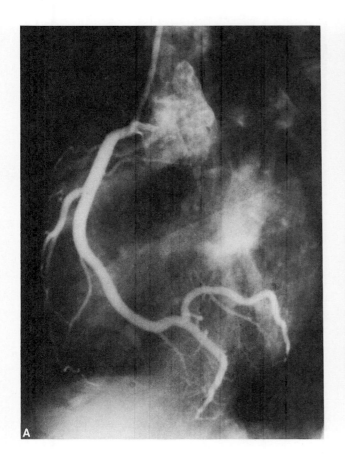
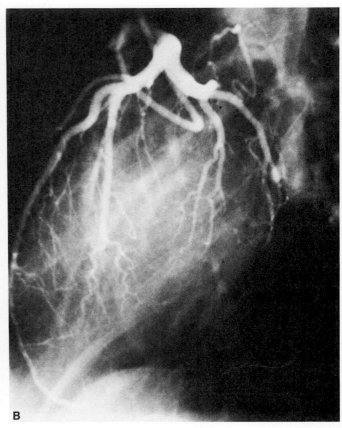

(A) Wolf-Parkinson-White syndrome
(B) aberrant origin of the left coronary artery
(C) acute coronary thromboembolism
(D) polyarteritis nodosa
(E) dominant left coronary circulation

---

511. Two weeks after cardiac transplantation, a patient develops widespread pulmonary infiltrates. The MOST likely causative agent is

(A) *Aspergillus*
(B) *Pneumocystis carinii*
(C) *Nocardia*
(D) Cytomegalovirus
(E) Pneumococcus

512. Of the following congenital syndromes, the ONE which is the LEAST commonly associated with a cardiovascular anomaly is

(A) Turner
(B) Down
(C) Ellis-van Creveld
(D) Apert
(E) Williams

513. Judging from the chest x-ray of this 55-year-old man (see the figure), what would you say is the MOST likely diagnosis?

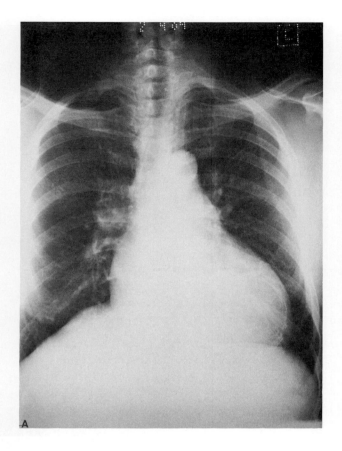 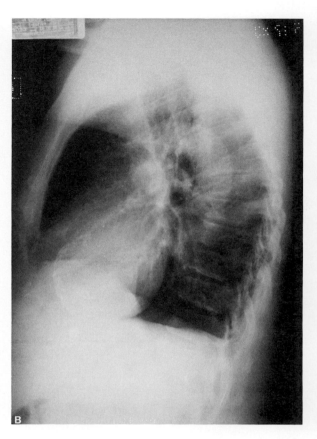

(A) Dressler syndrome
(B) Constrictive pericarditis
(C) False left ventricular aneurysm
(D) Endocardial fibroelastosis
(E) None of the above

514. Of the following collateral pathways, the ONE which is LEAST commonly found in occlusion of the right coronary artery is

(A) left anterior descending artery to posterior descending artery via septal branches
(B) Kugel's artery
(C) distal circumflex artery to distal right coronary artery
(D) conus artery
(E) left anterior descending artery branch to acute marginal branch of right coronary artery

515. Of the following primary cardiac neoplasms, the LEAST common is

(A) myxoma
(B) rhabdomyoma
(C) teratoma
(D) lymphoma
(E) sarcoma

516. A 67-year-old black woman presented to her family physician complaining of abdominal pain and irregular bowel movements. Her CT scan is shown in the figure at left. The contrast in the irregular vascular channels in the angiogram at right did not change appreciably with time. The MOST likely diagnosis is

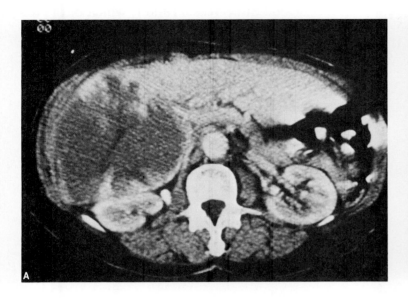
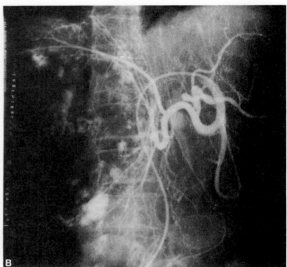

(A) hepatocellular carcinoma
(B) focal nodular hyperplasia
(C) focal fatty infiltration
(D) giant cavernous hemangioma
(E) regenerating nodule

517. A 74-year-old woman with a history of a left hemicolectomy for carcinoma had the follow-up studies shown in the figures. The MOST likely diagnosis is

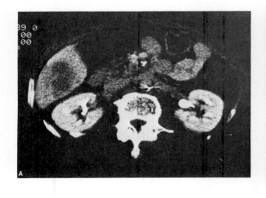
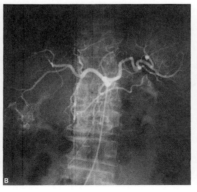
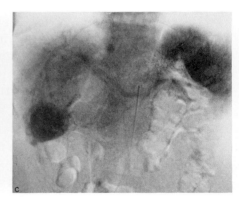

(A) hepatocellular carcinoma
(B) focal nodular hyperplasia
(C) colon carcinoma metastasis
(D) hepatic adenoma
(E) none of the above

518. The young man in the figure underwent angiography after being shot in the leg. The patient requires

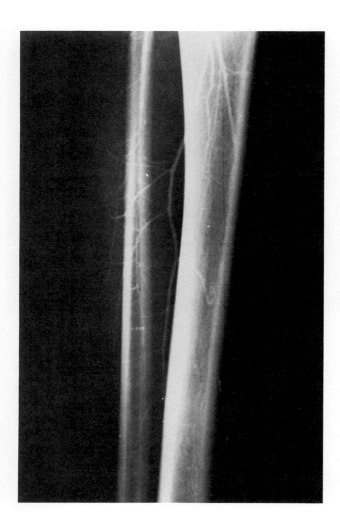

519. A 77-year-old diabetic man has had long-standing half-block claudication on the right and now complains of rest pain in the right foot. Based on the angiogram of the thigh (see figure) and given that there is good three-vessel runoff, which of the following treatments is/are MOST likely to be recommended?

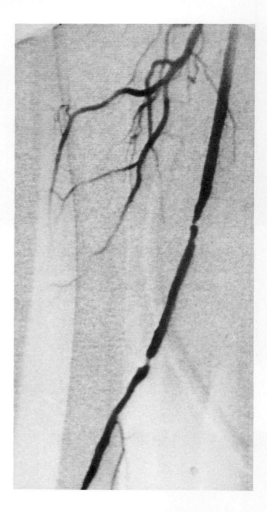

(A) surgical treatment of arterial injury
(B) intra-arterial nitroglycerin
(C) regional thrombolysis
(D) two- or four-compartment fasciotomy
(E) none of the above

(A) Transluminal angioplasty
(B) Femoropopliteal bypass graft
(C) Oral pentoxifylline (Trental) therapy and exercise
(D) Laser atherectomy
(E) Sympathectomy

520. Following uncomplicated treatment, the patient in Question 519 could anticipate a 3-year patency of up to

(A) 5%
(B) 20%
(C) 50%
(D) 70%
(E) 90%

521. The young woman whose angiogram is shown in the figure has been treated for chronic migraine headaches. She currently complains of numbness and weakness in both upper extremities. The LEAST likely diagnosis is

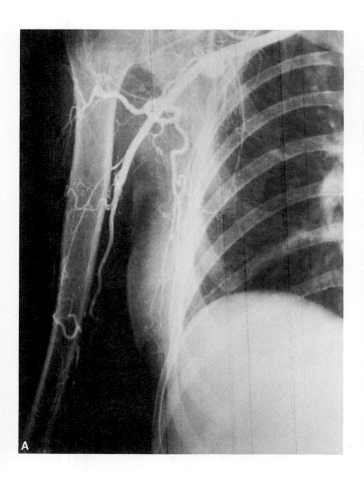
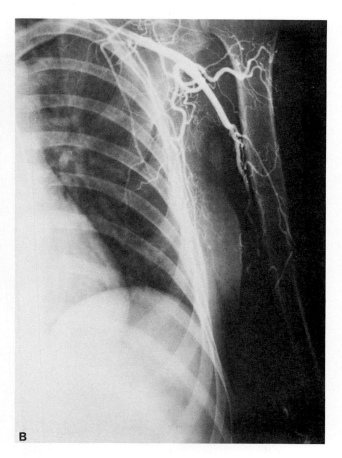

(A) ergotism
(B) giant cell arteritis
(C) Takayasu arteritis
(D) Buerger disease
(E) Raynaud phenomenon

522. A 60-year-old woman, who presented with disabling claudication (see arteriogram in the figure at left), had a lesion in the proximal left external iliac artery and good distal runoff. Another arteriogram was performed after percutaneous transluminal angioplasty (PTA) and is shown in the figure at right. Given no other changes, further treatment strategies might include ALL the following EXCEPT

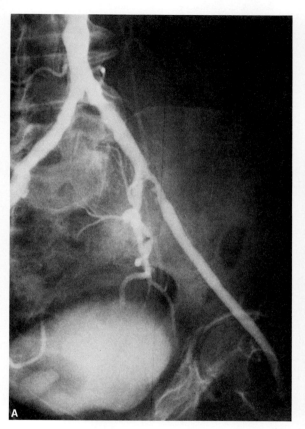 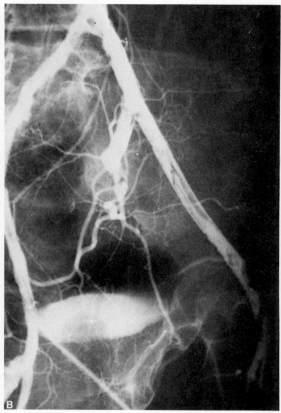

(A) thrombolysis
(B) transluminal atherectomy
(C) stent placement
(D) surgery
(E) anticoagulation and observation

523. If, following angioplasty, no further treatment were given to the patient in Question 522, the expected 3-year patency would probably be no higher than

(A) 10%
(B) 30%
(C) 60%
(D) 75%
(E) 90%

524. A 50-year-old man is being evaluated for transjugular intrahepatic portosystemic shunt (TIPS). The selective hepatic venogram shown in the figure reveals

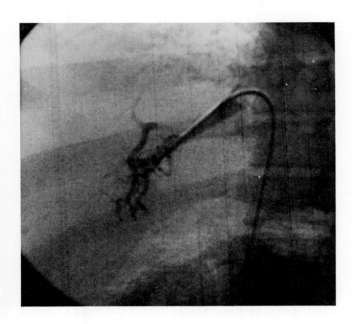

(A) hepatofugal portal blood flow
(B) presinusoidal portal hypertension
(C) Budd-Chiari syndrome
(D) portal vein thrombosis
(E) none of the above

525. First-order branches of the axillary artery include ALL the following EXCEPT

(A) lateral thoracic artery
(B) thoracodorsal artery
(C) supreme (superior) thoracic artery
(D) circumflex humeral artery
(E) subscapular artery

DIRECTIONS: Each group of questions below consists of lettered headings followed by a set of numbered items. For each numbered item select the **one** lettered heading with which it is **most** closely associated. Each lettered heading may be used **once, more than once,** or **not at all.**

Questions 526–529

For each of the following pathways described, select the eponym by which it is commonly known.

(A)   Arc of Riolan
(B)   Path of Winslow
(C)   Arc of Buehler
(D)   Marginal artery of Drummond
(E)   Arc of Barkow

526.   Ventral communication between celiac axis and superior mesenteric artery

527.   Vessel in root of mesentery linking superior and inferior mesenteric arteries

528.   Omental vessel which parallels the gastro-epiploic artery

529.   Common alternate blood supply to lower body in aortic occlusion

Questions 530–532

For each radiographic or angiographic sign or characteristic, select the cardiovascular anomaly with which it is most closely associated.

(A)   "Egg on its side" or "egg on a string"
(B)   "Gooseneck" deformity
(C)   "Waterfall" pulmonary hilum
(D)   "Figure eight" or "snowman"
(E)   Goetz sign

530.   Single ventricle with transposition of the great vessels

531.   Supracardiac total anomalous pulmonary venous return

532.   Endocardial cushion defect

Questions 533–537

For each of the following contrast agents, select the correct description of its molecular composition.

(A)   Nonionic monomer
(B)   Ionic monomer
(C)   Nonionic dimer
(D)   Ionic dimer

533.   Renograffin (diatrizoate meglumine)

534.   Sinograffin (iopamide meglumine)

535.   Omnipaque (iohexol)

536.   Hexabrix (ioxaglate meglumine)

537.   Isovue (iopamidol)

Questions 538–540

For each of the following patterns of chest x-ray and clinical presentation, select the cardiac condition with which it is most closely associated.

(A)   Increased pulmonary blood flow with cyanosis
(B)   Decreased pulmonary blood flow with cyanosis
(C)   Increased pulmonary blood flow without cyanosis
(D)   Decreased pulmonary blood flow without cyanosis
(E)   Normal pulmonary blood flow with cyanosis

538.   Complete transposition of the great vessels

539.   Sinus venosus atrial septal defect

540.   Ebstein anomaly

DIRECTIONS: Each group of questions below consists of four lettered headings followed by a set of numbered items. For each numbered item select

A	if the item is associated with	(A) **only**
B	if the item is associated with	(B) **only**
C	if the item is associated with	**both** (A) and (B)
D	if the item is associated with	**neither** (A) nor (B)

Each lettered heading may be used **once, more than once,** or **not at all.**

Questions 541–544

For each of the following corrective surgical procedures used for the treatment of congenital heart disease, select the eponym with which it is most closely associated.

- (A) Senning
- (B) Glenn
- (C) Mustard
- (D) Fontan
- (E) Jatene

541. Conduit connecting right atrium and pulmonary trunk

542. Division and switch of ascending aorta and main pulmonary artery

543. Anastomosis of superior vena cava to right pulmonary artery

544. Removal of interatrial septum and creation of baffles to redirect blood flow to the ventricles

Questions 545–547

- (A) Streptokinase
- (B) Urokinase
- (C) Both
- (D) Neither

545. Activates plasminogen

546. Immunogenic

547. Produces systemic fibrinolysis within 10–12 hours of starting local therapy

Questions 548–550

- (A) Polysplenia
- (B) Asplenia
- (C) Both
- (D) Neither

548. Pulmonic stenosis

549. Azygos continuation of the inferior vena cava

550. Bilateral hyparterial bronchi

Questions 551–553

- (A) Left-sided rib notching only
- (B) Right-sided rib notching only
- (C) Both
- (D) Neither

551. Postductal coarctation of the aorta

552. Aberrant right subclavian artery

553. Right-sided Blalock-Taussig operation

Questions 554–556

- (A) Calcification of the valve annulus
- (B) Calcification of the valve leaflets
- (C) Both
- (D) Neither

554. Correlates with hemodynamically significant mitral stenosis

555. Common in the mitral valve of elderly persons

556. Young patient with endocarditis of bicuspid aortic valve

DIRECTIONS: Each question below contains five suggested answers. For **each** of the **five** alternatives listed, you are to respond either YES or NO. In a given item, **all, some,** or **none of the alternatives may be correct.**

557. Regarding the lymphangiogram in the figure, TRUE statements include which of the following?

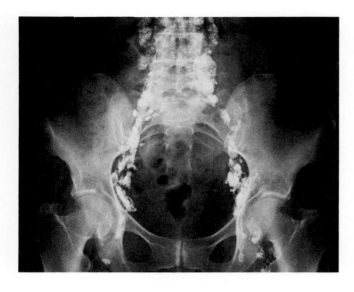

(A) In a 33-year-old female, the MOST likely diagnosis is lymphoma
(B) A gallium scan performed on this patient the following week would show diffusely increased lung activity
(C) Evaluation of the vascular phase is more important in a study for lymphoma than in a study for solid neoplastic metastasis
(D) A well-performed lymphangiogram can usually differentiate lymphomatous involvement from reactive hyperplasia
(E) Microscopic nodal metastases alter the normal architecture enough to make the lymphangiogram abnormal

558. Which of the following statements regarding ventricular septal defects (VSDs) are TRUE?

(A) More than half will close spontaneously during the first year of life
(B) The Maladie de Roger refers to the loud murmur that is heard in the larger membranous VSDs
(C) Patients who develop Eisenmenger physiology are cyanotic as a result of right-to-left shunting across the VSD
(D) High VSDs may produce aortic insufficiency if the right aortic cusp should prolapse into the VSD
(E) The hepatoclavicular view in cardiac angiography is the optimal method for visualizing a posterior VSD

559. Concerning anomalies of the aortic arch and great vessels,

(A) the "pulmonary sling" characteristically produces a posterior indentation on the esophagus, as seen on a lateral esophagram
(B) a double aortic arch usually occurs in association with other congenital heart disease
(C) a right aortic arch with mirror-image branching most frequently occurs in the setting of tetralogy of Fallot
(D) the aberrant right subclavian artery results from abnormal regression of a segment of the right fourth embryonic arch
(E) the most common arch anomalies involve maldevelopment or regression of elements of the sixth aortic arch

560. Concerning tetralogy of Fallot,

(A) the "coeur-en-sabot" shape of the heart refers to the prominent left ventricular contour

(B) a ventricular septal defect is necessary for life

(C) a right-sided aortic arch is present in 25% of cases

(D) "tetrad spells" are due to intermittent disturbances in the His-Purkinje system, leading to hypotension and loss of consciousness

(E) associated branch pulmonary stenosis occurs more commonly on the left

561. Regarding endocardial fibroelastosis (EFE),

(A) carcinoid syndrome can produce EFE which involves only the right side of the heart

(B) primary EFE is a disease of the elderly

(C) patients commonly develop congestive heart failure

(D) it is a cause of mitral valve insufficiency

(E) the left ventricle is usually small and thick-walled in primary EFE

562. Regarding echocardiography of the mitral valve,

(A) the presence of calcification improves visualization of the valve leaflets

(B) in mitral stenosis, the E-F slope is increased

(C) thickening of the valve leaflets is a prominent feature in patients with rheumatic heart disease

(D) during mitral valve prolapse, the tracing shows bowing of the leaflets into the left atrium

(E) vegetations produce disperse echoes which cannot be localized to the leaflet on which they originate

563. Regarding abnormalities of the pulmonary valve,

(A) the stenosis encountered in tetralogy of Fallot occurs at the level of the valve

(B) valvular pulmonic stenosis (PS) is diagnosed by upward "doming" of the fused valve leaflets during a right ventriculogram

(C) the most common type of valvular PS results from a dysplasia of the valve

(D) most cases of valvular PS have post-stenotic dilatation of the right and left pulmonary arteries

(E) most patients with PS are asymptomatic

564. Correct statements concerning Ebstein anomaly include which of the following?

(A) It is related to chronic maternal lithium intake

(B) Episodic paroxysmal atrial tachycardia is a common feature

(C) The degree of cardiomegaly evident on chest x-ray is often massive, even in the asymptomatic patient

(D) Cyanosis, present at birth, often spontaneously disappears in later life

(E) Cineangiography reveals the atrialized right ventrice contracting in synchrony with the right atrium

565. True statements concerning renal artery stenosis include which of the following?

(A) In patients with fibromuscular dysplasia, the cumulative patency rate at 10 years following angioplasty approaches 90%

(B) The percentage of hypertensive patients in the United States in whom renovascular disease is responsible for the stenosis is less than 5%

(C) The best screening test for renovascular hypertension is the radionuclide renal scan

(D) Failure of renal vein renin samples to lateralize is a predictor for a success rate for intervention of 50%

(E) The long-term success rate for angioplasty of ostial renal artery stenoses is less than 10%

566. Which of the following statements regarding percutaneous nephrostomy is/are TRUE?

(A) With the patient lying in the prone position, the anterior calyces typically appear en face

(B) Brödel's white line refers to the avascular plane which is optimal for nephrostomy access

(C) The renal pelvis normally angles anteriorly 30° with respect to the coronal plane

(D) Postobstructive diuresis following nephrostomy for obstruction should be treated by matching intravenous fluids to nephrostomy tube output

(E) Gross hematuria following nephrostomy often lasts 3 days or more

567. True statements concerning portal hypertension include which of the following?

(A) The most common cause of sinusoidal hypertension in the U.S. is Laennec cirrhosis

(B) The corrected sinusoidal pressure is calculated by taking the wedged hepatic venous pressure and subtracting the free inferior vena cava pressure

(C) Placement of a transjugular intrahepatic shunt is contraindicated in patients with ascites

(D) Blood flow in the portal vein remains hepatopetal even in severe cases of portal hypertension

(E) In bleeding esophageal varices, hemorrhage is related only to the degree of intrahepatic obstruction to portal blood flow.

568. True statements concerning deep venous thrombosis (DVT) of the lower extremity include which of the following?

(A) Thirty percent will resolve spontaneously within 72 hours

(B) Lack of filling of a vein by contrast venography, with filling of superficial collateral vessels, is a diagnostic criterion for DVT

(C) Superficial vein thrombosis, in the absence of DVT, has a 10% risk of pulmonary embolism

(D) Most DVT originates in the calf veins

(E) Over 75% of elderly patients with hip fractures will develop DVT

569. Indications for emergency arteriography of a limb that has sustained a penetrating injury include

(A) large hematoma

(B) multiple bone or gunshot fragments evident on x-ray

(C) distal ischemia

(D) proximity to major vessel

(E) pulsatile mass

570. Loss of the normal main pulmonary artery contour on a frontal chest x-ray occurs with which of the following?

(A) Ebstein anomaly

(B) Pulmonary atresia

(C) Persistent truncus arteriosus

(D) Pulmonary artery sling

(E) Complete transposition of the great vessels

571. True statements regarding persistent truncus arteriosus include which of the following?

(A) Types I to IV identify the various attachments of the pulmonary arteries to the ascending aorta

(B) A right aortic arch is present in 35–50% of cases

(C) The valve cusps are usually absent

(D) At least one ventricular septal defect is always present

(E) Ventriculography cannot distinguish this entity from severe tetralogy of Fallot

572. A patient in the angiography suite becomes hypotensive following contrast injection. Therapeutic measures might include which of the following?

(A) Atropine
(B) Epinephrine
(C) Lactated Ringer solution
(D) Oxygen
(E) Diphenhydramine

573. True statements about aortic stenosis include which of the following?

(A) A bicuspid aortic valve is the most common predisposing congenital factor
(B) Calcification of the valve which is visible on plain film correlates with symptomatic disease in adults
(C) Subvalvular aortic stenosis is a feature of Williams syndrome
(D) The dilatation of the ascending aorta is greater than that encountered in aortic regurgitation because of the jet effect and the turbulence it causes
(E) Valvular aortic stenosis is commonly associated with coarctation in the neonate

574. True statements regarding transposition of the great vessels include which of the following?

(A) Complete transposition is the most common cause of cyanosis in neonates
(B) A lesion which permits admixture is necessary for survival in patients with d-transposition
(C) In congenitally corrected transposition, there is atrioventricular concordance
(D) Treatment with prostaglandin E and a Rashkind procedure may successfully temporize an infant with complete transposition until definite surgery can be safely carried out
(E) The prognosis for congenitally corrected transposition is greater than 50% survival at 5 years

Cardiovascular and Interventional Radiology

Answers

505. The answer is E. *(Hurst, ed. 7, pp 701–706.)* The aortogram reveals a characteristic postductal coarctation, with collateral flow through large internal mammary and tortuous intercostal arteries. This is the most frequent location for a coarctation to occur in older children and adults. When coarctation is identified in a symptomatic infant, the stenosis is usually preductal or located across from the entrance of the ductus arteriosus. Histologically a form of tubular hypoplasia, this infantile form of the disease is associated with other congenital cardiac abnormalities, especially ventricular septal defect and bicuspid aortic valve. In adults, coarctation of the aorta is usually a discrete entity.

Clinically, congestive heart failure is a common presenting symptom in infants with coarctation. Upper-extremity hypertension and poor lower-extremity pulses are often presenting signs, but they may be less pronounced as collateral pathways develop. However, a significant pressure difference can always be found between the upper and lower extremities. Untreated, the median age at death is 31, which is usually due to the sequela of prolonged hypertension, most commonly aortic rupture or aneurysm formation around the circle of Willis and subsequent cerebral hemorrhage.

Regarding the other choices: Marfan syndrome is most commonly associated with aortic aneurysm and valvular incompetence; superior vena cava obstruction produces *venous* collaterals; the aortic arch in this case is continuous, though stenotic; and pulmonic stenosis would not be diagnosed on the basis of an aortogram. A pulmonary angiogram is required, although an aortogram may reveal intercostal and bronchial arterial collaterals.

506. The answer is E. *(Doroghazi, pp 33–34, 55–60. Hood, pp 227–229.)* The thoracic aortogram in the figure was taken in the left anterior oblique (LAO) projection. It reveals an abnormal aortic contour distal to the origin of the left subclavian artery. A transverse filling defect is located in the most stenotic portion, which represents a transection, or laceration, of the aorta. Also called *aortic rupture,* it involves a transverse injury to the vessel wall, usually following a deceleration type of accident. The mechanism of injury is currently felt to be due to compression of the thorax and deformation of the aorta, rather than the previous notion that attributed the injury to stress on the aorta at the point where it is fixed by the ligamentum arteriosum.

If the transection is transmural, the patient usually does not survive long enough to undergo angiography. If the patient survives, it is often because the adventitia has contained the leak. Nevertheless, if left untreated, mortality at 1 week remains as high as 60%.

An aortic *dissection,* on the other hand, occurs only rarely in the setting of deceleration injury. Rather, it results from degeneration of the medial layer of the aortic wall, often in the setting of hypertension. Repeated pulsation and motion with each cardiac cycle eventually results in a tear of the intima overlying the diseased media, which allows a dissecting hematoma to form and propagate along the length of the aorta, creating a "false" lumen. The false lumen may reestablish continuity with the "true" lumen through one or more fenestrations, or it may advance distally into the abdominal aorta and its branches. In the absence of a visible flap or opacification of the false lumen, frequently a clue to the presence of a dissection on an aortogram is narrowing of the true lumen, which represents compression by the false lumen.

507. The answer is D.   *(Spies, Radiology 166:381–387, 1988.)*   All the procedures mentioned, except for routine hepatic cyst aspiration, are performed with antibiotic prophylaxis. In any case where there is a suspicion of infection, therapeutic antibiotic blood levels should be reached before starting the procedure. In the absence of signs of overt infection, antibiotic coverage is also recommended for cases of biliary or renal obstruction.

Prior to nephrostomy, ampicillin (1 g IVSS) or similar coverage, such as cefoxitin (Mefoxin) or vancomycin (Vancocin), for gram-positive organisms, is given. Additionally, an aminoglycoside, usually gentamycin (Garamycin) (1.5 mg/kg bolus) is advised. Both should be given every 8 hours for 24 hours.

For biliary procedures, broad-spectrum coverage is required. Mezlocillin (Mezlin) (4 g IVSS, then q 6 h × 24 h) is the treatment of choice. Ampicillin or cefoxitin, and gentamycin are the second line of treatment.

Any patient for whom antibiotic prophylaxis is routinely used (such as a patient with a prosthetic cardiac valve) should receive antibiotic coverage prior to any invasive procedure.

508. The answer is B.   *(Gross, pp 293–334. Braunwald, ed. 4, pp 935–938. Kelley, pp 17–24.)*   The shunt depicted in the figure connects the descending thoracic aorta to the left pulmonary artery. This is the Potts procedure, which was originally developed in 1946 for patients with tetralogy of Fallot. Similarly, the Glenn, Blalock-Taussig, and Waterston shunts are all palliative methods for improving pulmonary blood flow.

The Glenn shunt is a connection between the superior vena cava (SVC) and the right pulmonary artery (RPA). The Waterston (Waterston-Cooley) shunt was devised in 1962, but is no longer used. It was an anastomosis of the ascending aorta to the RPA. As with the Glenn shunt, it was difficult to control the size of the shunt; patients often developed either congestive heart failure or pulmonary vascular obstruction. The Blalock-Taussig operation involved division of a subclavian artery, ligation of the distal segment, and an end-to-side connection of the proximal segment to the ipsilateral pulmonary artery. It was usually performed on the side opposite the aortic arch. Currently, the Blalock-Taussig shunt is preferred, which was a synthetic graft to connect the subclavian and ipsilateral pulmonary arteries.

509. The answer is A.   *(Silverman, pp 383–391. Hurst, ed. 7, pp 733–737. Kirks, ed. 2, p 454.)*   The most common causes of severe cyanosis in an infant during the first week of life include transposition of the great vessels, hypoplastic left or right heart, total anomalous pulmonary venous return (TAPVR) below the diaphragm (with obstruction of the abnormal draining vein at the diaphragm), Ebstein anomaly, and tricuspid atresia.

In contrast, infants with tetralogy of Fallot usually present *after* the first week of life. The majority do so within the first 6 months. Rarely, a mild case will present in adulthood. Of course, if the degree of pulmonary stenosis is severe enough, cyanosis may be present at birth or appear as the ductus arteriosus closes.

The age of presentation in tetralogy is a function of the degree of right ventricular outflow tract obstruction. Patients will become cyanotic and dyspneic when right ventricular outflow tract obstruction is severe enough to cause significant right-to-left shunting across the ventricular septal defect. The natural history is for the degree of infundibular stenosis to progress and right-to-left shunting to worsen. As a result, patients born with only mild pulmonary outflow tract stenosis may not become symptomatic until months or years after birth.

510. The answer is B. *(Hurst, ed. 7, pp 604–622. Cheitlin, Circulation 50:780–787, 1974.)* Sudden death may occur with Wolf-Parkinson-White syndrome (WPW), aberrant left coronary artery origin, acute coronary thromboembolism, or polyarteritis nodosa (PAN). The left coronary arteriogram in the figure at right, however, clearly shows the anomalous origin of the left coronary artery from the anterior sinus of valsalva. The lumen of the vessel becomes a thin ribbon as it passes between the aorta and pulmonary artery. With exercise, the increase in cardiac output and enlargement of the aorta and pulmonary artery further compromises left coronary blood flow, and ischemia and infarction may ensue. In a review of thirty-three otherwise healthy subjects with this anomaly, eight of them (24%) died suddenly after exercise. This is not the case with the other coronary artery anomalies.

Acute thromboembolism, from such sources as subacute bacterial endocarditis (SBE) and ulcerated aortic plaque, may cause sudden death, as may rupture of an aneurysm in patients with PAN. WPW and other arrhythmias may produce cardiac syncope, but sudden death usually occurs only in cases in which there is underlying myocardial instability or other heart disease.

The "dominant" coronary artery is the one that supplies the posterior and diaphragmatic portions of the interventricular septum and left ventricle. In 77–90% of the population, the right coronary artery is "dominant" and gives rise to the posterior descending artery (PDA) and posterior left ventricular (LV) branches. In 5–12% of the population, the left coronary artery gives rise to the PDA and posterior LV branches. Though this distribution puts more of the heart at risk in cases of severe left coronary artery disease, it is not associated with an increase in mortality.

511. The answer is A. *(Austin, Radiology 172:259–265, 1989.)* *Aspergillus* is the most common early pathogen to produce pneumonia in the immune-suppressed, posttransplant population, perhaps reflecting a particular deficiency of T-cell-mediated immunity. It typically appears between 2 weeks and 2 months following transplantation, and now occurs less frequently due to the use of cyclosporine.

Cytomegalovirus (CMV), *Pneumocystis carinii* pneumonia (PCP), herpes, and *Nocardia* tend to occur later, usually between 1 and 6 months. Of these, CMV has the worst outcome, with a 46% fatality rate. In patients with pneumonia appearing later than 6 months, PCP is a common cause and has a uniformly good outcome, unless accompanied by another organism. Interestingly, *Pneumococcus,* a common community-acquired organism, is rarely responsible for disease in the posttransplant population.

Radiographically, there is tremendous overlap, though *Aspergillus* often produces nodules which can cavitate and which have thick, shaggy walls. *Nocardia* also can appear as nodular infiltrates which may cavitate. PCP and CMV typically present as diffuse haziness.

512. The answer is D. *(Braunwald, ed. 4, p 1632. Silverman, pp 480–484.)* Numerous genetic disorders feature cardiac anomalies among their constellation of malformations. Apert syndrome, or acrocephalosyndactyly, is the least likely of the choices to have cardiac anomalies. Features include cranial synostosis, midfacial hypoplasia, "mitten" hands and feet, and occasionally mental retardation. Congenital heart disease (CHD) is *very* rare and includes pulmonic stenosis (PS), peripheral pulmonic stenosis (PPS), ventricular septal defect (VSD), and endocardial fibroelastosis.

Turner (XO) syndrome is characterized by webbed neck, shield-shaped chest, short stature, and short fourth metacarpals, as well as many other features. Coarctation of the aorta and aortic stenosis are common.

Down syndrome (trisomy 21) is associated with CHD in 40 to 70% of patients. Endocardial cushion defects, especially of the AV-canal type, atrial septal defects (ASD), and VSDs are common. Additional features include 11 rib pairs, hypersegmentation of the sternum, cleft palate, and duodenal atresia.

In the Ellis-van Creveld syndrome, or chondroectodermal dysplasia, patients have a high incidence of CHD. Single atrium, a type of ASD, and VSD occur commonly.

Patients with Williams syndrome, or idiopathic hypercalcemia, typically have supravalvular aortic stenosis and typical "elfin" facies. ASD, VSD, and PPS are common associations.

513. The answer is E. *(Hurst, ed. 7, pp 1073. Braunwald, ed. 4, pp 1260–1261.)* The chest x-ray in the figure shows cardiomegaly and a long arc of calcification conforming to the anterior and apical left ventricular contours. Approximately 80% of ventricular aneurysms occur in this location, and most are *true* ventricular aneurysms, which are the result of transmural infarction. Endomyocardial or myocardial calcification is also sometimes present. Roughly 10% of ventricular aneurysms occur in a posterolateral location and half of these are *false* aneurysms, which are also transmural infarctions, but with focal rupture of the ventricular wall which has been contained by adherent pericardium. In contrast to true aneurysms, the mouths of false aneurysms are usually small. On cineangiography, both types of ventricular aneurysm may paradoxically enlarge during systole.

False aneurysms have a tendency to rupture and should be treated surgically. True aneurysms may also require repair if the patient develops refractory angina, recurrent thromboembolism, congestive heart failure (CHF), or a tachyarrhythmia.

Dressler syndrome refers to an uncommon constellation of signs and symptoms occurring weeks to months following myocardial infarction. Characteristically, patients have fever and pain, with a pericardial friction rub and left pleural effusion discovered on examination. Its etiology is unknown, but it may be an autoimmune disorder.

Calcific pericarditis most commonly occurs over the right ventricular surface and the location is superficial. Endocardial fibroelastosis (EFE) may be found on a biopsy of the infarcted area, but is not associated with calcification when it occurs as a primary disease of myocardium.

514. The answer is E. *(Levin, Circulation 50:831–837, 1974.)* In a review of 200 coronary angiograms, the collateral circulation was identified in 74 of the 105 patients who had either right coronary artery (RCA) stenosis (>90%) or occlusion. Ten common pathways of collateral flow were identified.

The most common were left anterior descending (LAD) to posterior descending artery (PDA) through septal branches (38%); distal circumflex artery to distal RCA (32%), and obtuse marginal to posterior left ventricular branch of RCA (23%).

Kugel's artery, which connects either the right or the left coronary artery proximally to the A-V nodal branch of the distal RCA, occurs with equal frequency (12%) to collateral supply by the conus artery, which is a proximal acute marginal branch of the RCA.

Although the distal LAD supplied the distal PDA (by going around the cardiac apex) in equal frequency to Kugel artery and the conus artery pathways, connections between the LAD and RCA *over the right ventricular surface* were distinctly infrequent (3%).

515. The answer is D. *(Wilson, ed. 12, pp 988–989. Gomez, p 40.)* Of cardiac neoplasms, metastatic tumors are more common than primaries by several fold. Melanoma is the most frequent tumor type to metastasize to the heart, followed by lymphoma; *primary* lymphoma, however, is extremely rare. In absolute numbers, lung and breast metastases are the most common.

Three-fourths of primary cardiac neoplasms are histologically benign, but may nevertheless prove to be life-threatening. Myxomas are the most common cell type and are usually solitary. They typically arise from the interatrial septum, most frequently on the left side. They may prolapse into the atrium and obstruct the AV valve.

Sarcomas account for nearly 20% of primary malignancies and occur most frequently on the right. Rhabdomyoma and teratoma are less frequent. Rhabdomyoma and fibroma are the most common tumors in the pediatric age group. The former are usually multiple and develop in approximately 40% of patients with tuberous sclerosis.

516. The answer is D. *(Reuter, ed. 3, p 157–174.)* The abdominal CT scan in the figure at left reveals a large, irregular hypodense mass in the right lobe of the liver. There is no associated enhancement. The angiogram (at right) shows displacement of the surrounding vessels. There are irregular pools of contrast which persist well beyond the venous phase (not shown). This pattern is most consistent with a giant cavernous hemangioma, which this proved to be.

Cavernous hemangiomas are benign tumors of the liver and have a characteristic appearance on angiography. In the late arterial phase, small groups of dilated amorphous vascular spaces fill with contrast. They are well-defined, but have irregular walls. Since blood flow through a hemangioma is very slow, there is retention of contrast material into and usually well beyond the venous phase.

Focal nodular hyperplasia (FNH) is usually a hypervascular mass with a definable arterial supply that breaks up into small branches which permeate the mass. As a result, one can see a reticular or "spoke-wheel" pattern of vessels during the arterial phase. FNH does not usually have the irregular, dilated vascular spaces seen here. In further distinction, the hepatogram phase in cases of FNH often reveals a fine granular appearance to the lesion. However, in this case, only the dilated vascular channels stand out.

Hepatocellular carcinoma is typically hypervascular, with a dilated hepatic arterial supply and extensive neovascularity. However, the abnormal vascular spaces (or vessels) seen in hepatoma do not retain the contrast nearly as long as those of hemangiomas, and typically wash out during the venous phase.

Regenerating nodules are generally homogeneous and isodense as compared to normal liver parenchyma by CT and angiography, though they may appear hypodense, and/or exert a local mass effect. They would not be expected to contain pools of contrast such as those demonstrated by this angiogram.

517. The answer is A. *(Reuter, pp 135–138, 172–175.)* The contrast-enhanced CT scan in the figure at left reveals a hypodense, ill-marginated mass in the posterior segment of the right lobe of the liver. Arterial and hepatogram phase images (shown in the figures at center and at right) from a celiac injection demonstrate at least two hypervascular masses in the liver. The larger of the two has extensive neovascularity and arteriovenous (AV) shunting into the portal vein. Given the patient's age, history, and the imaging characteristics of the lesion, the diagnosis of malignancy is almost certain.

Vascular neoformation, or tumor neovascularity, is generally indicative of malignancy. However, abnormal channels around inflammatory masses can sometimes simulate neovessels, and contrast enhancement at CT is also nonspecific. The presence of AV shunting, however, implies an aggressive, invasive process. The early-draining veins should be followed to identify their connection to the hepatic or portal vein. Whereas hepatic vein shunting occurs with both benign and malignant processes, portal vein shunting indicates direct invasion by the tumor and is highly specific for hepatoma, although it is seen only in about 30% of cases.

518. The answer is D. *(Ernst, pp 652–655.)* The lower-extremity arteriogram in the figure demonstrates smooth tapering of all the calf vessels, which then occlude in the midcalf. There is no evidence of embolism. Given the history, the findings are most consistent with a compartment syndrome.

A compartment syndrome develops following penetrating trauma or massive soft-tissue injury to an extremity. Edema in the fascial compartment, following an ischemic or crush-type injury, gradually compromises the neurovascular supply to the extremity. It may also develop in patients who are undergoing endovascular or surgical recanalization of a limb after prolonged ischemia from emboli or occlusive peripheral vascular disease.

Early diagnosis and prompt surgical decompression by two- or four-compartment fasciotomy are critical, in order to prevent permanent functional disability, enhance limb salvage, and avoid potentially fatal conditions such as myonecrosis.

Most compartment syndromes can be diagnosed on clinical grounds. In alert patients, the most reliable early sign is a sensory deficit (specifically, two-point discrimination) in the distribution of nerves within the compartment. Pain out of proportion to the clinical situation, weakness and pain on passive stretch, and tense swelling are other indicators.

If there is any question as to the diagnosis, trans-needle tissue pressure measurement can be obtained. In the calf, there are anterior, lateral, and superficial and deep posterior compartments. Normal tissue pressure is approximately 0 to 10 mmHg. There is no single critical pressure for all individuals above which intervention is imperative, and some patients become symptomatic at much lower pressures than others. However, when the measured tissue pressure within a compartment is greater than 30 mmHg, fasciotomy is usually advised.

519. The answer is A. *(Becker, Radiology 170:921–940, 1989. Johnston, Radiology 183:767–771, 1992.)* The arteriogram of the right superficial femoral artery in the figure demonstrates two short-segment stenoses. The clinical evidence of rest pain and the nonhealing ulcer on the right foot are indications for a revascularization procedure. The focal nature of this patient's disease (<10 cm long) makes him an ideal candidate for percutaneous transluminal angioplasty (PTA). PTA and femoropopliteal bypass graft would both be expected to have similar long-term patency rates for the vessel demonstrated on this case. It is generally agreed that in patients with severe claudication who have good runoff in the affected leg, PTA and surgical revascularization have similar long-term success rates. Distal bypass is probably indicated for those with poor runoff (those with only one or with no tibial vessels). Overall, PTA has a lower morbidity and mortality, and also preserves the patient's veins for possible future coronary or other vessel bypass. It also does not preclude future surgical intervention on the affected limb.

520. The answer is D. *(Becker, Radiology 170:921–940, 1989. Johnston, Radiology 183:767–771, 1992.)* Technical success has been reported in nearly 90% of femoropopliteal angioplasties. The patency at both 2- and 5-year follow-up is 67%. Therefore, following uncomplicated treatment, the patient in Question 519 could anticipate a 3-year patency rate of approximately 70%.

Initial technical success rates for PTA of femoropopliteal atherosclerotic lesions range from 90 to 95%. The type of lesion (stenosis or occlusion) and indication for procedure (claudication or limb salvage) are two factors important in determining successful outcomes soon (1 month) after PTA. However, angiographic runoff and type of lesion are more significant factors for predicting long-term success.

Therefore, in patients with femoropopliteal atheromatous disease, long-term success rates are optimal when the patient presents with claudication, focal stenosis, and good distal runoff. As these parameters change for the worse, the long-term success of PTA is diminished, and surgical revascularization offers improved long-term success rates. PTA would be an option for those patients for whom there is a limited life expectancy, a high surgical risk, or insufficient bypass material.

An important limitation of PTA is post-PTA restenosis. One-third of atherosclerotic small- to medium-sized arteries will restenose in 1 year, though most of these respond well to a second dilatation. Restenosis following PTA can be divided into three types: acute, early, and late. Acute failures occur during or immediately following PTA, and are the result of dissection, elastic recoil, and/or spasm, which may be complicated by thrombosis. Endovascular stenting and thermal welding are currently being investigated as therapies for dissection. Spasm and thrombosis are treated intravenously with nitroglycerine and/or nifedipine, and heparin and/or urokinase, respectively.

Early stenosis occurs between 1 month and 1 year following PTA. It is thought to be caused by a fibrocellular response by myocytes which are exposed as the intima and media are injured during PTA. Late restenosis, occurring more than 1 year after PTA, is most often due to progression of the patient's underlying atherosclerotic disease.

521. The answer is E. *(Kadir [Angiography], pp 189–190. Abrams, ed. 3, p 1934. Taveras & Ferrucci, vol 2, chap 142, pp 10–12.)*   The upper-extremity arteriograms in the figure reveal smooth tapering and occlusion of the brachial arteries, with minimal collateral flow. This patient shows a complication of chronic ergotamine tartrate medication for her migraine headaches. The drug produces vasospasm which may have become irreversible at this point.

Buerger disease, or thromboangiitis obliterans, is a vasculitis of peripheral vessels. The diagnosis is based primarily on clinical and histologic examination. This condition is usually found in men, and has a high association with the use of nicotine. Typically, there are multiple segmental occlusions in the extremities, with tapering of proximal major vessels and "corkscrew" collaterals. The condition is usually seen in the tibial vessels, but has been reported to rarely involve the upper extremity.

Takayasu arteritis presents in the second and third decades and causes diffuse narrowing of the involved vessels, with occasional aneurysm formation. The aorta, its major branches, and the renal arteries are most commonly involved.

Giant cell arteritis typically occurs in older patients and causes multiple, segmental narrowings of the central medium-sized vessels.

Raynaud phenomenon is characterized by episodic vasoconstriction of small vessels of the extremities, causing digital pallor followed later by reactive hyperemia. Arteriographically, the proximal vessels are patent except for segmental vasospasm, and there are distal occlusions. Arterial involvement above the elbow virtually excludes Raynaud phenomenon, whereas all the other diseases discussed can produce the angiographic pattern shown in the case.

522. The answer is A. *(Becker, Radiology 170:921–940, 1989.)*   In percutaneous transluminal angioplasty (PTA), one hopes to create a "controlled" injury to the wall of a stenotic artery. The fracture may be superficial and penetrate only through an atherosclerotic plaque, or it may extend to involve the intima and media. The degree of penetration appears to be related to the incidence of restenosis; deeper tears elicit a more vigorous hyperplastic response.

The results of PTA can be immediately assessed by changes in the patient's symptoms and measurement of pressure gradients before and after treatment. Adjuvant administration of a vasodilator is often necessary to realize the full impact of a lesion. A systolic gradient of greater than 15% or a residual stenosis of greater than 30% is thought to be a significant risk for restenosis.

In an alert, cooperative patient, significant discomfort during balloon inflation suggests overdilatation and should be used as the endpoint for expansion. On the other hand, persistent pain following balloon angioplasty may indicate adventitial rupture. The treated vessel and runoff should be imaged for complications, such as extensive dissection or distal embolization. Persistent bleeding from a ruptured vessel, indicated by hypotension, may be temporized by reinflation of the angioplasty balloon in the ruptured segment awaiting surgical repair.

In this case, a dissection has occurred which has extended beyond the angioplasty site and compromised flow distally. A Palmaz (balloon-expanded) metal stent placed directly at the angioplasty site tacked the flap down. Often, as in this case, the distal dissection then collapsed down. If it had not, a series of overlapping stents could have been placed. The Wallstent, a self-expanding metal stent, is another type of stent which is currently under investigation for this purpose. Another possible treatment option is transluminal atherectomy of the flap.

523. The answer is C. *(Becker, Radiology 170:921–940, 1989.)*   Following uncomplicated percutaneous iliac angioplasty, the anticipated 3-year success rate is approximately 60%. A dissection may remodel and the lumen might be completely restored, or the vessel may go on to occlude. Given the complicated nature of the dissection in this case, the 3-year patency would probably be much less than 60%. The placement of a metal stent should improve the 3-year patency close to 90%, though there is not sufficient long-term experience with stents as yet to make an accurate prediction.

524. The answer is C. *(Reuter, pp 422–424. Murphy, AJR 147:9–15, 1986.)* The hepatic venogram reveals occlusions of the middle hepatic vein and numerous thready collateral vessels. There is a "spider web" appearance which is typical of hepatic vein thrombosis, or Budd-Chiari syndrome.

The Budd-Chiari syndrome occurs as a primary and/or secondary disorder of hepatic vein or inferior vena cava (IVC) obstruction. The primary form results from congenital webs or diaphragms which can be located in the hepatic veins or hepatic portion of the IVC. In the secondary type, tumor thrombus or trauma lead to obstruction. However, approximately two-thirds of cases are idiopathic. Ascites, hepatomegaly, and abdominal pain constitute the classic triad clinically, but these findings are nonspecific, and so the diagnosis is often overlooked.

Noninvasive imaging, such as ultrasound, CT, or MRI, may reveal thrombosis of the hepatic vein and/or IVC either directly or by its effect on flow within the veins and the presence of collateral channels. In addition, secondary signs such as an enlarged caudate lobe, ascites, hepatosplenomegaly, and abnormal hepatic parenchymal enhancement may be evident. Angiography can be used to measure the degree of portal hypertension and delineate the vascular anatomy prior to percutaneous or surgical shunting.

525. The answer is B. *(Kadir [Atlas], pp 57, 63–74. Cunningham, p 1284.)* The axillary artery originates at the level of the clavicle, just proximal to the pectoralis minor muscle. Its first branch is the superior, or supreme, thoracic artery, which supplies the uppermost intercostal arteries. As the vessel proceeds beneath the pectoralis minor muscle, it gives rise to the thoracoacromial artery, which further subdivides into acromial and pectoral branches. As it continues on, it gives off the lateral thoracic artery, which courses down along the chest wall and supplies the pectoralis minor, intercostal and subscapularis muscles and the lateral aspect of the mammary gland.

As the axillary artery emerges into the axilla, it gives off the subscapular artery, which rapidly subdivides into the circumflex scapular artery (which hooks back under the scapula), and a branch which proceeds down along the chest wall, known as the thoracodorsal artery. The circumflex humeral artery is the last branch of the axillary artery. It further divides into anterior and posterior divisions, which encircle the shoulder joint.

526–529. The answers are: 526-C, 527-A, 528-E, 529-B. *(Kadir [Atlas], pp 297–364. Abrams, ed. 3, pp 1068, 1074.)* The arc of Buehler represents persistence of the ventral anastomosis, which is a longitudinal vessel that parallels the embryonic aorta anteriorly. Each visceral artery can be thought of as rungs in a ladder, with the aorta and ventral anastomosis forming the siderails. The tenth, eleventh, and twelfth rungs will coalesce to form the celiac axis and the thirteenth rung will become the superior mesenteric artery (SMA). Just as with the formation of the aortic arch, as the ventral anastomosis regresses, the point at which it ultimately breaks determines the final branching pattern. For instance, the common or right hepatic artery may be on the SMA side when the break occurs, giving rise to "replaced" arteries. When the ventral anastomosis persists, the vestige is referred to as the arc of Buehler.

The arc of Riolan, described by the French anatomist in the early seventeenth century, lies in the mesentery. It is a connection between branches of the middle and left colic arteries that permits collateral blood flow between the SMA and inferior mesenteric artery (IMA). The marginal artery of Drummond lies more peripherally in the mesentery and runs along the length of the colon connecting the distal arcades.

The arc of Barkow is located in the greater omentum, paralleling the gastroepiploic artery. It may provide an alternative pathway for flow in the case of splenic artery occlusion. It also supplies small ascending branches to the transverse colon.

In the case of abdominal aortic occlusion, the path of Winslow becomes an important source of collateral blood flow to the lower abdomen, pelvis, and legs. Blood flows from the internal mammary and intercostal arteries through the anterior abdominal wall to reach the inferior epigastric branches of the common femoral arteries.

530–532. The answers are: 530-C, 531-D, 532-B. *(Taveras & Ferrucci, vol 2, chap 109. Amplatz, pp 280, 355–369.)* The anteroposterior chest radiograph in complete transposition of the great vessels (TOGV) reveals a narrow mediastinal shadow, created by the overlap of the aorta and pulmonary artery, and an ovoid, malpositioned heart. This appearance has been described as the "egg on its side" or "egg on a string."

In the rarer instance, when the transposition has been congenitally "corrected" by the additional anomaly of ventricular inversion, the heart shape becomes distinctive. The left heart border assumes a boxlike configuration formed by the straight lateral edge of the ascending aorta. The right pulmonary hilum is displaced medially and elevated, producing the "waterfall" appearance. Although this sign was described in reference to this specific entity, it may be seen with other anomalies that have a VSD and high pulmonary blood flow.

The "gooseneck" deformity that is seen with endocardial cushion defects results from the apparent elongation and narrowing of the left ventricular outflow tract that occurs from the deficiencies in the ventricular septum and a cleft in the anterior leaflet of the mitral valve.

The "Goetz sign" refers to a filling defect in the main pulmonary artery, seen during pulmonary arteriography, which results from a jet of unopacified blood from a patent ductus arteriosus.

The "figure eight" or "snowman" refers to the cardiomediastinal configuration on plain chest film of supracardiac total anomalous pulmonary venous return (TAPVR). The distinctive mediastinal contour is produced by the abnormal vertical vein in the left hemithorax.

533–537. The answers are: 533-B, 534-B, 535-A, 536-D, 537-A. *(Amis pp 43–44. Pollack pp 24–25.)* Currently used contrast agents are tri-iodinated derivatives of a benzoic acid salt. These salts dissociate in aqueous solution into two ions: an anion (diatrizoate, iothalamate, metrizoate, or iodamide), which contains the three iodine atoms, and a cation, which is either sodium or methylglucamine (meglumine), or a combination of both. These compounds are described as "ionic ratio 1.5 monomers" since the three iodine atoms are carried on a molecule that dissociates into two particles in solution. The above ionic monomers have osmolalities 5 to 6 times that of plasma, in order to have enough iodine to be visible. However, the high osmolality causes endothelial cell disruption, pain, and poor patient tolerance. In 1968, the concept of developing contrast material with lower osmolality was suggested, which could be achieved by increasing the relative number of iodine atoms per particle of contrast material molecule in solution. Ioxaglate meglumine (Hexabrix) is an ionic dimer with 6 iodine atoms for every 2 ions in solution (ratio of 3:1).

"Nonionic" contrast agents were developed in a further effort to reduce complications. Iohexol and iopamidol are also ratio 3 contrast media, by virtue of a polyhydroxylic group on the benzene ring, which allows them to be water-soluble enough to form only one osmotically active particle for every 3 iodine atoms. Therefore, they have the same amount of iodine and only half the osmolality. However, they still have an osmolality twice that of plasma. Contrast agents such as iodixanol, currently undergoing development, have osmolalities equal to or slightly greater than plasma.

538–540. The answers are: 538-A, 539-C, 540-B. *(Taveras & Ferrucci, vol 2, chap 94 and 109. Gedgaudas, chaps 5–9.)* When presented with a case in which congenital heart disease may be present, it is often helpful to focus the differential possibilities by addressing the presence or absence of cyanosis and the condition of the pulmonary vascularity.

Cyanosis with increased pulmonary blood flow is typical of the admixture lesions, in which deoxygenated blood is allowed to enter the systemic circulation. Typically, the shunt is bidirectional, and the pulmonic circulation receives greater-than-normal flow. The most common of these are the "T" lesions described by Elliott: transposition of the great vessels, truncus arteriosus, and total anomalous pulmonary venous return. In the latter, one-fourth of patients have obstruction of the abnormal vein, producing pulmonary venous congestion. However, many nonobstructed patients will develop congestive heart failure due to the increased demand on the right ventricle.

The condition of increased pulmonary blood flow, in the absence of cyanosis, indicates a left-to-right shunt. Most common are ventricular septal defect (VSD), atrial septal defect (ASD), and patent ductus arteriosus (PDA). To help differentiate these, determination of the left atrial size is the next step. If it is enlarged, then ASD and endocardial cushion defect can be excluded because the extra blood volume flows immediately into the lower-pressure right atrium. The next step is to evaluate the aorta. If the aortic knob is markedly diminished in size, this indicates that the shunt is intracardiac and a VSD is likely. An extracardiac shunt, such as a PDA, tends to equalize the size of the aorta and pulmonary artery.

Ebstein anomaly is one of several lesions which result in functional right ventricular (RV) outflow obstruction, and hence diminished pulmonary vascularity. These patients shunt right to left at the atrial level through a patent foramen ovale or ASD, producing cyanosis which is usually present shortly after birth. The most common cause of decreased pulmonary vascularity and cyanosis is tetralogy of Fallot. Tricuspid atresia, pulmonary stenosis, and Uhl anomaly (deficient RV myocardium) are other causes.

541–544. The answers are: 541-D, 542-E, 543-B, 544-C. *(Mustard, Surgery 55:469–472, 1964.)* The Glenn shunt and Fontan procedures were devised for the treatment of tricuspid atresia. The Glenn operation involved transecting the right pulmonary artery, ligating it proximally, and connecting the distal artery end-to-side to the superior vena cava (SVC). It is reserved for only those cases in which definitive surgery cannot be performed, because once created, it is nearly impossible to reverse. Additionally, should the shunt fail, an SVC syndrome (painful venous engorgement of the face, neck, and upper extremities) may result.

The Fontan procedure, introduced in 1971, has undergone an evolution since that time. Originally a conduit formed from the right atrial appendage, which was then connected to the pulmonary trunk, it is now most commonly constructed from prosthetic material. Also the link may vary between either the right atrium or right ventricle to the pulmonary trunk. A radioopaque sewing ring is often seen overlying the region of the pulmonary outflow tract.

The Mustard and Jatene operations are used for the treatment of transposition of the great vessels (TOGV). The Mustard procedure, introduced in 1964, consisted of first removing the interatrial septum and then using pericardium to construct channels to divert blood flow from the pulmonary veins to the right ventricle and from the systemic return to the left ventricle. The Senning operation is a similar concept, but uses synthetic material to form the baffles.

The Jatene operation, first performed in 1976, was created for the definitive treatment of TOGV. It is usually done within the first weeks of life. The aorta and pulmonary artery are transected and switched. The long-term results are as yet unknown.

545–547. The answers are: 545-C, 546-A, 547-A. *(Kadir [Interventional], pp 80–87. Kim, pp 421–439.)* Thrombolytic therapy is based on the activation of plasminogen to plasmin, which is a nonspecific proteolytic agent that has an affinity for fibrin. Alpha-2-antiplasmin is its most potent inhibitor, but many proteins on both sides of the thrombosis/lysis balance play key roles in maintaining homeostasis.

Streptokinase (SK), which is produced by Lancefield group C beta-hemolytic streptococci, was discovered in 1933. It binds to plasminogen, forming a combined molecule which activates circulating plasminogen and, to a lesser degree, plasminogen which has already bound to fibrin in clot. At high doses, a systemic lytic state is rapidly produced. In local infusions, a systemic effect is not usually achieved for 10–12 hours. Because humans often have had exposure to streptococcal organisms, many have antibodies to SK. These may occasionally produce an allergic reaction or even anaphylaxis. If not, they often develop them after SK therapy. Usually, though, these simply prevent the SK from binding plasminogen, neutralizing it.

Urokinase, whose lytic property was elucidated in 1951, is a protease that activates plasminogen by peptide bond cleavage. Being a product of human kidney cell culture, it is not antigenic. Though it has less selective affinity for fibrin-bound plasminogen than tissue plasminogen activator (tPA), it has less of a systemic effect than SK.

548–550. The answers are: 548-C, 549-A, 550-A.   *(Hurst, ed. 7, pp 758–759. Silverman, pp 459–461.)*
Though quite rare, the cardiosplenic syndromes have assumed a position of unusual visibility in radiology. The strong correlation between the syndromes of asplenia and polysplenia (also known as the *visceral heterotaxy syndromes*) and congenital malformations of the heart and lungs makes these entities particularly fascinating—and a favorite topic of examiners.

Asplenia, which was originally described by Ivemark in 1955, accounts for approximately 1–3% of all congenital heart disease. The anomalies are more severe than those of polysplenia; the patients therefore usually present in childhood and mortality is high. Also referred to as dextroisomerism, or bilateral right-sidedness (which is an embryologically false but useful concept), there is associated ASD in all cases. One can think of this as two right atria, and since the septum primum is a "left-sided structure," it is therefore absent. VSD is quite frequent, as is pulmonic stenosis or atresia (7890), TAPVR (72%), TOGV (72%), and single ventricle (44%). Whereas the SVC is often duplicate, the IVC is usually single and intact. The bronchi are both eparterial, typical of the right-sided configuration.

Polysplenia, or bilateral left-sidedness, has some features in common with asplenia. A few features, however, distinguish the two, such as interruption of the IVC (with continuation of the venous flow through the azygous vein). The two lungs are morphologically left lungs, with hyparterial bronchi. The anomalies are less severe, and patients tend to present later, usually in adulthood. ASD and VSD occur with less frequency than in asplenia, and although pulmonic stenosis occurs in both with equal frequency (33%), pulmonary atresia is much rarer (9%). Transposition of the great vessels (8%), single ventricle (8%), and total anomalous pulmonary venous return (TAPVR) (0%) are also much less common.

551–553. The answers are: 551-D, 552-D, 553-B.   *(Hurst, ed. 7, pp 258, 702. Hurst, ed. 6, pp 628. Kelley, pp 248–253.)*   Rib notching occurs if collateral flow through the intercostal arteries is recruited, such as in aortic coarctation. It may also occur due to venous collateral flow, as in a superior vena cava syndrome, or for a variety of nonvascular causes, such as neurofibromatosis. Though the entire length of the ribs may be involved, the posterior segments are usually best for evaluating notching on a chest x-ray.

In coarctation, rib notching does not usually develop before age 7 or 8 and is typically located along the undersurface of the middle and outer thirds of ribs 3 to 8. As the internal mammary arteries increase in size to supply collateral flow, the internal surface of the sternum may show similar waviness.

Postductal coarctation of the aorta is the most common type; it typically involves the ribs symmetrically. If the coarctation occurs in a patient with a left arch and an aberrant right subclavian artery (SCA), then the rib notching may be exclusively left-sided, because the right SCA is distal to the stenosis, and only the left side can develop collaterals. An aberrant right SCA does not of itself cause any significant hemodynamic alteration.

If rib notching occurs only on the right side, then the coarctation must be proximal to the origin of the left SCA by the same principle. The Blalock-Taussig operation, in which the subclavian artery was divided and the proximal end anastomosed to the pulmonary artery, would develop rib notching on the side of the procedure. The Blalock procedure, which does not interrupt subclavian flow, does not cause rib notching.

554–556. The answers are: 554-D, 555-A, 556-B.   *(Taveras & Ferrucci, vol 2, chap 1–5.)*   Congenital bicuspid aortic valve is the most common cause of acquired aortic stenosis. The calcification usually takes years to accumulate, except that it can be quite rapid in the case of infectious endocarditis. Calcification of the aortic valve nearly always signifies significant aortic stenosis. The most common symptoms are angina (50–70%), congestive heart failure, and syncope. The left ventricle becomes hypertrophied and poststenotic dilatation of the ascending aorta may occur, though it is usually less extreme than the dilatation that results from a regurgitant valve.

Although calcification commonly develops in the mitral annulus in the elderly (there is not a similar aortic annulus to calcify), the incidence of significant valvular disease is quite low. When mitral valve calcification *is* present in known rheumatic heart disease, there is no correlation with the degree of stenosis. Additionally, aortic valve calcification may be absent in that setting, and yet the patient has significant disease.

557. **The answers are: A-Y, B-Y, C-N, D-N, E-N.** *(Kadir, pp 627–634. Clouse, ed. 2, p 267.)* The nodal phase of the lymphangiogram in the figure demonstrates several enlarged paraaortic lymph nodes which have a foamy or lacy appearance that is highly suggestive, but not pathognomonic, of lymphoma. Other entities in the differential diagnosis would include sarcoidosis, metastases (especially seminoma), cat-scratch fever, dilantin-induced lymphadenopathy, and reactive hyperplasia. Reactive hyperplasia, a localized or generalized tumor-induced inflammatory response, can be very difficult to differentiate from lymphoma. Lack of nodal abnormality does not exclude disease, as early microscopic disease may not affect the lymphangiogram. The vascular phase of a lymphangiogram is less important during evaluation for lymphoma than for solid tumor metastases, since lymphoma seldom completely obstructs the lymph channels. Solid neoplastic metastases often completely replace lymph nodes and obstruct lymphatic channels, which may be overlooked if only the nodal phase is imaged.

During lymphography, contrast flows from the lymphatic channels into the nodal sinuses, but not into lymph follicles themselves, which appear as small filling defects and give the node a fine granular pattern. The contrast media for lymphography is fat-soluble ethiodol, with an iodine concentration of 37%. Ninety percent of the ethiodol is retained in the lymph nodes, whereas the remainder passes through the thoracic duct into the pulmonary circulation. Pulmonary embolization of ethiodol is seen in up to 55% of patients following lymphography. However, clinically significant pulmonary complications occur in less than 1% of patients. Individuals with severe compromise of pulmonary function are at greatest risk for developing clinically significant pulmonary embolisms.

Following lymphography, increased pulmonary activity on gallium scans can be seen in 50% of patients for at least 1 month. It results from pulmonary inflammation incited by the embolized ethiodol. Another potential complication of ethiodol use is an allergic reaction. Transient low-grade temperature elevation 6 to 18 hours following lymphography is reported as a minor complication and is not significant. However, high fever which persists may indicate the rarer complication of chemical pneumonitis.

558. **The answers are: A-N, B-N, C-Y, D-Y, E-Y.** *(Elliott, pp 17–18, 565–575.)* The interventricular septum (IVS) is convex anteriorly and also bulges into the right ventricular (RV) cavity. The anterior-cranial portion is viewed on edge using the long axis, or left anterior oblique (LAO), projection. The posterior-caudal portion of the septum is seen in profile on the hepatoclavicular (45°–50° LAO and 30° craniad angulation) view.

The incidence of VSD in all live births is approximately 1.5 to 2.5 per 1000. VSDs are the second most common congenital heart lesion, and although most occur as an isolated lesion, they are often part of more complex syndromes.

Most VSDs are of the perimembranous type, and involve both the membranous and muscular portions of the septum. These are best appreciated in the LAO projection. Muscular VSDs may occur as isolated muscular defects or as multiple perforations—the "swiss cheese" septum.

VSDs which are located in the portion of the IVS that forms the anterior aspect of the left ventricular outflow tract (this same portion of the septum also forms the posterior wall of the pulmonary infundibulum) are situated beneath the right aortic valve cusp. When associated with aortic valve override, as in patients with tetralogy of Fallot, these VSDs are called *anterior,* or *conal,* VSDs. When the aortic valve remains in its normal position and the VSD exits above the crista supraventricularis, it is referred to as a supracristal VSD.

A posterior VSD, which involves the AV-canal, occurs just anterior to the anterior leaflet of the mitral valve. This defect is best identified by the hepatoclavicular view.

Most VSDs close spontaneously, though not within the first year of life. Two of the possible complications of VSD are prolapse of the right aortic valve cusp, resulting in aortic insufficiency, and the development of high pulmonary vascular resistance (Eisenmenger physiology).

559. **The answers are: A-N, B-N, C-Y, D-N, E-N.** *(Gedgaudas, pp 184–193.)* Aortic arch anomalies arise from abnormal regression of the fourth embryonic arches during fetal development. The pulmonary arteries are formed from remnants of the sixth aortic arches, which are much less likely to have congenital anomalies. The "pulmonary sling" is the most significant sixth-arch anomaly, wherein the left pulmonary artery arises from the right (instead of the main) pulmonary artery and crosses between the trachea and esophagus as it enters the left hemithorax. The result is a "nutcracker" compression of the trachea and right mainstem bronchus between the arteries and an anterior indentation on the esophagus. Consequently, respiratory compromise usually develops in infancy.

The double aortic arch represents persistence of both fourth embryonic arches. The trachea and esophagus are trapped by the vascular ring that results, with an anterior indentation on the trachea (made by the left arch) often visible on a lateral chest x-ray and a posterior indentation on the esophagus (produced by the right arch), which may be seen on a lateral esophagram. The aorta usually descends on the left, but the right arch is usually larger.

Although arch anomalies are commonly associated with other defects, the double aortic arch is more often an isolated finding. The right aortic arch results from abnormal regression of the left arch and can occur in two forms. If the left arch becomes atretic proximal to the origin of the left subclavian artery, the latter will maintain a connection to the right arch and pass behind the esophagus to form an "aberrant" left subclavian artery. Should the primitive left arch "break" beyond the origin of the left subclavian artery, mirror-image branching occurs; that is, all the arteries arise from the right arch, so that everything is reversed from the normal left arch configuration. This form is associated with congenital heart disease in nearly all cases. Nearly 90% of the time, patients have tetralogy of Fallot. Less common associations include truncus arteriosus, transposition of the great vessels, and tricuspid atresia.

560. **The answers are: A-N, B-N, C-Y, D-N, E-Y.** *(Gedgaudas, pp 147–152. Elliott, pp 7–9.)* The tetralogy of Fallot, described nearly a hundred years ago by the French physician for whom it is named, consists of (1) infundibular pulmonic stenosis, (2) right ventricular hypertrophy, (3) a large membranous ventricular septal defect (VSD), and (4) an aorta which straddles the VSD. The VSD allows admixture of deoxygenated blood into the systemic circulation, which causes cyanosis. The degree of pulmonic stenosis directly affects the amount of shunting. The anomaly, which accounts for about 10% of all congenital heart disease, can be thought of as a failure of the normal development of the crista supraventricularis, which is a muscular sheet that forms the posterior portion of a muscular ring that divides the right ventricle into an inflow tract and an outflow tract (the infundibulum). The crista also forms part of the interventricular septum. It supports the right side of the aortic root where the right sinus of valsalva is located. In tetralogy of Fallot, the normal crista fails to grow, resulting in a conal VSD and a rightward shift of the aortic root that causes the aorta to straddle the VSD.

Chest radiographs reveal the classic "boot-shaped" heart (coeur-en-sabot), which is caused by the prominent, hypertrophied *right* ventricle. In 25% of patients, there is a right aortic arch, which typically has mirror-image branching.

"Tet," or "tetrad," spells are paroxysmal episodes of sudden cyanosis due to increased shunting, presumably due to a sudden increase in pulmonary resistance. The children often squat, which is thought to be an instinctive means of increasing systemic resistance in order to reduce shunting.

The VSD is not only *not* necessary for life, it is part of the patient's problem and it requires closure. In addition to the main pulmonary artery being stenotic (usually the infundibular portion), the more peripheral branches may be stenotic as well, which is more common on the left. As the degree of pulmonic obstruction increases, the size and number of bronchial collaterals also increase.

561. The answers are: A-Y, B-N, C-Y, D-Y, E-N. *(Braunwald, ed. 4, pp 994–995, 1424.)* Endocardial fibroelastosis (EFE) is characterized by a shiny, thickened endocardium due to a proliferation of elastic tissue. Primary EFE presents in infancy (typically between 2 and 12 months), usually with clinical signs of left ventricular dysfunction and congestive heart failure. Chest radiographs reveal marked four-chamber cardiac enlargement, with normal or congested pulmonary vasculature. Angiography typically shows a markedly dilated, poorly contractile left ventricle and mitral regurgitation. Pompe disease (type II, glycogen storage disease), cystic medial necrosis of the coronary arteries, viral myocarditis, and primary EFE are all included in the differential diagnosis of nonobstructive cardiomyopathy in the infant.

In secondary EFE, focal areas of fibroelastic thickening of the endocardium occur in association with obstructive cardiac anomalies, such as aortic stenosis, coarctation of the aorta, and hypoplastic left heart syndrome. Although no definite cause of the condition has been identified, endocardial ischemia has been proposed as an etiologic mechanism or cofactor of both primary and secondary EFE.

The deposition of fibroelastic plaques in the endocardium has also been described in patients with carcinoid syndrome. Cardiac abnormalities are seen in over two-thirds of patients with carcinoid syndrome and are felt to be related to circulating humeral substances (serotonin or a degradation product) secreted by the tumor. Gastrointestinal carcinoid, metastatic to the liver, can result in right-sided EFE. In this situation, the left heart is protected by inactivation of the humeral substances by the lungs. However, pulmonary carcinoid can cause carcinoid syndrome and EFE which involves primarily the left heart.

562. The answers are: A-N, B-N, C-Y, D-Y, E-N. *(Elliott, pp 511–513, 522, 534. D'Cruz, pp 28, 82.)* Rheumatic endocarditis results from an antigen-antibody reaction following an attack of rheumatic fever. The leaflets are susceptible to fibrin and platelet deposition, which produces "vegetations" along the margins. Eventually, the leaflets become thickened, the commissures fuse, and the chordae become matted together, which restricts the mobility of the leaflets and narrows the valve orifice.

In M-mode echocardiography, the normal tracing of the anterior mitral valve leaflet resembles the letter M. The posterior leaflet mirrors this motion and the tracing is shaped like a W. The point at which the mitral valve starts to open is called the D point. The E and F points represent the maximal and minimal points of the initial opening, respectively. A second opening of the mitral valve occurs with atrial systole. The maximal and minimal points are labeled A and C, respectively.

The echocardiogram in patients with mitral stenosis reveals thickened and scarred leaflets, a *decreased* E-F slope (because of decreased flow across the stenotic valve), an abnormal anterior motion of the posterior mitral leaflet, and a fixed separation of the two leaflets during diastole of no greater than 15 mm. The left parasternal, short-axis view is used to calculate the valve area. The presence of calcification on the valve leaflets scatters the sound beam and often obscures them.

Mitral valve vegetations should be detectable by echocardiography if they are 3 mm or larger. They are seen as areas of focal, nodular thickening on the leaflet, but the leaflet appears and moves otherwise normally. This should be easily differentiated from the thickened, sclerotic valve of rheumatic heart disease.

In mitral valve prolapse, redundant valvular tissue and "billowing" of the leaflets into the left atrium occurs during systole.

563. The correct answers are: A-N, B-Y, C-N, D-N, E-Y. *(Elliott, pp 235–243.)* Valvular pulmonic stenosis (PS) is most commonly congenital; 10% of patients with congenital heart disease have PS. Depending on the severity of the stenosis, patients may be asymptomatic and may be shown to have a cardiac murmur during routine physical examination, or they may present with cyanosis and decreased pulmonary vascularity.

Pulmonary valve stenosis is characterized by thickening of the pulmonary valve leaflets and fusion of the commissures. The valve is often bicuspid, and poststenotic dilatation of the main pulmonary artery and proximal left pulmonary artery results. A key to recognizing valvular PS is the asymmetrical dilatation of the left pulmonary artery, as turbulent flow distal to the obstruction follows a straight line into the left pulmonary artery.

By 2-D echocardiography, most patients have poststenotic dilatation of the proximal left and main pulmonary arteries, while the size of the right heart chambers remains normal. The development of right ventricular (RV) hypertrophy follows increasing severity and duration of the obstruction. Right ventriculography will show a domed, thickened pulmonic valve, and hypertrophy of the crista supraventricularis and ventricle.

Uncommonly, pulmonic stenosis can result from a dysplastic valve where the leaflets and commissures do not fuse. The valve tissue is myxomatous, thickened, and redundant, and it encroaches on the valve orifice. This type of PS causes the "stuffed shirt" form of obstruction.

In tetralogy of Fallot, obstruction to the flow of blood out of the right ventricle can occur at one or more anatomic sites. Although a combination of both subpulmonic infundibular stenosis and pulmonary valve stenosis occurs in many cases, by definition there is always at least obstruction of the outflow tract.

564. The answers are: A-Y, B-Y, C-Y, D-Y, E-N. *(Gedgaudas, pp 162–165. Hurst, ed. 7, pp 748–749. Braunwald, ed. 4, pp 940–941.)* Ebstein anomaly is a congenital displacement of the posterior and septal leaflets of the tricuspid valve downward, into the right ventricular chamber. As a result, a portion of the ventricle is "atrialized" and the remaining ventricular chamber is small. Forward flow is reduced, and depending on the degree of tricuspid insufficiency, a right to left shunt is almost always present through a patent foramen ovale or an atrial septal defect. The anomaly is found more frequently in infants whose mothers were receiving lithium during pregnancy.

Conduction disturbances are common. Most typically, the EKG shows giant peaked P waves and a right bundle branch block. About 10% of patients have the Wolff-Parkinson-White syndrome. Although the most common symptom is dyspnea on exertion, palpitations from episodes of supraventricular tachyarrhythmia are not uncommon.

The chest radiograph often reveals marked cardiomegaly and decreased pulmonary vasculature. Although half of those with Ebstein malformation will present with cyanosis and congestive heart failure in infancy, the remainder who do not have associated anomalies may not present until early adulthood. Occasionally, cyanosis that is present at birth will disappear as pulmonary vascular resistance falls, but, eventually, almost all patients come to medical attention.

Cineangiography is diagnostic. The right ventricle is small and contracts out of phase with the atrialized portion, producing a "paradoxical" motion. The regurgitant tricuspid valve and right to left shunt are also evident.

Management is symptom-oriented; digitalis and diuretics are used to treat cases of congestive heart failure. When medical therapy is no longer effective, replacement of the tricuspid valve and/or plication of the atrialized portion of the RV is performed.

565. The answers are: A-Y, B-Y, C-N, D-Y, E-Y. *(Pickering, Circulation 83(I):147–154, 1991. Tegtmeyer, Circulation 83(I):155–161, 1991. Sos, Circulation 83(I):162–166, 1991. Sellars, J Hypertens 3(2):177–181, 1985. Cicuto, AJR 137:599–601, 1981.)* Renovascular hypertension (RVHTN) is the term applied to a condition in which correction of renal artery stenosis results in lowered blood pressure; it should not be applied to renal artery stenoses that are discovered incidentally and which coexist with hypertension. The prevalence of RVHTN is unknown, but it accounts for less than 5% of all patients with hypertension.

Clinical features that suggest RVHTN include an abrupt onset of hypertension, hypertension in individuals less than 30 years old, or onset after age 50. However, given the low prevalence of the condition, these clinical predictors have low positive predictive values and have been reported to be present in only one-third of patients with RVHTN.

There are two simple screening tests for the detection of RVHTN that can be performed in a physician's office: (1) the measurement of peripheral plasma renin activity and (2) the captopril test. The peripheral plasma renin activity is useful as a negative predictor of RVHTN, since a low plasma renin level in an untreated patient virtually excludes the possibility of RVHTN. Presently, the most sensitive screening test for the RVHTN is the plasma renin activity response to captopril. The sensitivity and specificity for this test have been reported to be as high as 95%. Captopril-stimulated peripheral renin activity has been shown to be more sensitive than even captopril radionuclide renal scans.

The measurement of the renal vein renin ratio has been used in an attempt to predict the response to surgery in patients with RVHTN. A review of these ratios, however, has revealed a false positive rate of 39% and a false negative rate of 71% in predicting a successful outcome. Therefore, renal vein renin ratios are thought to be of little help.

In patients in whom fibromuscular dysplasia (FMD) is the cause of RVHTN, there is a predicted cumulative patency rate at 10 years of 87% following angioplasty. It has also been observed that renal artery FMD is often successfully redilated, should the lesion(s) recur.

Ostial renal artery stenoses are due to aortic wall atherosclerotic plaques which overhang the renal ostium and cause a decrease in renal blood flow. True renal artery stenoses are usually located within the proximal third of the renal artery proper and are defined as beginning after 2 to 3 mm from the angiographic origin of the renal artery. This distinction is an important one to make, since the success of PTA is less for ostial lesions, with worse long-term results as well. In a recent series, a 60% initial success rate for ostial renal artery PTA was noted. This experience is atypical and may be related to differences in lesion classification.

566. The answers are: A-N, B-N, C-Y, D-N, E-N. *(Uflacker, pp 504–509, 535.)* The long axis of the human kidney parallels the ipsilateral psoas muscle, angling approximately 13° away from the midline. The upper pole is also more posterior and medial than the lower pole, and the coronal axis is tilted 30° posteriorly to the coronal plane of the body. As a result, the renal pelvis lies anteriorly; radiographically, the posterior calyces usually project medially and en face, whereas the anterior calyces lie laterally and are viewed in tangent.

Brödel's *white line* is a surface landmark that lies over a highly vascularized zone at the lateral margin of the kidney. Brödel's *avascular plane* is located 1 to 2 cm posterior to the kidney's lateral margin and is the ideal plane for puncture in nephrostomy placement.

Following uncomplicated percutaneous nephrostomy, gross hematuria usually resolves completely during the first 24 hours. If hematuria persists beyond 48 hours, the cause should be investigated.

Unilateral renal obstruction does not result in significant fluid and electrolyte derangement if the contralateral kidney can maintain homeostasis. With bilateral renal obstruction, relief of one or both kidneys often results in a postobstructive diuresis that usually lasts several days. Matching intravenous fluids to urine output during this period only increases an already large urine output, which may be as much as 5 liters per day.

567. The correct answers are: A-Y, B-Y, C-N, D-N, E-N. *(Reuter, pp 382–383, 394–395.)* Cirrhosis ultimately produces diffuse hepatic fibrosis. During the course of disease, however, the processes of hepatocellular necrosis, fibrosis, and hepatic regeneration are occurring simultaneously. The most common type is Laennec cirrhosis, which typically occurs in the setting of alcoholism and malnutrition.

Progressive hepatic fibrosis obstructs normal *hepatopetal* (L., "liver-seeking") portal venous flow. During periods of elevation of sinusoidal or absolute portal venous pressures, the direction of flow may oscillate. Eventually, with end-stage disease, the flow remains *hepatofugal* (L., "liver-fleeing") and large gastric, esophageal, and/or hemorrhoidal varices carry the entire portal venous circulation.

The wedged hepatic venous pressure (WHVP) and splenic pulp pressure (obtained by spleno-portography) reflect the total portal venous pressure which should normally be less than 12 mmHg (156 cm saline). The pressure in the portal vein is affected by both the resistance of the hepatic sinusoids and the transmitted pressure from the inferior vena cava (IVC). Therefore, the degree of intrahepatic obstruction, or corrected sinusoidal pressure, is obtained by taking the WHVP and subtracting the transmitted IVC pressure. However, a patient with stable intrahepatic portal obstruction from cirrhosis can still develop esophageal variceal bleeding if the central venous pressure becomes elevated.

Current indications for placement of transjugular intrahepatic portosystemic shunts include catastrophic variceal bleeding, which can be temporized only by a Blakemore-Sengstaken or Minnesota tube, esophageal varices which can no longer be treated by sclerotherapy, and refractory ascites.

568. The answers are: A-Y, B-N, C-Y, D-Y, E-Y. *(Abrams, pp 1893–1894, 1903–1906.)* Venographic manifestations of deep vein thrombosis (DVT) reflect both the presence of the thrombus itself and the flow alterations that result. The direct demonstration of one or more constant intraluminal filling defect(s) is conclusive evidence of DVT. Signs which are suggestive, but not *diagnostic,* of DVT include failure to opacify a vein or veins, and the diversion of contrast flow from the deep into the superficial veins. These are nonspecific and may also be caused by marked leg edema, cellulitis, muscle rupture, hematoma, or periarticular cysts. In patients with DVT, failure of a vein to opacify indicates that thrombus and edema have prevented any contrast from flowing into the vein at all. This sign is found in up to 80% of patients with extensive DVT. In such instances, the superficial veins tend to be densely opacified and somewhat dilated, since they are draining most of the blood volume from the leg.

The etiology of DVT involves a triad that was originally described by Virchow: stasis of blood flow, intimal damage, and an underlying tendency to form blood clots. Malignancy, obesity, and increasing age are known to predispose to the development of DVT, possibly by affecting one or more of the arms of Virchow's triad. Other predisposing factors include trauma, surgery, prolonged immobilization, recent myocardial infarction, and the use of oral contraceptives. Several studies have shown that DVT occurs in 25 to 30% of abdominal surgery patients and 40 to 60% of hip fracture patients. At extremely high risk are the elderly with hip fractures; the incidence of DVT in this group is as high as 85%.

Studies of the natural history of DVT have shown that it most commonly originates in the calf, especially the peroneal veins. In approximately one-third of patients, calf vein thrombi lyse spontaneously within 72 hours. In about another half of patients, they persist, but do not propagate. In the remaining 20 to 30%, thrombi propagate proximally into the popliteal, femoral, and iliac veins, and these are the patients who are at risk for clinically significant pulmonary embolism.

In patients with documented pulmonary embolism, venography demonstrated lower-extremity DVT in only 70%. Therefore, in the remainder, the pulmonary embolism did not originate in a lower extremity vein or all of the thrombus from the lower extremities was embolized into the lungs. The experience with ultrasound documentation of DVT in patients with PE is similar.

Thrombosis of the superficial veins, a relatively common condition, extends to involve the deep veins in only 17% of cases. Of these, only 10% are associated with pulmonary embolism. Clinically serious pulmonary embolism from *isolated* superficial vein thrombosis has been reported, but is very rare.

569. **The answers are: A-N, B-Y, C-Y, D-N, E-Y.** *(Frykberg, J Trauma 29:1041–1049, 1989. McCorkell, Am J Roentgen 145:1245–1247, 1985.)* Clinical evaluation of patients that have sustained penetrating trauma to an extremity strives to triage those who require emergency surgical exploration and repair of arterial injuries. In most patients that are hemodynamically stable, arteriography is performed preoperatively to detail the extent of injury. Patients that require emergency surgical exploration are those with "hard" clinical evidence of arterial injury, which include absent distal pulse(s), distal ischemia, neurologic deficit, expanding hematoma, active hemorrhage, or a bruit or thrill in the area of injury.

"Soft" clinical signs, such as proximity to major vessel, large hematoma, or hypotension are associated with arteriographically demonstrable major arterial injury in only 10% of cases, and only 1.8% of these require surgery.

Therefore, in cases of penetrating extremity trauma, where there are no "hard" signs of arterial injury, arteriography can be safely delayed for up to 24 hours. However, angiography should probably not be delayed in patients that have multiple (e.g., shotgun fragments), severely comminuted fractures, or wounds to the thoracic outlet.

570. **The answers are: A-Y, B-Y, C-Y, D-N, E-Y.** *(Taveras & Ferrucci, chaps 90–97, 103–105, 114–116; Gedgaudas, pp 191–193.)* Loss of the main pulmonary artery contour results from lesions which restrict the normal flow of blood to the heart or from abnormalities of position or rotation of the heart and great vessels. Only pulmonary artery (PA) sling fails to alter the normal mediastinal silhouette. The left PA arises from the proximal right and passes between the trachea and esophagus.

Ebstein anomaly, in which a right-to-left shunt is produced at the atrial level by the abnormal tricuspid valve, causes a loss of the normal PA contour because of decreased pulmonary flow. Pulmonary atresia is the severest form of decreased flow. Interestingly, if the PA is only stenotic, poststenotic dilatation frequently produces an enlarged main PA contour, with accentuation of the left PA created by a jet effect through the stenotic valve.

In half of patients with persistent truncus arteriosus (PTA), the pulmonary arteries arise directly from the aorta in such a way that they lose the normal PA contour. In those patients with type I PTA, however, the abnormal common pulmonary stem mimics the normal main PA. By definition, corrected transposition of the great vessels has reversal of the normal aortic and pulmonary artery outflow tracts, producing an abnormally narrow mediastinum on chest x-ray.

571. **The answers are: A-N, B-Y, C-N, D-Y, E-N.** *(Gedgaudas, pp 112–117. Elliott, p 693.)* Persistent truncus arteriosis (PTA) is the embryologic result of a failure of the conotruncus to properly divide into the aorta and pulmonary artery. A single semilunar truncal valve is usually present and has three cusps, though occasionally there are two or four cusps. The pulmonary arteries arise from the ascending aorta in one of three ways, classified as types I, II, and III.

In type I PTA, they arise from the left inferior base of the common arterial trunk via a short "pseudopulmonary trunk" vessel. In type II, the pulmonary arteries arise independently from the posterior aspect of the common trunk. They originate separately from the sides of the truncus in type III PTA. However, the most common type involves a hybrid of these (types I and II), causing many to abandon this system. Type IV PTA involves the descending thoracic aorta and is actually thought to be a severe form of tetralogy of Fallot, in which large bronchial collateral vessels have arisen to supply the pulmonary circulation.

Angiography is needed to outline the truncal and pulmonary arterial anatomy, as well as to evaluate the interventricular septum, which often has multiple defects. The conus is absent, distinguishing this entity from tetralogy of Fallot with pulmonary atresia. In over one-third of patients, there is a right aortic arch.

572. The answers are: A-Y, B-Y, C-Y, D-Y, E-N. *(Cohan, AJR 151:263–270, 1988.)* Initial evaluation of a hypotensive patient following contrast injection should include eliciting a brief description of symptoms and determining blood pressure and pulse. Hypotension with bradycardia indicates a vasovagal reaction, unless the patient is receiving beta-blockers. Vasovagal reactions should be treated by positioning the patient in the Trendelenberg position, giving them intravenous fluids, and possibly administering intravenous atropine (0.6 mg IV).

Hypotension with tachycardia indicates that the patient is suffering from an anaphylactoid or cardiogenic reaction, which is an emergency. Epinephrine (0.3–0.5 mg; 1:1000 subcutaneously), an alpha- and beta-adrenergic stimulator, is the cornerstone of therapy for all anaphylactoid reactions.

Volume replacement constitutes the most important therapy for all patients who develop hypotension. Large bore intravenous lines for the administration of crystalloid or colloid solutions are essential in patients undergoing intravenous or intraarterial contrast injection. Dyspnea may accompany hypotension, and patients with any respiratory compromise should receive oxygen during the procedure.

Diphenhydramine, an H_1-antihistamine, is used for the treatment of hives and pruritus, and are not used for therapy of hypotension. In fact, rapid intravenous administration of diphenhydramine can cause hypotension.

There have been case reports of H_2 blockers, such as cimetidine, being used for treatment of anaphylactoid reactions. However, neither H_1 nor H_2 blockers should be used as first-line therapy for any contrast reaction associated with hypotension.

573. The answers are: A-Y, B-Y, C-N, D-N, E-Y. *(Elliott, pp 244–245, 264–268, 459.)* Aortic stenosis (AS) is the third-most-frequent cardiac condition that is associated with a fatal outcome, preceded only by coronary artery disease and hypertensive heart disease. AS can be classified into three groups: congenital, rheumatic, and degenerative. More than 95% of patients with congenital aortic stenosis have a bicuspid or, less commonly, unicuspid valves. These patients will usually present before 65 years of age. Patients with rheumatic aortic stenosis will also have mitral stenosis and/ or regurgitation related to rheumatic disease. Degenerative aortic stenosis manifests itself after the age of 65 and is associated with aortic valve calcification, without commissural fusion. Since the diagnosis of degenerative aortic stenosis can be easily overlooked clinically, it is very important to remember that aortic valve calcification on plain film correlates well with hemodynamically significant AS.

By angiography, the degree of dilatation of the ascending aorta in aortic insufficiency is greater than that seen with aortic stenosis. This is because aortic regurgitation occurs in the setting of conditions that often directly dilate the ascending aorta, such as syphilitic aortitis or anuloaortic ectasia.

The time at which valvular aortic stenosis presents is a function of the degree of aortic obstruction. Symptomatic aortic stenosis at birth is indicative of severe obstruction and often manifests as left ventricular failure. In this setting, it is frequently associated with coarctation of the aorta. *Supra*valvular aortic stenosis is one of several cardiac anomalies in Williams syndrome, or idiopathic hypercalcemia of infancy, which is also characterized by mental retardation, neonatal hypercalcemia, and "elfin" facies.

574. The answers are: A-Y, B-Y, C-N, D-Y, E-N. *(Gedgaudas, pp 101–112.)* Transposition of the great vessels may occur in one of two ways. The most common form, and the most common cause of cyanosis in the neonate, is "complete" transposition. Because the bulbus cordis normally forms through looping to the right (*dextro-*, or *d-looping*), it is often referred to as *d-transposition*. The abnormality is not a failure of looping, but is the result of the conotruncal septum failing to spiral as it divides the ventricular outflow tracts. The result is that the systemic and pulmonary circulations become isolated circuits.

Congenitally corrected transposition, which is much rarer, is a combination of the above process *and* abnormal looping of the bulbus cordis to the left (*levo-*, or *l-transposition*), which corrects the hemodynamic problem by inverting the ventricles. The atria maintain their normal position and hence are "discordant" with the ventricles. Though the hemodynamic problem is corrected, unfortunately the high incidence of other cardiac anomalies in congenitally corrected transposition reduces the 5-year survival to less than 30%.

In both cases, ventricular septal defects are common, but in complete transposition, an admixture lesion (VSD, PPA, or patent foramen ovale) is necessary for survival. Temporizing a neonate with prostaglandin E may keep the ductus arteriosus open, and often a Rashkind procedure (balloon atrial septostomy) is done to allow admixture. The Rastelli operation is a definitive repair, but is usually delayed a year or more, to improve the chances for success. There are other definitive procedures, but only the Jatene ("switch") operation is performed in the neonatal period.

Mammography

DIRECTIONS: Each question below contains five suggested responses. Select the **one best** response to each question.

575. The calcifications depicted in the figure MOST likely represent

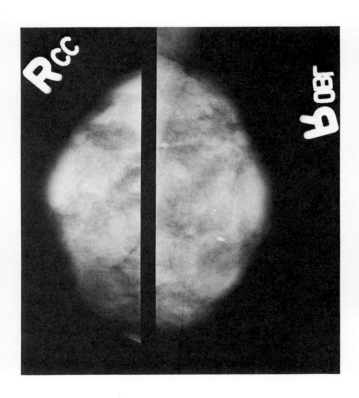

(A) invasive carcinoma
(B) ductal carcinoma in situ (DCIS)
(C) cystic disease
(D) sclerosing adenosis
(E) fat necrosis

576. The MOST likely diagnosis in the figure is

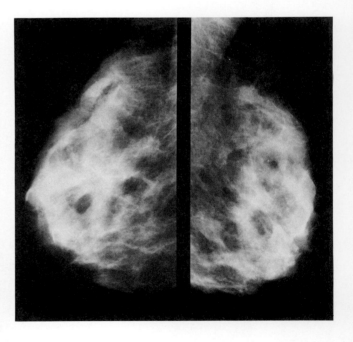

(A) radial scar
(B) invasive ductal cancer
(C) fat necrosis
(D) two invasive cancers
(E) normal breast tissue

577. The calcifications depicted in the figure are MOST likely due to

[full-width left mammogram image]

(A) secretory disease
(B) intraductal carcinoma
(C) papillomatosis
(D) plasma cell mastitis
(E) fat necrosis

578. The number of new cases of breast cancer annually in the United States is estimated to be

(A) 24,000
(B) 80,000
(C) 140,000
(D) 175,000
(E) 210,000

579. The estimated number of deaths from breast cancer in 1991 was

(A) 20,000
(B) 34,000
(C) 64,000
(D) 98,000
(E) 140,000

580. The bilateral process depicted in the figure is most likely

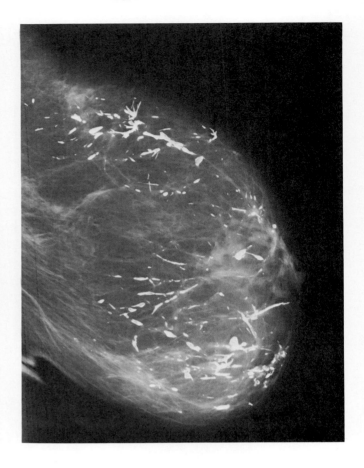

(A) papillomatosis
(B) sclerosing adenosis
(C) intraductal carcinoma
(D) vascular calcification
(E) secretory disease

581. The percent reduction in mortality from screening mammography, based on several studies, is approximately

(A) 2%
(B) 6%
(C) 10%
(D) 30%
(E) 41%

582. The mammogram and ultrasound of the 55-year-old woman in the figure at left and right, respectively, MOST likely depict

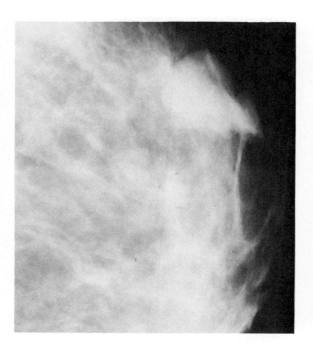
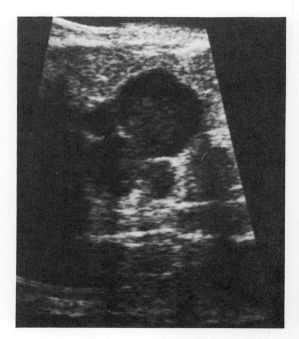

(A) a fibroadenoma
(B) an invasive ductal carcinoma
(C) an intracystic papillary carcinoma
(D) a benign papillary neoplasm
(E) a cyst with debris

---

583. Modern mammography requires an exposure of _____ rad per breast.

(A) 0.01
(B) 0.20
(C) 0.5
(D) 1.0
(E) 2.0

584. The theoretical risk for developing breast cancer from a screening mammography exposure of 1 rad will produce _____ additional cancer(s) per million women per year (after a 10- to 15-year latent period).

(A) 1
(B) 6
(C) 12
(D) 20
(E) 28

585. Magnification technique, as compared to standard mammography, will

(A) decrease dose in proportion to focal spot size
(B) have no overall effect on dose
(C) increase dose 2 to 3 times
(D) increase dose 4 to 5 times
(E) require the use of a higher grid ratio

586. The optical magnification ratio for best sharpness and detail is

(A) 1:1
(B) 1.5:1
(C) 3:1
(D) 5:1
(E) 10:1

587. Judging from the figure, what would you say is the MOST likely diagnosis?

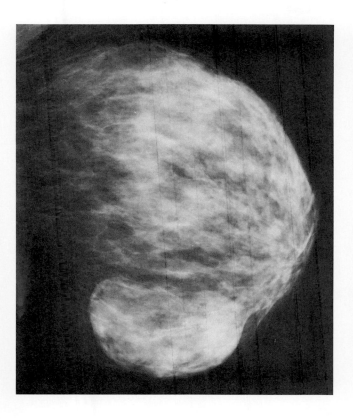

(A) Comedocarcinoma
(B) Phylloides tumor
(C) Fat necrosis
(D) Cyst
(E) Fibroadenolipoma

588. Which ONE of the following statements is TRUE?

(A) mammographic detail is most dependent on keV
(B) peak keV for a molybdenum target occurs at 17.9 and 19.5 keV
(C) peak keV for a tungsten target is 25.1 keV
(D) optimal contrast for mammography occurs at 15 to 20 keV for a molybdenum target
(E) tungsten produces more low keV photons than molybdenum, which improves contrast.

589. The lesion depicted in the figure is MOST likely a

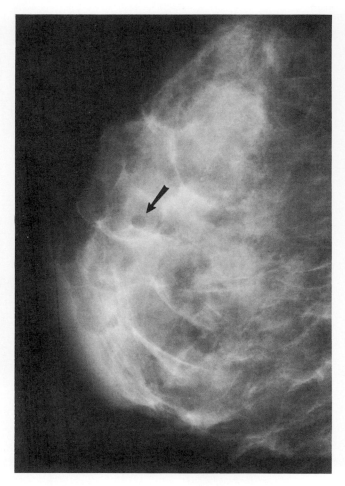

(A) granular cell myoblastoma
(B) galactocele
(C) hamartoma
(D) fibroadenoma
(E) papilloma

590. The false negative rate for mammography is

(A) 1%
(B) 6%
(C) 12%
(D) 21%
(E) 29%

591. The MOST likely diagnosis in the figure is

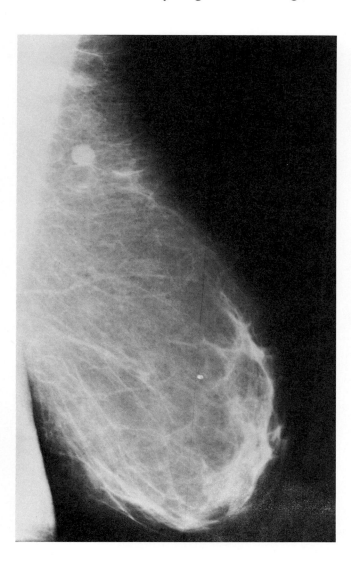

(A)   multiple sebaceous cysts
(B)   fibroadenomatosis
(C)   fat necrosis
(D)   granular cell myoblastomata
(E)   lipomas

592. If a focal cluster of microcalcifications is biopsied, the chances of malignancy are

(A)   5%
(B)   10%
(C)   20%
(D)   50%
(E)   80%

593. Referring to the figure, what would you say is the LEAST likely diagnosis?

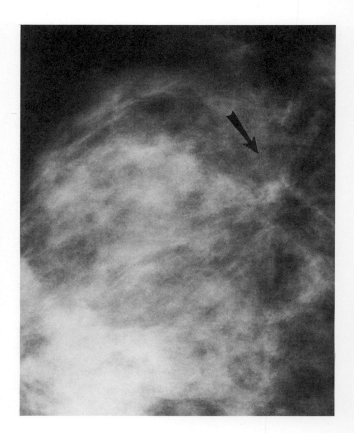

(A)   A surgical scar
(B)   Fibroadenoma
(C)   Carcinoma
(D)   Plasma cell mastitis
(E)   Fibroelastosis

594. The highest risk for developing breast cancer occurs in women whose

(A)   father and uncle develop breast cancer
(B)   mother develops bilateral breast cancer premenopausally
(C)   mother and sister develop postmenopausal breast cancer
(D)   daughter develops unilateral premenopausal breast cancer
(E)   mother and maternal aunt develop postmenopausal breast cancer

595. The MOST important finding in the mammogram shown in the figure is

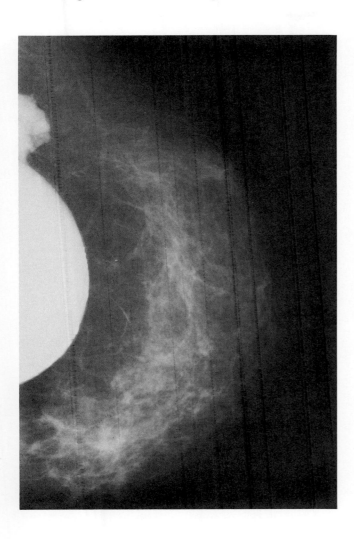

(A) ruptured breast prosthesis
(B) fat necrosis
(C) probable intraductal carcinoma
(D) sclerosing adenosis
(E) fibrous encapsulation of breast prosthesis

596. The prognostic index is based on

(A) tumor site, lymph node status, and histologic grade
(B) presence of microcalcification
(C) tumor marginal characteristics
(D) size of lymph nodes
(E) histologic grade of tumor alone

597. Breast tissue is embryologically derived from

(A) endoderm
(B) mesoderm
(C) ectoderm
(D) neural crest
(E) none of the above

598. The terminal duct lobular unit consists of the

(A) extralobular duct and its lobule
(B) main duct and sinus lactiferi
(C) sinus lactiferi and the acini
(D) main duct and myoepithelium
(E) none of the above

599. ALL the following are included in the differential diagnosis of a stellate mass EXCEPT

(A) granular cell myoblastoma
(B) biopsy scar
(C) infiltrating ductal carcinoma
(D) tubular carcinoma
(E) cystosarcoma phylloides

DIRECTIONS: Each group of questions below consists of lettered headings followed by a set of numbered items. For each numbered item select the **one** lettered heading with which it is **most** closely associated. Each lettered heading may be used **once, more than once,** or **not at all.**

Match each of the following entities with the clinical feature that is MOST commonly associated.

- (A)   Spontaneous nipple discharge
- (B)   Does not originate in the terminal ductal lobular unit
- (C)   Premalignant
- (D)   Frequently associated with calcification
- (E)   More common in men

600.   Solitary papilloma

601.   Multiple papillomas

602.   Papillomatosis

Match the following lesions with the clinical or radiographic feature with which it is MOST commonly associated.

- (A)   May mimic a benign lesion
- (B)   Biopsy is contraindicated
- (C)   Usually rapidly fatal
- (D)   More common in men
- (E)   Diffusely dense breast

603.   Inflammatory carcinoma

604.   Lymphoma

605.   Medullary carcinoma

DIRECTIONS: Each question below contains five suggested answers. For **each** of the **five** alternatives listed, you are to respond either YES or NO. In a given item, **all, some,** or **none of the alternatives may be correct.**

606. A halo around a lesion

    (A) occasionally occurs with a malignant lesion
    (B) is probably caused by a Mach phenomenon
    (C) is also known as *la ligne de sécurité*
    (D) is not seen with intracystic carcinoma
    (E) is typical of tubular carcinoma

607. The accepted criteria for "minimal" breast cancer include which of the following?

    (A) Lobular carcinoma
    (B) Ductal carcinoma in situ (DCIS)
    (C) Invasive carcinoma less than or equal to 0.5 cm in size
    (D) Node negative invasive cancer
    (E) Bilateral invasive carcinoma, no lesion greater than 1.5 cm in size

608. Components of the fibrous stroma of the breast include which of the following tissues?

    (A) Retinaculum cutis
    (B) Lobules
    (C) Ductal cells
    (D) Myoepithelium
    (E) Cooper ligaments

609. Which of the following calcifications arise in the lobules?

    (A) Milk of calcium
    (B) Comedocarcinoma
    (C) Degenerating fibroadenoma
    (D) Liponecrosis microcystica calcificans
    (E) Secretory

610. Concerning extraabdominal desmoids,

    (A) they are usually related to striated muscle
    (B) they usually contain myoepithelial cells
    (C) the treatment of choice is radiation
    (D) they metastasize hematogenously
    (E) they represent an unusual form of infiltrating duct cancer

611. Tubular carcinoma of the breast

    (A) is highly aggressive
    (B) is characterized pathologically by an irregular radiating pattern
    (C) is readily distinguishable mammographically from a radial scar
    (D) has a 5-year survival rate of 60%
    (E) is treated by modified radical mastectomy

612. Mammographic patterns after reduction mammoplasty include

    (A) skin thickening
    (B) transposition of breast tissue from a low to a high position
    (C) high nipple
    (D) retraction of the lower breast
    (E) fat necrosis

613. Which of the following statements are TRUE regarding a rapid throughput mammography screening practice?

    (A) Sensitivity is greater than 90%
    (B) Specificity is greater than 90%
    (C) The positive predictive value is approximately 10%
    (D) Most cancers have spread to the axillary lymph nodes at the time of discovery by mammography
    (E) Median cancer size at discovery is 5 mm

614. Concerning the male breast,

    (A) gynecomastia may be accompanied by skin thickening
    (B) axillary node enlargement in a patient with gynecomastia is an ominous sign
    (C) approximately 5% of all breast cancers occur in males
    (D) male breast cancer differs histologically from female breast cancer
    (E) the most common location for breast tissue to appear in gynecomastia is the subareolar region

615. Concerning detection of recurrent cancer in the lumpectomized and irradiated breast,

(A) mammography is superior to physical examination in its detection of recurrence

(B) recurrent disease may be manifest as microcalcification and/or a mass

(C) recurrent malignancy is usually heralded by skin thickening

(D) an enlarging mass may represent a developing hematoma

(E) mammography should be performed yearly after a follow-up baseline is obtained

616. Common complications of augmentation mammoplasty with prosthetic devices which can be detected radiographically are

(A) malignant change

(B) fat necrosis

(C) fibrous encapsulation

(D) prosthesis rupture

(E) silicone granulomata

617. Concerning phylloides tumor,

(A) it usually presents mammographically as a round or lobulated "benign-appearing" lesion

(B) it has an appearance which is diagnostic on ultrasound

(C) benign and malignant phylloides tumor are distinguishable mammographically

(D) local recurrence is common

(E) in cases of malignant phylloides tumor, metastases are to the axillary nodes

618. Concerning lobular carcinoma in situ,

(A) it is a marker for an increased risk of cancer

(B) it has a characteristic mammographic appearance

(C) it spreads via dermal lymphatics

(D) it is the same entity as lobular neoplasia

(E) it is usually bilateral

619. True statements regarding plasma cell mastitis include which of the following?

(A) It is premalignant

(B) It is considered a lobular process

(C) Calcifications may be linear and/or contain lucent centers

(D) Skin retraction or thickening may be associated

(E) Serosanguinous nipple discharge from a solitary duct is a common manifestation

620. Which of the following statements regarding ductal carcinoma in situ is/are TRUE?

(A) It is mammographically occult

(B) The typical mammographic appearance is that of granular or cast-type ductal calcifications

(C) Most cases are asymptomatic

(D) Invasion of the basement membrane is a late finding

(E) It accounts for less than 5% of all breast cancers

Mammography

Answers

575. The answer is C. *(Kopans, pp 93–95.)* The craniocaudad (CC) and oblique views of the breast shown in the figure demonstrate calcifications which are amorphous on the CC view, but which layer out on the oblique view, resembling a teacup.

Cysts in the breast may contain "granulations" or "milk of calcium" which settle dependently on an erect view and form a dense crescent along the inferior margin of the cyst. In the CC view, the calcifications become uniformly dense and sometimes mistaken for a malignant process. An erect view (lateral or mediolateral oblique) is pathognomonic, however, and helps to avoid unnecessary biopsy.

576. The answer is D. *(Kopans, p 186.)* The area of architectural distortion seen at the 12 o'clock position on the craniocaudad (CC) (at left) is too posterior to be the same lesion as the spiculated density seen in the subareolar region on the mediolateral oblique view (at right). Closer inspection of the CC view shows that the smaller, more posterior lesion is approximately 2 cm posterior and slightly lateral to the larger one. Two solid masses were detected by ultrasound, one in the subareolar region at 1 o'clock, and one at the 12 o'clock position, approximately 6 to 7 cm from the nipple. Both were invasive ductal carcinoma.

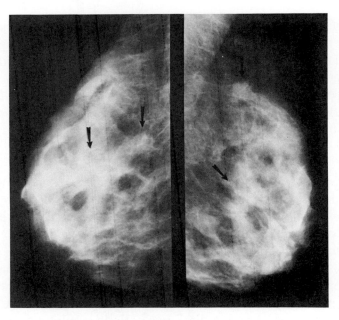

The phenomenon of multicentric cancer highlights the need for preoperative mammography, since mastectomy is usually the treatment of choice for multifocal disease.

577. The answer is B. *(Kopans, pp 289–290.)*   The calcifications in the close-up view of the breast in the figure have a linear configuration, resembling rods. Smudgy and beaded, these malignant-appearing calcifications are a manifestation of intraductal carcinoma, which is the ill-defined mass in the center of the image.

Intraductal carcinoma refers to cancers of ductal origin which may remain in situ or which may infiltrate beyond the duct. A mammogram often reveals small (0.5–1.0-mm) calcifications. A mass with irregular borders reflects the invasive tumor elements, and the calcium may result from secretion into the ducts by tumor cells or from cell necrosis.

578. The answer is C. *(American Cancer Society, pp 19–36, 1991.)*   Breast cancer has now reached epidemic proportions. The incidence of breast cancer has steadily risen in the past century, with little change in mortality. However, early detection by mammography and heightened awareness of the disease by women has started to slow the increase in the death rate. In 1991, 140,000 new cases of breast cancer were expected. The figures for 1992 are not yet available.

579. The answer is B. *(American Cancer Society, pp 19–36, 1991.)*   The mortality rate for female breast cancer has kept pace with the steady increase in incidence of breast cancer, despite earlier detection and newer treatment modalities. There were approximately 34,000 deaths from breast cancer in 1991. In the U.S., breast cancer deaths among women are exceeded only by deaths from lung cancer.

580. The answer is E. *(Kopans, pp 89–90.)*   The oblique view of this breast shows solid, coarse, rod-shaped calcifications which radiate toward the nipple. When they occur diffusely and bilaterally, they represent a frequent incidental mammographic finding which is of no clinical concern; they are the result of an inflammatory reaction involving the ducts, which ultimately can calcify. The ducts are often dilated, yielding large, tubular calcifications, some with hollow centers. A coincidental cancer can sometimes be difficult to detect, but should be sought. Absent are the beading and irregularity that reflect the malignant behavior of intraductal carcinoma.

581. The answer is D. *(Tabár, Radiology 174:655–656, 1990.)*   Two large studies are cited in discussions of reduction in mortality from breast cancer by screening mammography. The first is the HIP (Health Insurance Plan of New York) study, begun in 1963, which included 64,000 healthy women. It demonstrated a significant reduction in mortality (approximately 30%), even in the much-debated 40- to 49-year-old group. The later study was begun in Sweden in the late 1970s, and is ongoing. At the point at which 134,000 women were enrolled, there was a 31% reduction in deaths when screening was done by film-screen mammography.

582. The answer is C. *(Knelson, JCAT, 11(6):1074–1076, 1987.)*   The craniocaudad image in the figure at left shows a well-defined mass near the nipple. The ultrasound study in the figure at right demonstrates a cyst which contains fluid and a papillary soft-tissue mass within it. This patient has an intracystic papillary carcinoma.

Papillary carcinoma is relatively rare, accounting for only 2 to 5% of all breast carcinoma. It occurs in the intracystic form even more rarely (0.3%). It may mimic a simple cyst, and is often quite indolent. The presence of malignancy is suggested mammographically when a portion of the cyst wall becomes indistinct, indicating invasion. Ultrasound reveals both the cystic and solid components of the lesion, and often papillary projections can be discerned.

583. The answer is B. *(Kopans, p 14.)*   Several methods can be used to measure exposure from mammography to the breast. Skin exposure is misleading, because there is rapid absorption of the low kV spectrum used, even though exit dose may be as high as 90% of the entrance (skin) dose. Therefore, a more reliable indicator is the mean glandular (absorbed) dose (MGD), which averages 200 mR (0.2 rad) per breast.

A grid will increase the MGD to the breast threefold. Molybdenum filtration (a 30-μm thickness = 3 to 4 mm A1) significantly reduces the dose to the breast, and careful columnation further reduces the dose by decreasing scatter.

584. The answer is B. *(BEIR Report, Natl Acad Sci, 1980.)*   Questions concerning the safety of mammography are constantly raised. In fact, at one time it was alleged that more breast cancers might be produced than would be detected by mammography. Since risks and benefits are age-related, careful analysis was necessary in order to ascertain the safety and efficacy for each age group. Based on best current estimates, it appears that the theoretical risk to the screened population of 1 rad exposure to the breast will produce six excess cancers per million women per year after a 10- to 15-year latent period.

The mean glandular dose to the breast during mammography averages 200 mR. The incidence of breast cancer in the general population is estimated at 800 cases per million at age 40, 1800 per million at age 50, and 2500 cases per million at age 65. The risk of developing cancer from a mammogram is therefore extremely small over the age of 40.

585. The answer is C. *(Sickles, Radiology 131:599–607, 1979.)*   Even using an air gap and long subject-to-image distance (SID), the dose to the breast using magnification technique increases approximately 2 to 3 times that of a conventional mammogram, albeit, to a more focal area. However, since it is an ancillary technique for clarifying a specific question, the increased dose should not dissuade the radiologist from employing this useful tool. Obviously, the increase in dose mitigates against its routine use. The usefulness of magnification has been well-established by Sickles, who demonstrated that 60% of initially equivocal cases were reduced to 23% after the use of magnification technique. Magnification technique is helpful for evaluating microcalcifications and small masses, and improves one's ability to define marginal characteristics. A grid should not be used for regular or magnification mammography, as the air gap will clean up scatter sufficiently, and it significantly raises the radiation dose.

586. The answer is B. *(Sickles, Radiology 125:69–77, 1977.)*   Magnification has become an indispensable tool for the mammographer. It is useful for both characterizing microcalcifications and better evaluating lesion borders. Occasionally, it reveals an otherwise-hidden stellate mass.

It should be used with a compression cone, to decrease scatter and motion unsharpness. It is imperative that the smallest focal spot be used to minimize geometric unsharpness. Presently, the smallest available focal spot for magnification mammography is 90 to 100 μm with a 1.5:1 to 2:1 magnification ratio. This can easily be done with a 150-μm focal spot by using a 60-cm subject-to-image distance. A grid is not used, as it needlessly increases the radiation dose. The air gap between the object and film reduces scatter.

587. The answer is E. *(Kopans, pp 283–284.)*   The mediolateral oblique view of the left breast shown in the figure demonstrates an encapsulated mass which contains stromal elements and fat; it is a typical *fibroadenolipoma*.

Also called *hamartomas* of the breast, fibroadenolipomas are encapsulated lesions which contain fibrous and glandular elements in addition to fat. They are very rare, benign tumors which are difficult to detect because of their similarity to normal breast tissue. Occasionally, they are palpable. Finding the capsule is the key to distinguishing them from normal breast tissue. Phylloides tumor may have a capsule, but it is typically dense.

588. The answer is B. *(Price, Br J Radiol, 58:99–100, 1985.)* In order to best image the low-contrast densities found in the breast, it is necessary to utilize x-rays at the low-energy end of the spectrum. Molybdenum is an ideal target since the K edge produces characteristic x-rays at 17.9 and 19.5 keV. If the energy drops below the K edge, there are too few photons to make a useful radiograph. In order to filter out energies below 15 keV, a 20-μm (.03-mm) molybdenum filter is used. Contrast decreases, however, as kVp increases.

Tungsten targets produce photons from bremsstrahlung, rather than by characteristic x-rays, and the mammogram has less contrast than one made with a molybdenum target. Mammographic detail is more dependent on other factors—such as source-to-image distance, focal-spot-receptor combination, and processing—rather than on kVp.

589. The answer is B. *(Kopans, pp 282–284.)* The figure shows a rounded, lucent lesion of less than 1 cm in diameter superiorly in the right breast. It is a galactocele, which is a lesion that develops during lactation. It may represent an obstructed duct which contains milk. Clinically, it presents as a palpable round mass. Because milk has a high fat content, it is relatively radiolucent, and is indistinguishable from other fat-containing breast masses. Occasionally, a galactocele may be distinguished by a fat-fluid level demonstrated on an erect view. When large, they may be aspirated, usually with complete resolution.

The remaining choices—granular cell myoblastoma, hamartoma, fibroadenoma, and papilloma—do not appear as purely lucent lesions.

590. The answer is B. *(Martin, AJR 132:737–739, 1979. Kalisher, Radiology 133(2):397–401, 1979.)* False negatives are expected with any examination, and efforts are always being made to minimize them. Analysis of false negatives has shown that approximately 6% of breast cancers will not be seen on technically adequate mammograms. This is often due to lack of fat around the dense cancer to contrast it from the surrounding parenchyma. For this reason, a palpable lesion with a negative mammogram should not dissuade further evaluation, including biopsy. Placing a small marker such as a B-B over a palpable mass and using coned-down spot magnification views may be helpful in better localizing such a lesion. It is also imperative that faintly visible cancers are not overlooked. Therefore, the mammograms must be read without extraneous ambient light and in a quiet atmosphere. A careful search using a magnifying glass and bright spotlight is very important. Previous mammograms should be viewed in comparison, and it is often helpful to look at the oldest films, if they are technically comparable.

591. The answer is A. *(Aboody, Invest Radiol 27:329–330, 1992.)* The figure reveals several rounded lesions in the left breast. This patient has a familial disorder which is called steatocystoma multiplex. It occurs in both men and women, and is characterized by multiple sebaceous cysts on the upper torso, especially over the breasts, axillae, and upper back. The cysts may appear dense or lucent mammographically, with thin capsules. They are most prominent in the axillary portion of the breast. Many more lesions are often found mammographically than are apparent clinically.

592. The answer is C. *(Egan, Radiology 137:1–7, 1980.)* When all lesions with microcalcifications are biopsied, the proportion which is cancerous is 20 to 30%. Certain characteristics suggest malignancy such as pleomorphism, casting, and multiplicity. Some calcifications are obviously benign, such as the coarse rim type (eggshell) or the amorphous, large and rounded, or layered types. Analysis of these features helps decrease the false positive rate to an acceptable level. Unfortunately, it is often not possible for mammography to differentiate benign from malignant microcalcifications, and needle localization and specimen radiography are necessary. The radiologist's role is not complete even after documentation of removal of microcalcification, since follow-up mammography must be done according to accepted guidelines.

593. The answer is B. *(Kopans, p 288.)* The mammogram in the figure reveals an architectural distortion, but minimal central density. Radial scar, fibroelastosis, indurative mastopathy, and sclerosing duct hyperplasia are all terms to describe this entity. It is a benign, naturally occurring scar within the breast. The typical appearance of radiating streaks without a central mass is characteristic, but the differentiation from malignancy is not absolute, and biopsy is still warranted. A history of surgery at this site would favor the diagnosis of a scar, and comparison could be made to previous examinations to assure stability. Plasma cell mastitis may also give this appearance.

Carcinomas often elicit an intense desmoplastic reaction causing architectural distortion, which occasionally is the only clue to the presence of cancer. However, there is more often a mass at the center.

Fibroadenomas are benign lesions which appear as well-circumscribed round or oval nodules that usually maintain their size over time. They arise in the young breast and may develop a characteristic dense calcification as they degenerate. They do not appear after menopause. The intense fibrotic reaction and lack of a mass in this case make a fibroadenoma the least likely choice.

594. The answer is B. *(Anderson, Cancer 34:1090–1097, 1974. Sattin, JAMA 253:1908–1913, 1985.)* Risk factors for breast cancer development have been identified which may be useful for directing more vigorous screening at a selected population. For example, in women whose mothers had bilateral premenopausal breast cancer, the risk is 47 times higher than for women with no prior family history. Similarly, if there is a history of a mother and sister who developed postmenopausal breast cancer, a daughter who developed unilateral premenopausal breast cancer, or a mother and maternal aunt who developed postmenopausal breast cancer, the risk is approximately 2 to 4 times greater. For women whose male relatives have developed breast cancer, there is no increased risk.

595. The answer is C. *(Silverstein, Ann Plast Surg 25:210–213, 1990.)* The figure depicts a breast prosthesis which has a surrounding fibrous capsule that has calcified. There has been extravasation of silicone, which is visible superiorly. The patient had come for a routine preoperative evaluation for removal of the prosthesis.

The location of the prosthesis can be determined by its position relative to the pectoralis muscle. It may be placed anterior to the muscle (retromammary) or posterior to it (subpectoral). The subpectoral position is preferable, as it is less likely to become encapsulated. When a prosthesis is removed, the fibrous capsule is usually densely adherent and remains behind.

As an incidental finding, there is a cluster of microcalcifications anterior to the prosthesis, which most likely represent an intraductal carcinoma. Although readily visible on the mammogram of this patient, it has been estimated that silicone implants may obscure up to 83% of the breast on a mammogram. The "pinch" technique, whereby the prosthesis is displaced posteriorly as the breast is drawn forward, is credited for reducing the amount obscured to less than 25%, while improving the image quality. Some still advocate application of standard technique as well to optimize imaging of the posterior breast.

596. The answer is A. *(Todd, Br J Cancer 56:489–492, 1987.)* The prognostic index, as described by Todd, is a mechanism for determining the long-term risk for metastases or recurrence from breast cancer. The presence or absence of microcalcifications has no relevance as a prognosticator, which is supported by the fact that purely intraductal comedocarcinoma may have myriad calcifications and is yet quite indolent. Marginal characteristics may also be misleading: for example, medullary and colloid cancers, in spite of their smooth, well-defined margins may metastasize and recur. Lymph node size is even less important, since fatty-replaced benign nodes can approach 6 cm in size, whereas nodes under 1 cm in diameter may contain significant amounts of tumor. The prognostic index is based on the combination of tumor size, histologic grade, and lymph node status.

597. The answer is C.   *(Knight, J Reprod Fertil 65:521–536, 1982.)*   Breast tissue in mammals first appears as two parallel strips of ectoderm during the 5th week of fetal development. They extend from the axilla to the groin. In humans, only the tissue over the chest further develops into breast tissues. Lactiferous ducts begin to invade the ectodermal ridge and dichotomously begin branching at 24 weeks of gestation. Approximately ten to fifteen ductal systems are present at birth, surrounded by support stroma and subcutaneous fat.

598. The answer is A.   *(Wellings, JNCI, 50:1111, 1973.)*   The terminal duct lobular unit is an extremely important structural component of the breast, as it is the site of cancer formation. It is considered the basic functional unit of the breast, and is composed of an end duct surrounded by a lobule made up of many acini. Under hormonal control, the acini produce colostrum and, later, milk.

599. The answer is E.   *(Kopans, pp 302–303.)*   A stellate lesion is a very significant finding and should be considered a malignancy unless proved otherwise. Some factors may mitigate against biopsy, such as a history of previous trauma or scar, but suspicion should remain high, as carcinomas sometimes arise in areas of scarring. With time (usually by 6 months), a biopsy scar should flatten and lose its mass effect.

Granular cell myoblastoma is an extremely rare entity which is more commonly found in the tongue. Clinically, it may mimic cancer, being hard, irregular, and often fixed. Radiographically, it appears as a mass with irregular margins, sometimes in a stellate configuration. However, the biological behavior is benign.

Tubular carcinoma is a well-differentiated, slow-growing tumor which tends to form ductlike areas microscopically and may look mammographically similar to a radial scar.

Cystosarcoma phylloides has a well-defined lobulated or smooth contour, looking much like a giant fibroadenoma. It does not take the form of a stellate mass.

600–602. The answers are: 600-A, 601-C, 602-D.   *(Cardenosa, Radiology 181:751–755, 1991. Homer, pp 86–87. Haagensen, ed. 3, pp 136–191.)*   Solitary papillomas of the breast are usually subareolar in location and arise within the major ducts. The most common presentation is spontaneous nipple discharge. They are rarely bilateral and are most often mammographically occult. Galactography is frequently helpful for investigating spontaneous nipple discharge. The involved duct is usually dilated and the papilloma appears as an intraluminal filling defect. Preoperative staining of the duct with methylene blue may be performed to aid the surgeon.

By contrast, multiple papillomas arise from the periphery of the breast in the terminal ductal lobular units. They are usually discovered by mammography, typically as bilateral small round or oval nodules which are relatively well-defined. Haagensen and others have described a 25–30% risk of carcinoma in these patients. Pathologically, atypical ductal hyperplasia and lobular carcinoma in situ (LCIS) have been found in association.

Papillomatosis represents a peripheral epithelial disorder which occurs within the ducts as opposed to the lobules. It often appears mammographically as diffuse, bilateral microcalcifications. Alternatively, the disease may be more focal, and there may appear only a solitary cluster of calcifications or an irregular mass.

603–605. The answers are: 603-C, 604-E, 605-A.   *(Meyer, Radiology 170:79–82, 1989. Droulies, Ann Surg 184:217–222, 1976. Kopans, pp 305–307.)*   Inflammatory carcinoma is a virulent form of cancer with a 5-year survival of less than 5%. About 90% of patients have metastatic disease at the time of diagnosis. Inflammatory carcinoma is a clinical diagnosis; the skin of the breast is typically red or purple, indurated, tender, and warm. An underlying mass or fullness may be palpable. The differential diagnosis includes cellulitis, mastitis, locally advanced noninflammatory carcinoma, radiation change, or edema (anasarca). Currently, palliation is the only treatment and is best achieved by supervoltage irradiation.

Lymphoma is unusual in the breast. It is very rarely primary; more commonly it accompanies disease elsewhere in the body. Clinically, there is a discretely palpable mass or masses of similar size, which appear mammographically as well-defined nodules. Occasionally, they are ill-defined, but without spiculation. Sometimes the only sign is a diffuse increase in breast density. When a mammogram reveals large axillary nodes (greater than 2 cm in size) and similarly sized intramammary nodules, the diagnosis of lymphoma should be considered.

Medullary carcinoma is an uncommon tumor (less than 5%), appearing mammographically as a round or oval, well-defined mass. Since this tumor has a high water content, ultrasound may reveal enhanced through transmission, which was shown to be the case in all twenty-four lesions in a recent series.

606. The answers are: A-Y, B-Y, C-Y, D-N, E-N. *(Swann, AJR 149:1145–1147, 1987.)* Marginal characteristics are often useful, but occasionally may be misleading. When the lucent halo around a well-defined margin was first described, it was believed to be a manifestation of fat compressed by a slow-growing (benign) lesion. Later it was ascribed to the Mach effect, due to the sharp interface between the density of the lesion and its less dense surroundings. Gros called this halo *la ligne de sécurité,* as it was believed to ensure that a lesion was benign. However, rare tumors have demonstrated well-formed halos; specifically, colloid, intracystic, and medullary carcinoma. Any area of smudging or loss of marginal detail should be looked upon with suspicion. Tubular carcinomas typically have irregular, spiculated margins without a lucent halo.

607. The answers are: A-N, B-Y, C-Y, D-N, E-N. *(Martin, Cancer 28:1519, 1971.)* Gallagher (a pathologist) and Martin (a radiologist) first specifically defined the term *minimal cancer* and discussed the significance of breast cancers falling into this category. Early stage, or minimal, breast cancer includes lobular carcinoma in situ (LCIS), ductal carcinoma in situ (DCIS), and invasive carcinoma no larger than 0.5 cm in diameter.

LCIS is believed to be a high-risk marker for cancer, but may not necessarily develop into infiltrative *lobular* cancer. The Breast Cancer Detection Demonstration Project (BCDDP) later redefined the term to include tumors up to 1 cm in diameter.

There has been some confusion because of the BCDDP definition. Current concepts favor the Gallagher-Martin definition.

608. The answers are: A-Y, B-N, C-N, D-N, E-Y. *(Mitchell, p 4.)* The fibrous stroma is the supporting structure that surrounds lobules. It sweeps posteriorly to condense into Cooper's ligaments and passes from the dermis into the parenchymal cone as the retinaculum cutis. Desmoplastic processes will often foreshorten the retinaculum cutis, causing tethering and retraction of the skin.

The lobules themselves are not made of fibrous stroma, but the interdigitation of perilobular fibrous tissue makes blunt dissection of the separate lobules impossible. Ducts are surrounded by periductal collagen and are invested in fibrous tissue, but are not included in the tissues considered to be fibrous stroma. The myoepithelial cells are contractile units which surround the lobules and function in the mechanical expression of milk from the acini.

609. The answers are: A-Y, B-N, C-N, D-N, E-N. *(Millis, Br J Radiol 49:12–26, 1976. Sickles EA, Radiology 141:655–658, 1981.)* Milk of calcium occurs in lobules rather than ducts, and is often seen as dependent, teacup-shaped calcific collections on an upright view, while being smudged and poorly visible in a craniocaudad view (see figure, top left).

Comedocarcinoma is a type of intraductal malignancy with a propensity for branched, irregular calcifications described as "casting." It results from calcium depositing in the ducts, which are lined by irregular, heaped-up epithelium (top middle).

A degenerating fibroadenoma often has characteristic "popcorn" or amorphous calcifications. The calcium often begins near the periphery of the fibroadenoma and tends to coalesce (top right).

Liponecrosis microcystica calcificans produces a round, smooth calcification sometimes with a central lucency and thick calcific rim. They are small, usually less than 2 mm in diameter, and represent a minor form of fat necrosis (bottom left). They are of no clinical significance.

Secretory calcifications (bottom right) are ductal or periductal and may be linear or rounded, often mimicking phleboliths. They are related to plasma cell mastitis and probably represent end-stage duct ectasia.

All these calcifications, except those associated with comedocarcinoma, are benign.

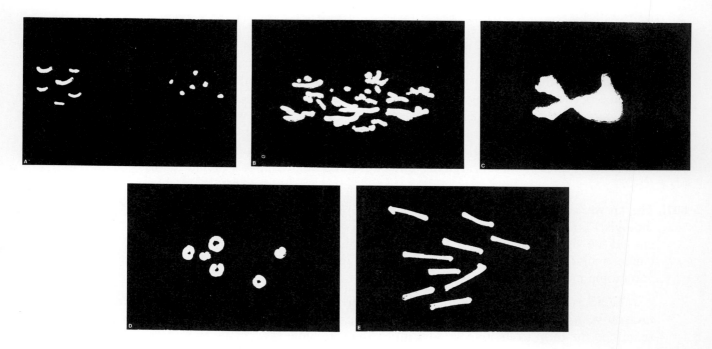

610. The answers are: A-Y, B-N, C-N, D-N, E-N. *(Kalisher, AJR 126:903, 1976.)* Extraabdominal desmoids are very rare lesions and are usually found in the breast or axilla, adjacent to the pectoralis muscles. They may be related to prior trauma. They are slow-growing lesions which do not metastasize, but rather infiltrate locally and have a high rate of recurrence after removal. They have irregular, spiculated margins, mimicking infiltrating ductal cancers. Histologically, they look like fibrous tissue which is invading the striated muscle. Treatment is wide local excision.

611. The answers are: A-N, B-Y, C-N, D-N, E-N. *(Feig, Radiology 129:311–314, 1978.)* Tubular carcinoma is a well-differentiated tumor which grows slowly. Histologically, it consists of elongated tubules lined by a single epithelial layer, which are arranged in an irregular irradiating pattern. If there is a pronounced desmoplastic reaction, it may produce a stellate mass or resemble a radial scar. It may also contain clusters of microcalcification. The prognosis is excellent, with a 5-year survival of 85 to 100%.

612. The answers are: A-Y, B-N, C-Y, D-Y, E-Y. *(Miller, AJR 149:35–38, 1987.)* The changes in the breast following mammoplasty are characteristic. They include skin thickening and retraction of the lower portion of the breast. There is a linear vertical scar inferiorly. The breast tissue is transposed from a high to a low position. The nipple is moved to a position which is high relative to the relocated breast cone. Fat necrosis may occur.

613. The answers are: A-Y, B-Y, C-Y, D-N, E-N. *(Sickles, Radiology 175:323–327, 1990.)* Audits of several practices have recently been published, which address the sensitivity, specificity, and positive predictive value of mammography. The study by Sickles et al. found a 93% sensitivity and a 94% specificity of initial mammography interpretation. The positive predictive value was 10%, which means that of all positive results, 10% were truly cancer cases [PPV = TP/(TP + FP)].

Biopsies prompted by screening mammography yielded a diagnosis of malignancy in 32% of cases. Of the 170 breast cancers that were identified, 114 (67%) underwent needle localization. The median mammographic cancer size was 12 mm, and the axillary nodes were positive in 17 (11%) cases. Systemic metastatic disease was discovered in 2 (1.2%).

614. The answers are: A-Y, B-N, C-N, D-N, E-Y. *(Kopans, pp 342–350.)* Gynecomastia is a proliferation of normal breast tissue in the male; it may be unilateral or bilateral. Skin thickening and axillary node enlargement may accompany it as a benign phenomenon. The usual location is subareolar, though it may extend to the upper outer quadrant. The ducts may hypertrophy.

Causes of gynecomastia include liver disease (cirrhosis), drugs (e.g., digoxin, cimetidine, spironolactone, thiazides, and marijuana), testicular tumors, and hormonal therapy, such as that for prostate carcinoma.

Male breast cancer accounts for less than 1% of all breast cancers. Risk factors include radiation exposure and increased estrogen states. Histologically, it is indistinguishable from female breast cancer. The poor prognosis associated with it may be due to the fact that it is often diagnosed at a later stage.

615. The answers are: A-N, B-Y, C-N, D-N, E-Y. *(Stomper, AJR 148:39–43, 1987.)* Mammography and physical examination are complementary in the detection of recurrent disease in the posttreatment breast. In a recent series of 23 recurrences, 35% were detected by mammography alone, 39% were detected by physical examination alone, and 26% were detectable by both.

Local recurrence of cancer, like the primary tumor, may manifest as microcalcifications, microcalcifications associated with a mass, or a soft-tissue mass alone. The risk for recurrence is approximately 2% per year for the first 14 years.

Benign changes after treatment include skin thickening due to radiation therapy, architectural distortion, and/or a mass representing a hematoma. These changes stabilize at 3 to 6 months. Coarse, dystrophic calcifications typically develop over a longer course. At 6 to 12 months, a baseline mammogram should be obtained.

Enlargement of a parenchymal scar should be regarded as suspicious for recurrence, since hematomas usually attain their maximum size immediately after operation and then remain the same size or decrease thereafter.

616. The answers are: A-N, B-Y, C-N, D-Y, E-N. *(Kopans, pp 110–112.)* Malignant change is not considered to be an association of augmentation mammoplasty, but can occur in any breast. Prostheses which are inserted behind the breast core (retromammary) are subject to fibrous encapsulation, as compared to those placed beneath the pectoralis major muscle (subpectoral). The capsule, if not calcified, is mammographically occult but obvious clinically, as it results in extremely hard breasts. The motion of the pectoralis major muscle may account for the protective effect of subpectoral prostheses against this complication.

Prosthesis rupture is the most common complication that is detected radiographically. It is evident as a focal bulge in the prosthesis or elongation of its contour. It may be detected clinically as a palpable mass.

The calcifications of fat necrosis are fairly common after augmentation mammoplasty, just as with any surgical or other traumatic insult to the breast. The posttraumatic "oil cyst" is characteristic in its mammographic appearance as a lucent lesion with a capsule, which may be calcified. Other manifestations of fat necrosis include neodensity, architectural distortion, and calcium deposition.

Silicone granulomata typically result from the injection of free silicone into the breast. The silicone can migrate throughout the entire body and form granulomata anywhere. The injection of free silicone is now illegal in the United States.

617. The answers are: A-Y, B-N, C-N, D-Y, E-N. *(Buchberger, AJR 157:715–719, 1991.)* Phylloides tumor is rare, accounting for less than 1% of all breast neoplasms. It is usually large, round, and well-defined, mammographically, giving it a "benign appearance." It may be so large as to occupy the entire breast. Calcification is not a feature. Clinical evaluation may suggest the diagnosis, as the tumor is often quite large. The age of presentation is variable, usually in the fifth or sixth decade, but patients occasionally present under age 20.

The diagnosis is usually made histologically, after wide local excision. Ultrasound may show cystic spaces or low-level echoes, but the appearance is generally that of a nonspecific, solid mass. Aspiration cytology is difficult to interpret because of similarity between phylloides tumor and fibroadenoma. Additionally, even with malignant phylloides tumor, not all aspirates contain malignant cells. Thus, differentiation of benign versus malignant must be made by frozen section.

Local recurrences are common. The recurrence rate is approximately 16 to 28% after mastectomy or wide resection and 28 to 46% after removal of the tumor nucleus only. Distant metastasis occurs via the vascular route; the tumor does not spread through lymphatic channels. About two-thirds of metastases are to lung; other sites include bone, liver, and myocardium.

618. The answers are: A-Y, B-N, C-N, D-Y, E-Y. *(Beute, AJR, 157:257–265, 1991. Sonnenfeld, Radiology 181:363–367, 1991.)* Lobular carcinoma in situ (LCIS) is a controversial entity which is presently believed to be a high-risk marker for cancer. It is also called lobular neoplasia (LN), though it does not necessarily progress to an invasive lobular cancer. In fact, there is no significantly increased risk for invasive *lobular* cancer, but the risk of intraductal carcinoma is approximately 15% over 10 to 15 years. Since LCIS is usually bilateral, the same risk applies to both breasts.

It occurs primarily in premenopausal women and seems to regress after menopause. The risk of cancer, however, persists beyond and into the postmenopausal years. LCIS has no characteristic mammographic features, and is an incidental finding at biopsy. Many have noted associations of clusters of microcalcifications with LCIS, but these have recently been demonstrated to occur more frequently within benign lobules which are adjacent to areas of LCIS.

The cancer risk associated with LCIS has prompted some to suggest bilateral mastectomy as a prophylactic measure. Unilateral mastectomy is *not* an option. Close clinical and mammographic follow-up of both breasts is generally the accepted practice.

619. The answers are: A-N, B-N, C-Y, D-Y, E-N. *(Bassett, Rad Clin No Am [Breast Imaging], 30(1):100, 1992.)* Plasma cell mastitis, a type of secretory disease, is a chronic inflammatory process which has no known malignant potential. Pathologically, it appears to be due to duct ectasia and the accumulation of inspissated grumous material. As it progresses, periductal inflammation and breakdown of the duct wall occur, with calcifications developing in both intraductal and periductal locations. Therefore, the process is primarily *ductal,* rather than lobular, and is usually bilateral. Periductal calcifications tend to develop lucent centers while the intraductal calcifications are smooth, solid, and linear, occasionally with needlelike ends. Fibrosis, induration, and skin or nipple retraction during the late stages is termed *mastitis obliterans.* Clinically, it may be mistaken for carcinoma. Nipple discharge from plasma cell mastitis is not uncommon, but several ducts are often involved, and the color of the discharge is not red, but rather varies from white to yellow to green. Serous, serosanguineous, or sanguineous discharge from a solitary duct usually indicates an intraductal papilloma.

620. The answers are: A-N, B-Y, C-Y, D-N, E-N. *(Stomper, Radiology 172(1):235–241, 1989.)* Ductal carcinoma in situ (DCIS) is a malignant proliferation which is confined to the ducts. By definition, it does not invade the basement membrane. DCIS accounts for 22 to 32% of all clinically occult breast cancers. Detected 3 to 4 times more frequently in a screened (as compared to an unscreened) population, DCIS has been treated by mastectomy, with survival rates approaching 100%. Currently, breast-conserving options are being explored.

Most DCIS is nonpalpable. In a recent large series, 72% of cases had microcalcifications, but only 12% had calcifications associated with a mass. Only 10% had a soft-tissue mass only, and 6% were incidentally discovered during microscopic analysis.

Bibliography

Chest Radiology

Armstrong P, Wilson AG, Dee P: *Imaging of the Diseases of the Chest*. Chicago, Year Book Medical, 1990.

Fraser RG, Paré JAP, Paré PD, Fraser RS, Genereux GP: *Diagnosis of Diseases of the Chest*, 3d ed. Philadelphia, WB Saunders, 1991.

Goodman PC: *Pneumocystis carinii* pneumonia. *J Thor Imag* 6(4):16–21, 1991.

Lee JKT, Sagel SS, Stanley RJ: *Computed Body Tomography with MRI Correlation*, 2d ed. New York, Raven Press, 1989.

Mayo JR: The high-resolution computed tomography technique. *Sem Roentgen* 26(2):104–109, 1991.

Petasnick JP: Radiologic evaluation of aortic dissection. *Radiology* 180(2):297–305, 1991.

Stitik FP: Staging of lung cancer. *Radiol Clin N Am* 28:619–630, 1990.

Templeton PA: Magnetic resonance imaging in lung cancer. *Cont Diag Radiol* 14(11):1–6, 1991.

Webb WR: High-resolution computed tomography of the lung: Normal and abnormal anatomy. *Sem Roentgenol* 26(2):110–117, 1991.

Westcott JL: Percutaneous transthoracic needle biopsy. *Radiology* 169(3):593–601, 1988.

Gastrointestinal Radiology

Eisenberg RL: *Gastrointestinal Radiology*, 2d ed. Philadelphia, JB Lippincott, 1990.

Friedman AC: *Radiology of the Liver, Biliary Tract, Pancreas and Spleen*. Baltimore, Williams & Wilkins, 1987.

Lee JKT, Sagel SS, Stanley RJ (eds): *Computed Body Tomography*, 2d ed. New York, Raven Press, 1989.

Levy DW, Rindsberg S, Friedman AC, et al: Thorotrast-induced hepatosplenic neoplasia: CT identification. *AJR* 146:997–1004, 1986.

Margulis AR, Burhenne HJ (eds): *Alimentary Tract Radiology*, 4th ed. St. Louis, CV Mosby, 1989.

Megibow AJ, Balthazar EJ, Hulnick DH: Radiology of nonneoplastic gastrointestinal disorders in AIDS. *Sem Roentgenol* 22(1):31, 1987.

Moss AA, Gamsu G, Genant HK: *Computed Tomography of the Body*, 2d ed. Philadelphia, WB Saunders, 1992.

Taveras JM, Ferrucci JT (eds): *Radiology: Diagnosis-Imaging-Intervention*. Philadelphia, JB Lippincott, 1990.

Genitourinary Radiology

Amis ES Jr, Newhouse J: *Essentials of Uroradiology*. Boston, Little, Brown, 1991.

Davidson AJ: *Radiology of the Kidney*. Philadelphia, WB Saunders, 1985.

Hunt RB, Siegler AM: *Hysterosalpingography: Techniques and Interpretation*. Chicago, YearBook Medical Publishers, 1990.

Pollack HM: *Clinical Urography*. Philadelphia, WB Saunders, 1990.

Wilson JD (ed): *Harrison's Principles of Internal Medicine*, 12th ed. New York, McGraw-Hill, 1991.

Bone Radiology

Chen C, Chandnani VP, Kang HS, et al.: Scapholunate advanced collapse: A common wrist abnormality in calcium pyrophosphate dihydrate crystal deposition disease. *Radiology* 177(2):459–461, 1990.

Moore SG, Dawson KL: Red and yellow marrow in the femur: Age-related changes in appearance art MR imaging. *Radiology* 175:219–223, 1990.

Resnick D, Niwayama G: *Diagnosis of Bone & Joint Disorders,* 2d ed. Philadelphia, WB Saunders, 1988.

Scott WW, Riley LH Jr, Dorfman HD: Focal lytic lesions associated with femoral stem loosening in total hip prosthesis. *AJR* 144:977–982, 1985.

Neuroradiology

Atlas SW (ed): *Magnetic Resonance Imaging of the Brain and Spine.* New York, Raven Press, 1991.

Banna M: *Clinical Radiology of the Spine and Spinal Cord.* Rockville, MD, Aspen Systems Corporation, 1985.

Barkowich AJ: *Pediatric Neuroimaging.* New York, Raven Press, 1990.

Brant-Zawadzki M, Norman D (eds): *Magnetic Resonance Imaging of the Central Venous System,* 1st ed. New York, Raven Press, 1987.

Friedman DP, Rao VM: MR and CT of squamous cell carcinoma of the middle ear and mastoid complex. *Am J Neuroradiol* 12:872–874, 1991.

Harnsberger HR: *Head and Neck Imaging,* 1st ed. Chicago, YearBook Medical, 1990.

Huston J III, Rufenacht DA, Ehman RL, et al: Intracranial aneurysms and vascular malformations: Comparison of time-of-flight and phase-contrast MR angiography. *Radiology* 181(3):721–730, 1991.

Latchaw RE (ed): *MR and CT Imaging of the Head, Neck, and Spine,* 2d ed. St. Louis, Mosby-YearBook, 1991.

Newton TH, Potts DG (eds): *Radiology of the Skull and Brain.* St. Louis, CV Mosby, 1974.

Osborn AG: *Introduction to Cerebral Angiography.* Philadelphia, Harper & Row, 1980.

Schnitzlein HN, Murtagh FR: *Imaging Anatomy of the Head and Spine,* 2d ed. Baltimore, Urban & Schwarzenberg, 1990.

Som PS, Bergeron RT (eds): *Head and Neck Imaging,* 2d ed. St. Louis, CV Mosby, 1991.

Williams AL, Haughton VM: *Cranial Computed Tomography.* St. Louis, CV Mosby, 1985.

Nuclear Medicine

Biello DR, Mattar AF, McKnight RC, et al: Interpretation of ventilation perfusion studies in patient with suspected pulmonary embolism. *AJR* 133:189–194, 1979.

Bonte F, Hom J, Tintner R: Single photon tomography in Alzheimer's disease and the dementia. *Sem Nucl Med* 20(4):344–345, 1990.

Devous M, Leroy E, Homan R: Single photon emission tomography in epilepsy. *Sem Nucl Med* 20(4):325–341, 1990.

Freeman L: *Freeman & Johnson's Clinical Radionuclide Imaging,* 3d ed. Orlando, FL, Grune & Stratton, 1986.

Freeman L: *Nuclear Medicine Annual.* New York, Raven Press, 1991.

Iskandrian AS: *Nuclear Cardiac Imaging: Principles and Application,* 1st ed. Philadelphia, FA Davis, 1987.

Kramer E, Sanger J: Brain imaging in acquired immune deficiency syndrome dementia complex. *Sem Nucl Med* 20(4):353–363, 1990.

Mettler F, Guiberteau M: *Essentials of Nuclear Medicine Imaging,* 3d ed. Philadelphia, WB Saunders, 1991.

PIOPED Investigators: Value of the ventilation/perfusion scan in acute pulmonary embolism: Results of the prospective investigation of pulmonary embolism diagnosis (PIOPED). *JAMA* 263:2753–2759, 1990.

Sorenson J, Phelps M: *Physics in Nuclear Medicine,* 2d ed. Philadelphia, Harcourt Brace Jovanovich, 1987.

Taylor A, Datz F: *Clinical Practice of Nuclear Medicine,* 1st ed. New York, Churchill Livingstone, 1991.

Thrall J: *Nuclear Radiology Test and Syllabus,* 4th series. Reston, VA, American College of Radiology, 1990.

Pediatric Radiology

Edeiken J: *Edeiken's Roentgen Diagnosis of Diseases of Bone,* 4th ed. Baltimore, Williams & Wilkins, 1989.

Felman AH: *Radiology of the Pediatric Chest.* New York, McGraw-Hill, 1987.

Lee SH, Rao K: *Cranial Computed Tomography and MRI,* 2d ed. New York, McGraw-Hill, 1983.

Kirks DR: *Practical Pediatric Imaging,* Boston/Toronto, Little, Brown, 1984.

Sarti DA: *Diagnostic Ultrasound Text and Cases,* 2d ed. Chicago, YearBook Medical, 1987.

Silverman FN: *Caffey's Pediatric X-Ray Diagnosis,* 8th ed. Chicago, YearBook Medical, 1985.

Silverman FN, Kuhn JP: *Essentials of Caffey's Pediatric X-Ray Diagnosis.* Chicago, YearBook Medical, 1990.

Stringer DA: *Pediatric Gastrointestinal Imaging.* Philadelphia, BC Decker, 1989.

Torrisi JM, Haller JO, Velcek FT: Choledochal cyst and biliary atresia in the neonate: Imaging findings in five cases. *AJR* 155(6):1273–1276, 1990.

Ultrasonography

Appelman PT, De Jong TE, Lampmann LE: Deep venous thrombosis of the leg: US findings. *Radiology* 163:743–746, 1987.

Callen PW (ed): *Ultrasonography in Obstetrics and Gynecology,* 2d ed. Philadelphia, WB Saunders, 1988.

Comstock CH, Kirk JS: Arteriovenous malformations: Locations and evolution in the fetal brain. *J Ultrasound Med* 10:361–365, 1991.

Dachman AH, Ros PR, Olmsted WW, Lichtenstein JE. Nonparasitic splenic cysts: Report of 52 cases with radiologic-pathologic correlation. *AJR* 147:537–542, 1986.

Estroff JA, Mandell J, Benacerraf BR: Increased renal parenchymal echogenicity in the fetus: Importance and clinical outcome. *Radiology* 181:135–139, 1991.

Federle MP: A radiologist looks at AIDS: Imaging evaluation based on symptom complexes. *Radiology* 166:553–562, 1988.

Filly RA, Goldstein RB, Callen PW: Fetal ventricle: Importance in routine obstetric sonography. *Radiology* 181:1–7, 1991.

Friedman AC, Lichtenstein JE, Dachman AH: Cystic neoplasms of the pancreas: Radiologic-pathologic correlation. *Radiology* 149:45–50, 1983.

Friedman AC, Lichtenstein JE, Goodman Z, Fishman EK, Siegelman SS, Dachman AH: Fibrolamellar hepatocellular carcinoma. *Radiology* 157:583–587, 1985.

Georg CG, Schwerk WB: Splenic infarction: Sonographic patterns, diagnosis, follow-up and complications. *Radiology* 174:803–807, 1990.

Haney PJ, Yale-Loehr AJ, Nussbaum AR, Gellad FE: Imaging of infants and children with AIDS. *AJR* 152:1033–1041, 1989.

Jackson V: The role of ultrasound in breast imaging. *Radiology* 177:305–311, 1990.

Kirks DR (ed): *Practical Pediatric Imaging,* 1st ed. Boston, Little, Brown, 1984.

Mittelstaedt CA: *Abdominal Ultrasound.* New York, Churchill Livingstone, 1987.

Nelson TR, Pretorius DH: The Doppler signal: Where does it come from and what does it mean? *AJR* 151:439–447, 1988.

Pollack HM (ed): *Clinical Urography.* Philadelphia, WB Saunders, 1990.

Radin DR, Baker EL, Klatt EC, Balthazar EJ, Jeffrey RB, Megibow AJ, Ralls PW: Visceral and nodal calcification in patients with AIDS-related *Pneumocystis carinii* infection. *AJR* 154:27–31, 1990.

Reuther G, Wanjura D, Bauer H: Acute renal vein thrombosis in renal allografts: Detection with duplex doppler US. *Radiology* 170:557–558, 1989.

Ros PR, Moser RP, Dachman AH, Murari PJ, Olmsted WW: Hemangiomas of the spleen: Radiologic-pathologic correlation in ten cases. *Radiology* 162:73–77, 1987.

Rosado-de-Christenson ML, Stocker JT: Congenital cystic adenomatoid malformation. *Radiographics* 11:865–886, 1991.

Sanders R, James AE Jr. (eds): *The Principles and Practice of Ultrasonography in Obstetrics and Gynecology,* 3d ed. Norwalk, CN, Appleton-Century-Crofts, 1985.

Taveras JM, Ferrucci JT (eds): *Radiology-Diagnosis-Intervention.* Philadelphia, JB Lippincott, 1990.

Taylor KJW, Holland S: Doppler US. *Radiology* 174:297–307, 1990.

Wilson JD (ed): *Harrison's Principles of Internal Medicine,* 12th ed. New York, McGraw-Hill, 1991.

Cardiovascular and Interventional Radiology

Abrams HL: *Abrams Angiography,* 3d ed. Boston, Little, Brown, 1983.

Amis E, Newhouse J: *Essentials of Uroradiology.* Boston, Little, Brown, 1991.

Amplatz K, Moller J, Castañeda-Zuñiga W: *Radiology of Congenital Heart Disease.* Philadelphia, Thieme Medical, 1986.

Austin JHM, Schulman LL, Mastrobattista JD: Pulmonary infection after cardiac transplantation: Clinical and radiologic correlations. *Radiology* 172:259–265, 1989.

Becker G, Katzen B, Dake M: Noncoronary angioplasty. *Radiology* 170:925–928, 1989.

Braunwald E: *Heart Disease: A Textbook of Cardiovascular Medicine,* 4th ed. Philadelphia, WB Saunders, 1992.

Cheitlin MD, DeCastro CM, McAllister HA: Sudden death as a complication of anomalous left coronary artery originating from the anterior sinus of valsalva: A not-so-minor congenital anomaly. *Circulation* 50:780–787, 1974.

Cicuto KP, McLean GK, Oleaga JA: Renal artery stenosis: Anatomic classification for percutaneous transluminal angioplasty. *AJR* 137:599–601, 1981.

Clouse M, Wallace S: *Lymphatic Imaging: Lymphography, Computed Tomography and Scintigraphy,* 2d ed. Baltimore, Williams & Wilkins, 1985.

Cohan R, Dunnick N, Bashore T. Treatment of reactions to radiographic contrast material. *AJR* 151:263–270, 1988.

Cunningham DJ: *Textbook of Anatomy.* London, Oxford University Press, 1951.

D'Cruz I: *Echocardiographic Diagnosis.* New York, Macmillan, 1983.

Doroghazi RM: *Aortic Dissection.* New York, McGraw-Hill, 1983.

Elliott LP: *Cardiac Imaging in Infants, Children and Adults.* Philadelphia, JP Lippincott, 1991.

Ernst CB, Stanley JC: *Current Therapies in Vascular Surgery,* 2d ed. Philadelphia, BC Decker, 1991.

Frykberg E, Crump JM, Vines FS: A reassessment of the role of arteriography in penetrating proximity extremity trauma. *J Trauma* 29:1041–1049, 1989.

Gedgaudas E, Moller JH, Castaneda-Zuniga WR, Amplatz K: *Cardiovascular Radiology.* Philadelphia, WB Saunders, 1985.

Gomez MR: *Neurocutaneous Disorders: A Practical Approach.* Boston, Butterworths, 1987.

Gross GW, Steiner RW: Radiographic manifestations of congenital heart disease in the adult patient. *Radiol Clin N Am* 29:293–317, 1991.

Hood RM, Boyd AD, Culliford AT: *Thoracic Trauma.* Philadelphia, WB Saunders, 1989.

Hurst JW (ed): *The Heart,* 6th ed. New York, McGraw-Hill, 1986.

Hurst JW (ed): *The Heart,* 7th ed. New York, McGraw-Hill, 1990.

Johnston KW: Femoral and popliteal arteries: Reanalysis of results of balloon angioplasty. *Radiology* 183:767–771, 1992.

Johnston KW, Rae M, Hogg-Johnston SA: Five-year results of a prospective study of percutaneous transluminal angioplasty. *Ann Surg* 206:403–413, 1987.

Kadir S: *Atlas of Normal and Variant Angiographic Anatomy.* Philadelphia, WB Saunders, 1991.

Kadir S: *Current Practice of Interventional Radiology.* Philadelphia, BC Decker, 1991.

Kadir S: *Diagnostic Angiography.* Philadelphia, WB Saunders, 1986.

Kelley MJ, Jaffe CC, Kleinman CS: *Cardiac Imaging in Infants and Children.* Philadelphia, WB Saunders, 1982.

Kim D: *Peripheral Vascular Imaging and Intervention.* St. Louis, Mosby, YearBook Medical, 1992.

Kirks D: *Practical Pediatric Imaging,* 2d ed. Boston, Little, Brown, 1991.

Levin DC: Pathways and functional significance of the coronary collateral circulation. *Circulation* 50:831–837, 1974.

McCorkell SJ, Harley JD, Morishima MS: Indications for angiography in extremity trauma. *AJR* 145:1245–1247, 1985.

Murphy F, Steinberg HV, Shires GT: The Budd-Chiari syndrome: A review. *AJR* 147:9–15, 1986.

Mustard WT: Successful 2-stage correction of TOGV. *Surgery* 55:469–472, 1964.

Pickering T: Diagnosis and evaluation of renovascular hypertension. *Circulation* 83(suppl I):147–154, 1991.

Pollack H: *Clinical Urography.* Philadelphia, WB Saunders, 1990.

Reuter SR, Redman HC, Cho KJ: *Gastrointestinal Angiography,* 3d ed. Philadelphia, WB Saunders, 1986.

Sellars L, Shore AC, Wilkinson R: Renal vein renin studies in renovascular hypertension—Do they really help? *J Hypertens* 3(2):177–181, 1985.

Silverman F, Kuhn J: *Essentials of Caffey's Pediatric X-ray Diagnosis.* Chicago, YearBook Medical, 1990.

Sos TA: Angioplasty for treatment of azotemia and renovascular hypertension in atherosclerotic renal artery disease. *Circulation* 83(suppl I):162–166, 1991.

Spies JB, Rosen RJ, Lebowitz AS: Antibiotic prophylaxis in vascular and interventional radiology: A rational approach. *Radiology* 166:381–387, 1988.

Taveras JM, Ferrucci JT (eds): *Radiology: Diagnosis-Imaging-Intervention.* Philadelphia, JB Lippincott, 1989.

Tegtmeyer CG, Selby JB, Hartwell GD: Results and complications of angioplasty in fibromuscular disease. *Circulation* 83(suppl I):155–161, 1991.

Uflacker R, Wholey M, *Interventional Radiology.* New York, McGraw-Hill, 1991.

Wilson JD (ed): *Harrison's Principles of Internal Medicine,* 12th ed. New York, McGraw-Hill, 1991.

Mammography

Aboody L, Asch T, Estabrook A: Breast masses in two women with steatocystoma multiplex. *Invest Radiol* 27:329–330, 1992.

American Cancer Society. *Ca—A Cancer Journal for Clinicians.* New York, JB Lippincott, 41(1):19–36, 1991.

Anderson DE: Genetic study of human breast cancer identification of a high risk group. *Cancer* 34:1090–1097, 1974.

Bassett LA. Mammographic analysis of calcifications. *Radiol Clin N Am* 30(1):100–105, 1992.

BEIR Report, National Academy of Sciences Advisory Committee on the Biological Effects of Ionizing Radiation: *The Effects on Population of Exposure to Low Levels of Ionizing Radiation.* Washington, National Academy of Sciences, 1980.

Beute BJ, Kalisher L, Hutter RVP: Lobular carcinoma in situ. *AJR* 157:257–265, 1991.

Buchberger W, Strasser K, Heim K, et al: Phylloides tumor: Findings on mammography, sonography and aspiration cytology in 10 cases. *AJR* 157:715–719, 1991.

Cardenosa G, Eklung GW: Benign papillary neoplasms of the breast: Mammographic findings. *Radiology* 181:751–755, 1991.

Droulies C, Sewell C, McSweeney B: Inflammatory carcinoma of the breast. *Ann Surg* 184(2):217–222, 1976.

Egan RL, McSweeney MB, Sewell GW: Intramammary calcifications without an associated mass in benign and malignant disease. *Radiology* 137:1–7, 1980.

Feig S, Shaber G, Patchefsky A: Tubular carcinoma of the breast. *Radiology* 129:311–314, 1978.

Haagensen CD: *Diseases of the Breast,* 3d ed. Philadelphia, WB Saunders, 1971.

Homer MJ: *Mammographic Interpretation: A Practical Approach.* New York, McGraw-Hill, 1991.

Kalisher L: Factors influencing false negative rates in xeromammography. *Radiology* 133(2):397–401, 1979.

Kalisher L, Long J, Peyster RG: Extra-abdominal desmoid of the axillary tail mimicking breast carcinoma. *AJR* 126:903, 1976.

Knelson MH, EL Yousef S, Goldberg R: Intracystic papillary carcinoma of the breast: Mammographic, sonographic, MR appearance with pathologic correlation. *JCAT* 11(6):1074–1076, 1987.

Knight CH, Peaker M: Development of the mammary gland. *J Reprod Fertil* 65:521–536, 1982.

Kopans DB: *Breast Imaging,* 1st ed. Philadelphia, JB Lippincott, 1988.

Martin JE, Gallagher HS: Mammographic diagnosis of 'minimal' breast cancer. *Cancer* 28:1519, 1971.

Martin JE, Moskowitz M, Milbrath JR: Breast cancer missed by mammography. *AJR* 132:737–739, 1979.

Meyer J, Amin E, Lindfors K: Medullary carcinoma of the breast: Mammographic and ultrasound appearance. *Radiology* 170:79–82, 1989.

Miller C, Feig S, Fox J: Mammographic changes after reduction mammoplasty. *AJR* 149:35–38, 1987.

Millis RR, Davis R, Stacey AJ: The detection and significance of calcifications in the breast. *Br J Radiol* 49:12–26, 1976.

Mitchell GW, Bassett CW. *The Female Breast and Its Disorders*. Baltimore, Williams & Wilkins, 1990.

Price JL, Gamble J, Pierce P: Film screen combination in mammography. *Br J Radiol* 58:99–100, 1985.

Sattin EW, Rubin GL, Webster LA: Family history and the risk of breast cancer. *JAMA* 253:1908–1913, 1985.

Sickles EA: Microfocal spot magnification using xerographic and screen film recording systems. *Radiology* 131:599–607, 1979.

Sickles EA, Doi K, Genant HK: Magnification film mammography: Image quality and clinical studies radiology. *Radiology* 125:69–77, 1977.

Sickles EA: Medical audit of a rapid throughput mammography screening practice: Methodology and results of 27,114 exams. *Radiology* 175:323–327, 1990.

Sickles EA, Abele JS: Milk-of-calcium within tiny benign breast cysts. *Radiology* 141:655–658, 1981.

Silverstein M, Gamagami P, Handel N: Missed breast cancer in an augmented woman using implant displacement mammography. *Ann Plast Surg* 25:210–213, 1990.

Sonnenfeld M, Frenna T, Weidner N: Lobular carcinoma in situ: Mammographic-pathologic correlation of results of needle-directed biopsy. *Radiology* 181:363–367, 1991.

Stomper PC: Clinically occult ductal carcinoma-in-situ detected with mammography: Analysis of 100 cases with pathologic correlation. *Radiology* 172(1):235–241, 1989.

Stomper PC, Recht A, Berenberg A: Mammographic detection of recurrent cancer in the irradiated breast. *AJR* 148:39–43, 1987.

Swann CA, Kopans DB, Koerner FC: The halo sign and malignant breast lesions. *AJR* 149:1145–1147, 1987.

Tabár L: Control of breast cancer through screening mammography. *Radiology* 174:655–656, 1990.

Todd JH, Dowle C, Williams MR: Confirmation of a prognostic index in primary breast cancer. *Br J Cancer* 56:489–492, 1987.

Wellings SR, Jensen HM: On the origin and progression of ductal carcinoma in the human breast. *JNCI* 50:1111, 1973.